Promoting Health Through Organizational Change

Related Benjamin Cummings Health Titles

Promoting Health Through Organizational Change

Harvey A. Skinner, PhD

University of Toronto

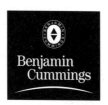

San Francisco   Boston   New York
Cape Town   Hong Kong   London   Madrid   Mexico City
Montreal   Munich   Paris   Singapore   Sidney   Tokyo   Toronto

Publisher: Daryl Fox
Acquisitions Editor: Deirdre McGill
Publishing Assistant: Michelle Cadden
Managing Editor: Wendy Earl
Production Editor: Janet Vail
Copy Editor: Carla Briedenbach
Cover and Text Designer: Brad Greene
Cover Photographer: David Bradford
Illustrator: Richard Sheppard
Manufacturing Buyer: Megan Cochran
Marketing Manager: Sandra Lindelof

Library of Congress Cataloging-in-Publication Data
Skinner, Harvey A., 1949-
    Promoting health through organizational change / Harvey A. Skinner.
       p. cm.
    Includes bibliographical references and index.
    ISBN 0-205-34159-4
    1. Health promotion. 2. Health services administration. 3. Organizational change.
  I. Title.

    RA427.8 .S58 2001
    613--dc21

                                           2001047045

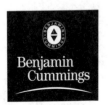

ISBN 0-205-34159-4

1 2 3 4 5 6 7 8 9 10–DVA–05 04 03 02 01

www.aw.com/bc

Benjamin Cummings

FOR PEARL

&

the memory of my father,
William A. Skinner

Contributors

Richard J. Botelho, MD, University of Rochester *(Chapters 9,10,12,16)*

Pearl Bader, MSW, MHSc, Centre for Addiction and Mental Health *(Chapter 4)*

Martin Sommerfeld, MD, University of Toronto *(Chapter 6)*

Eileen deVilla, MD, University of Toronto *(Chapter 12)*

Shawna Mercer, PhD, Centers for Disease Control, Atlanta *(Chapter 12)*

G. Ross Baker, PhD, University of Toronto *(Chapter 13)*

Wayne Velicer, PhD, University of Rhode Island *(Chapter 16)*

James Prochaska, PhD, University of Rhode Island *(Chapter 16)*

Oonagh Maley, MIS, University of Toronto *(Chapter 17)*

Eudice Goldberg, MD, Hospital for Sick Children, Toronto *(Chapter 17)*

Louise Smith, BA, University of Toronto *(Chapter 17)*

Meg Morrison, MEd, Inspire Foundation, Australia *(Chapter 17)*

Cameron Norman, MA, University of Toronto *(Chapter 18)*

Shawn Chirrey, MA, MHSc, University of Toronto *(Chapter 18)*

Reviewers

Dr. David Anspaugh, University of Memphis

Dr. Robert Bensley, Western Michigan University

Donald Barr, MD, PhD, Stanford University

Contents

Preface

The "Monday Morning Question"

Where did the idea for this book begin? The project was anything but a linear process. Instead, it resembles the chronicle of detective Dirk Gentley in *The Long Dark Tea-Time of the Soul* by Douglas Adams. Dirk had an unusual method called 'Zen navigation' for finding his way. Whenever he got lost, Dirk would follow a car that looked like it knew where it was going—and Dirk inevitably ended up where he should be. Following Zen navigation, *this is not the book that I set out to write, but it is definitely a book that needed to be written!*

In the mid-1990s, I began working with my colleague Richard Botelho on a project aimed at helping practitioners learn about new approaches for addressing patient resistance and building motivation for health behavior change. Numerous workshops were conducted at national and international conferences.

At the close of each workshop, a discussion was typically held regarding 'next steps.' *"What will you do differently on Monday morning as a result of this workshop?"* This became known as the **"Monday Morning Question."** Participants would begin with ideas about how they would use some of the strategies for dealing with resistance and enhancing patient motivation. Often, the discussion would shift to expressions of frustration by participants about hitting the system back home, that is: too little time, inadequate reimbursement, lack of resources and backup, and questionable support from their clinical chief.

We all know these frustrations. This Monday Morning Question stimulated, indeed propelled, my journey into organizational improvement. The further I ventured along this path, the more I was convinced of a central premise. Success in changing health behavior requires a focus on BOTH the individual (practitioner, patient) and the organization…but address the organization first!

While working on the early stages of this book in the winter of 1997, I relaxed with my daughter Ana over a meal at the South China restaurant in Toronto. My fortune cookie read: *"You emerge victorious from the maze you've been traveling in."* The Monday Morning Question this book asks is how to do just that.

My aim is that this book will help you emerge victorious from the maze of organizational change through which you are traveling.

Harvey Skinner
Toronto, Canada

Acknowledgments

A number of people were instrumental in helping me complete this project: colleagues, friends and family.

First, I thank my colleagues who made important contributions to several chapters in this book. The ideas and tools in the Five Step Model were refined through many fruitful interactions with Rick Botelho. Also, Martin Sommerfeld was invaluable in helping edit the final version of each chapter. His insight and enthusiasm made our work together quite enjoyable.

Allan Graham provided encouragement in the early stages and detailed feedback on a full draft of the book. Robert (Tommy) Thompson and his leadership at the Group Health Cooperative of Puget Sound provided much inspiration. Tommy gave many insightful comments on a full draft of the book.

Several colleagues provided inspiration at various stages throughout this project: Arnie Aberman, Fred Glaser, John Hastings, Jerry Mings, David Naylor, Arnie Noyek, Irv Rootman and Chan Shah. Each of you is a leader in your unique way and I have learned many valuable lessons. Also, Randy Gangbar, Karl Loszak and Keith Norton played a special role in helping shape my path in life.

The concepts and tools in this book have evolved and been polished through interaction with students in my graduate course on Health Behaviour Change. I thank my colleagues Curtis Breslin and Joan Brewster who co-teach this course with me for their invaluable feedback.

At various stages of this project, the following individuals helped with the research and many details of production: Susan Alexander, Sherry Biscope, Shawn Chirrey, Eileen de Villa, Oonagh Maley and Meg Morrison. The difficult and valuable job of cross checking all references was performed by Louise Smith, Anushuya Parameswaralingam and Veronique Michelli. Also, I would like to thank Rosie Luisi for her administrative and secretarial support.

This book profited invaluably from my close friend and fellow sailor, Steve Manley. He kept asking a very important question until I got the answer clear: *"Harvey: who are you writing this book for?"* Also, thanks to Ann Vanderhoof for her warm encouragement of my project. Steve and Ann truly know publishing from the 'inside out.'

David Korn, my close friend, colleague and running partner, provided ongoing support, shrewd advice and a wacky sense of humour. *"Don't take the project TOO seriously."* Many of the ideas in this book were honed through early morning conversations with David as we ran together through rain, snow and shine!

My family expressed ongoing interest in this project, although they sometimes wondered if I ever would finish the "BOOK." Yet, my son Mark and daughter Ana believed in dad from the start. Thanks. I am so proud to watch you excel in achieving your own goals in life.

As well, my stepchildren Russell and Jeffrey Bader help make life fun and ever interesting. It is great to share our passion for sports.

I also want to acknowledge gratitude to my mom Noreen and my brother Charlie. This book reflects the Skinner work ethic.

My greatest thanks is to my wife Pearl Bader for her love and inspiration, not the least of which is being my marathon running partner. I am so very fortunate to have met you on that winter day as we ran together through the snow. We immediately bonded in our life journey together. Through the ups and downs you give me unwavering support. Although I do not always appreciate it at the time, you push me to get below the surface and understand the root causes. Therein lies the way forward.

Zen Art of Navigation

My own strategy is to find a car ... which looks as if it knows where it's going and follow it. I rarely end up where I was intending to go, but often I end up somewhere that I needed to be.

Douglas Adams—*The Long Dark Tea-Time of the Soul*

CHAPTER 1

About Promoting Health

There is one thing stronger than all the armies in the world, and that is an idea whose time has come.

—Victor Hugo

Overview

We are in the midst of what is arguably the biggest advance in health care thinking in the past 25 years—the transition from reacting to disease to preventing health problems through behavior change. Most health care organizations now recognize the need to expand their efforts beyond changing the individual behavior of patients and practitioners to changing the behavior of the organization itself. But, changing organizational behavior takes time, adequate support and—most important—the guidance of trained professionals.

This is where *Promoting Health* can help you. It successfully integrates patient, practitioner and organizational change into a practical Five-Step Model. It is designed to be used effectively by health practitioners at different stages of their careers: from students in training, to early career practitioners, to more senior practitioners and managers in leadership roles. The Five-Step Model provides a framework for understanding the complexities of health care organizations, and it directs this understanding to learning the practical skills necessary for effective change and renewal.

The Impetus for Promoting Health

Until recently, our approach to health care was primarily reactive. Someone gets sick or injured, and the system springs into action. We know that people continue to get sick from the same preventable causes but have been unable to move beyond our focus on reactive acute care. Over the past ten years, with the formidable and rising cost of health care, the system finally sat up and took notice.

Analysis shows that fully 70% of the health care system's burden of disease and the associated cost is due to preventable illness (Koop, 1995). Furthermore, risk behaviors such as smoking, excessive drinking, poor diet, lack of exercise, and their associated social conditions—the prime factors in preventable illness—account for 50% of premature deaths (McGinnis and Foege, 1993). This recognition, that these illnesses—and much of the attendant costs—are indeed preventable, has led to a new and proactive approach to health care. We are finally shifting our attention to the behavior that affects health and, even more, to the behavior of the health care organizations and the system itself. This proactive approach has become a prime focus of the major governing and professional accreditation bodies in North America and internationally.

Behavior change directed at patients and practitioners has long been recognized as a means of improving the quality of traditional, acute care medicine. A recent analysis by the Institute of Medicine (Kohn et al.,1999) raised serious questions about the U.S. health care system and, by implication, health care systems in other countries. The study estimated that between 44,000 and 98,000 Americans die each year because of adverse events that are preventable. Three types of problems were identified (Chassin et al., 1998): l) *underuse*: failure to identify conditions or offer treatments of known effectiveness (e.g., failure by practitioners in primary care to diagnose and treat depression in almost half of cases: Wells et al., 1989); 2) *overuse:* subjection of patients to tests, procedures or medications that are unnecessary or of questionable value on scientific grounds (e.g., 21% antibiotic prescriptions given to adults or children in 1992 were inappropriate: Gonzales et al., 1997; Nyquist et al., 1998); 3) *misuse:* errors in dispensing medication and poorly executed tests and procedures (e.g., a Harvard Medical Practice Study of hospitalizations found adverse medical events in over 3% of patients: Brennan et al., 1991).

However, lecturing patients for failing to adhere to a treatment protocol or blaming practitioners for failing to identify cases or indeed the health care organization for inadequate support will not bring about the kind of positive change that is needed. To achieve desired improvements, we need to take account of the complex interactions among patients, practitioners and health care organizations (i.e., complex adaptive systems). Our approach recognizes these interactions and offers tools for integrating the change of individuals and organizations.

Two Areas of Health Behavior Change

Two parallel aspects of behavior change have been recognized not only as instrumental in the health care process but also as focal points for improvement: the individual and the organization. Both demand an informed and educated approach by the health care system.

The need for individual (patient/practitioner) behavior change. Practitioners are faced daily with patients who ought to change their behaviors. Behavior change is vital for reducing costs, preventing disease or injury, promoting wellbeing and ensuring that treatment and medication instructions are followed. Although this form of health behavior change is easy to understand, it is difficult to address in practice.

The need for organizational behavior change. Before there can be effective strategies and solutions for dealing with patient behavior, it is necessary for health care organizations to change their own behaviors and to adapt to the new proactive, preventive approach. This major step is essential for health care quality improvement.

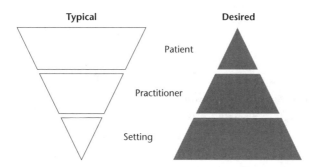

Figure 1.1 Comparison of current versus desired emphasis regarding change in patients, practitioners and health organizations (settings).

Our Priorities for Behavior Change Are Upside Down

The traditional focus for change is on patients (Figure 1.1). Patients are given advice and expected to change their health behaviors. To achieve this, practitioners are trained to provide health education and advice. However, most practitioners lack sufficient time, resources and managerial support for addressing either risk behavior change or self-care of chronic disease. This has been termed 'The Practitioner's Dilemma' by Becker and Janz (1990, p.14):

> ... *either suffer professional and public criticism for inattention to preventive health care or attempt to provide such services in the face of powerful impediments.*

Organizational change in the practice setting is largely ignored. Emphasis needs to be redirected to transforming health settings in ways that truly support practitioners and patients in changing health behavior. According to a quality management adage, approximately 85% of opportunities for improvement lie with the system or organization and 15% with individuals. Often, a straightforward modification in an organizational process can produce significant improvements. This could involve a change in patient scheduling or the re-assignment of responsibilities and roles among the health care team. For example, physicians were almost five times as likely to examine the feet of diabetic patients when patients were barefoot (70%) versus wearing shoes (15%) in the examination room. This demonstrates the impact of a simple organizational change, in this case having the receptionist instruct the patient to remove his or her shoes and socks (Cohen, 1983).

Adapting to the Pace of Change

The rapid transformation underway in health care has greatly accelerated both the amount and rate of change. Stress and burnout are common among practitioners, managers and caregivers (e.g., family). Many are struggling with the question: "How do we get through the next 12 months?"

At times of major transition, organizations place members under immense pressure to accelerate the pace of change. We tend to operate most effectively and efficiently at a specific pace (Conner, 1995). When we assimilate less change than our optimum speed allows, we fail to live up to our potential. When we try to assimilate more than our optimum speed permits, we behave in a dysfunctional way and again fail to live up to our potential. This results in staff absenteeism, low morale, poor performance and errors (Kohn et al., 1999). The concepts and practical tools described in this book help practitioners and managers to be more resilient and to produce organizations that shift gears and adapt effectively to change.

Practitioners' Need for Accreditation

National bodies in medical education have deemed health behavior change and organizational improvement a necessary 'basic science' for practice and accreditation. Also, these competencies are increasingly emphasized in nursing, public health, psychology and rehabilitation sciences. Emphasis is such that this new basic science is seen as a necessary competency for licensure and maintenance of certification. For example: the U.S. Accreditation Council for Graduate Medical Education has mandated that residency programs require residents to develop competencies in six major areas: patient care, medical knowledge, practice-based learning and improvement, systems-based practice, interpersonal and communication skills, and professionalism. *Promoting Health* directly addresses two of these areas, practice-based learning and improvement and systems-based practice. Similarly, the American Association of Medical Colleges is placing increased emphasis on behavior change, quality improvement and organizational skills in the undergraduate medical education curriculum.

How Promoting Health Works

Promoting Health is intended to serve as a primary text for undergraduate, graduate and postgraduate education of health care professionals. It can be used effectively with medical and health science students as well as practitioners engaged in continuing education. This book prepares practitioners to develop effective health promotion and disease management programs. It directly covers key competencies in organizational change, quality improvement and systems-based practice that are mandated by professional accreditation bodies in medicine and other health professions. And, it is designed to work in traditional educational formats (courses, workshops and case-study rounds), as well as in new approaches that use information technology (IT) for distance education and self-directed learning.

The Five-Step Model (Figure 1.2) successfully bridges the gap between patient and organizational change. Although several books have been written on organizational change and improvement, most are aimed at management (executives and consultants). On the other hand, books on health promotion and behavioral medicine typically take a clinical or community health perspective. *Promoting Health* integrates these domains. The Five-Step Model addresses how practitioner and organizational change work together to affect patient outcomes at both individual and population levels. The book goes several steps further by focusing on what practitioners need to know about their own roles in organizational improvement. It provides a structure for understanding organizational behavior from macro- through to micro-levels: both 'top down' and 'bottom up'.

The Five-Step Model is presented in an engaging manner with learning exercises, case studies and practical tools for organizational analysis. The case studies and examples are composites (to preserve anonymity) adapted

Figure 1.2 Five-Step Model for improving health organizations in behavior change.

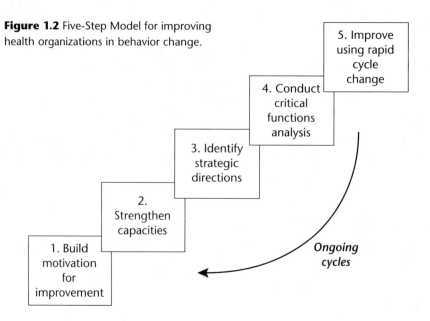

from real-life organizations and experiences. The approaches and tools have undergone extensive trials over the past seven years in professional and continuing education sessions throughout North America and internationally. The Model is distinctive as an effective learning tool in several respects:

- **Integrative:** Rather than dealing with isolated issues, the Model links key concepts and opportunities for improvement spanning all levels of an organization.

- **Practical:** Each step of the way, the Five-Step Model provides practical tools for implementing and testing change; it provides methods for the student and practitioner to turn theory into reality.

- **Team Work:** Like 'real life', the Model encourages team approaches using top down and bottom up strategies for improvement. Everyone has a role to play.

- **Comprehensive:** The Five-Step Model addresses a wide variety of behavior change, prevention and disease management programs.

- **Adaptable:** The Five-Step Model can be applied to a range of health organizations and settings. It will satisfy the needs of a variety of educational institutions and continuing education programs.

- **Convenient and Ongoing Learning:** The Five-Step Model can be learned in an incremental and interactive way using the book's tools and the author's website (*www.HealthBehaviorChange.org*).

A Walk Through Promoting Health

Part One. Re-Orienting Health Care Organizations

This section addresses the major challenges and forces driving change in health care and health promotion, and it sets the context and impetus for new approaches.

Chapter 2. Problems and Solutions. Root causes of the health care crisis versus myopic cost cutting: An analysis of the health care delivery system demonstrates how current and increasingly costly methods contribute only minor improvements to the overall health status of the population.

Chapter 3. Beyond Clinical Care. Addressing behavioral and population determinants of health: A discussion about the benefits of dealing proactively (rather than merely reactively) with health behavior at individual and population levels in health care organizations.

Chapter 4. Improving the Organization. The need for change beyond patients and practitioners: A look at why organizations rather than practitioners and patients are often at the root of failures to achieve health behavior change. Emphasis is given to the need for improving organizational support systems.

Chapter 5. Putting Prevention into Practice. Working proof: This chapter goes beyond the theory of the previous chapters to provide an in-depth example of an organization, the Group Health Cooperative of Puget Sound, which has successfully implemented prevention and behavior change programs at both clinical and population levels.

Chapter 6. Physicians' Perspectives on Organizational Change. Physicians are in a unique position of responsibility and influence in health care, yet they are facing increased stress and workloads along with encroachments upon professional autonomy. Many are participating with reluctance in organizational change. This chapter focuses on these pressures and considers proactive approaches that physicians can take for improving the quality of health care, prevention and health promotion.

Chapter 7. What Motivates People to Change. Sooner or later, initiatives for organizational change and system improvement are determined at an individual level. Understanding what underlies resistance and how to motivate positive change are critical for success. The forces of change for individuals are integrated into a ten-step *Likelihood of Action Index*. This will help you design approaches for lowering resistance and increasing motivation for organizational improvement among key stakeholders (e.g., physicians, clinical unit staff).

Part Two. Five Steps for Improving Organizations

Part II describes the practical Five-Step Model for improving organizations through behavior change. The Model integrates 'top down' and 'bottom up' approaches to organizational improvement.

Chapter 8. The Five-Step Model. *Getting a clear start:* A comprehensive yet practical approach is described for understanding complex health care organizations and for improving their effectiveness in prevention and disease management. The Model emphasizes the practical as well as the theoretical. Its assessment tools allow both teams and individuals to analyze, measure and test their performance.

Chapter 9. Step 1: Developing Motivation for Change. *Dealing with different organizations:* This chapter distinguishes 'reactive' from 'high performing' organizations and shows how to build commitment to improvement within each. A self-study tool is provided: *Your Organizational Prototype* is used to contrast individual and team evaluations of how an organization is currently performing with how it should perform. The chapter then demonstrates how the magnitude of this discrepancy can be used as a catalyst for change.

Chapter 10. Step 2: Strengthening Capacities for Improvement. *Establishing the basics:* Recognizing that organizations vary widely in their resiliency and capacity for change, five essential capacities are described for strengthening the resolve and improving performance (ACTSS: Affective, Cultural, Technical, Structural, Strategic). A study tool is provided for assessing the organization's readiness for change and for strengthening its ability to change.

Chapter 11. Step 3: Identifying Strategic Directions in Behavior Change. *Giving a shape to change:* This chapter shows how high–performing organizations achieve success by identifying and concentrating efforts on a small number of strategic directions. These directions shape what the organization is, where it is going, and why. Five interrelated activities are described: *Stakeholder Analysis; Environmental Scans; SWOT Analyses* (Strengths, Weaknesses, Opportunities, Threats); *Issue Identification;* and *Payoff Matrix Analysis.*

Chapter 12. Step 4: Conducting a Critical Functions Analysis. *Assessing the impact:* This chapter builds on the knowledge that badly organized systems are stronger than individual practitioners; it focuses on an analysis of the organization. A *Critical Functions Analysis (CFA)* identifies opportunities for improvement and generates a data base for assessing the impact of improvement initiatives. It describes seven critical functions that support practitioners and patients in health behavior change:

- **Professional Development in Behavior Change:** both individual (patient, practitioner) and organizational levels

- **Priming Patients and Practitioners:** addresses prevention and behavioral risk factors

- **Identification of Risk Behaviors:** case-finding in clinical encounters and screening at the community and population levels

- **Continuing Care:** monitoring, re-assessment, provision of additional care

- **Links and Networks Among Services and Resource Options**: both within and outside the health care setting

- **Help Options:** making use of professional assistance, professionally led support groups, self-help groups and community resources

- **Information Management**: system design and maintenance to support behavior initiatives

Chapter 13. Step 5: Improvement Using Rapid Cycle Change. Assessing the available tools: A variety of new methods and tools offer practical assistance to enable practitioners and organizations to make 'rapid cycle improvements.' Emphasis is placed on making limited trials of change. These changes are based on ideas from the *Critical Functions Analysis*, comparative practices in other clinics, and an analysis of the literature. Several tools and practices are discussed.

Chapter 14. Sustaining the Momentum for Positive Change. How to maintain a proper course: This chapter outlines an eight-stage process for leading and sustaining change and describes how to apply the Five-Step Model through successive iterations. The goal is to keep the organization focused on improvement and maintenance of gains. Attention is paid to an oft-neglected area: avoiding slippage or motivational drift.

Part Three: e-Health: The New Role of Information Technology

This section investigates the rapid developments and emerging opportunities in information technology and their use for health behavior change.

Chapter 15. Information Technology to Support Practitioners and Patients. New and wide-ranging opportunities are explored for organizational improvement by using the Internet in professional development, telemedicine and telehealth applications. Other revolutionary technologies including interactive voice and 'telephone-linked care' are also discussed.

Chapter 16. Computer Systems That Motivate Behavior Change. Expert systems and programs can effectively apply an individual-based intervention to a population. A profile is given of the 'Pathways To Change' system for smoking cessation.

Chapter 17. TeenNet: Using the Internet for e-Health. The Internet offers untold opportunities for health promotion and clinical care. Practical examples of e-Health are given from the TeenNet Project websites for engaging youth. A parallel site provides guidelines and skill-based learning for practitioners in health and educational settings. What makes the Teen-Net Project unique for organizational change is the interweaving of 'high tech' website development with community involvement to produce websites that directly meet consumer needs.

Chapter 18. Consumer Perspectives on e-Health. Information technology is revolutionizing the way consumers and practitioners interact with the health care system. Questions remains about whether enhanced access to information will result in more informed decisions and better health outcomes. This chapter examines circumstances in which e-Health will help answer consumer's health questions or create confusion and anxiety; ways in which technology can be used for self-help and mutual aid, and the impact that e-Health is having on the quality of the patient-practitioner relationship.

Part Four: Afterword

Chapter 19. Initiating Your Personal and Organizational Learning Plan. Promoting Health goes beyond its one-time use as a textbook by forming the vital link to an ongoing, interactive learning process via the Internet. Students and practitioners are encouraged to develop their personal and organizational change plans and continue learning using the tools and education modules on the web site *www.HealthBehaviorChange.org*. In particular, this website provides an ongoing discussion forum for interaction with the author and others engaged in organizational change.

Part One

Re-Orienting Health Care Organizations

The physician's function is fast becoming social and preventative, rather than individual and curative. Upon him, society relies to ascertain and through measures essentially educational, to enforce the conditions that prevent disease and make positively for the physical and moral well-being.

—Abraham Flexner (1910)

CHAPTER 2

Problems and Solutions

The American public has come to expect more from medicine than it can deliver and less from public health than it can accomplish.

—Robbins and Freeman (1999, p.120).

Overview

Health care is in the midst of a major transformation. Indeed, many would say crisis. These changes are driven by a number of compelling forces. Escalating health care costs have galvanized media attention and exercised policy makers, especially in North America and other developed countries. Both costs and concerns are fuelled by rapid advances in biomedical and information technology, 'heroic' measures for extending life, as well as enhanced often unrealistic public expectations (patient consumerism). In addition, our population is aging with a concomitant shift in health care needs, morbidity patterns, and emphasis on chronic disease and disability. The general public is increasingly concerned about the health of the health care system, and debates over access, quality, and effectiveness are common. Can we continue 'business as usual' with incremental refinements in health care, or do we rethink our present situation and work toward a more fundamental change?

This chapter reviews the forces affecting health care. We propose a substantial shift in emphasis from acute care to a coordinated effort at putting prevention and behavioral health care into practice at clinical, community and population levels. This rebalancing builds on an integration of medical care and public health approaches.

Imperatives for Health Care Reform

"That's not the way I want to practice," exclaimed a frustrated physician. Advances in biomedical technology are creating major frustrations for practitioners and health care organizations. For example, consider the use of 'stents', heralded as the biggest advance in opening clogged arteries in more than a decade. They don't look like much—just tiny tubes of wire mesh used as miniature scaffolding, shoring up the narrowed area of a diseased blood vessel.

"It sure made a big difference in my life," said a 52-year-old patient. The patient suffered 90% blockage in two of his coronary arteries and was treated with stents. Within a week, he was out playing golf with his friend. *"I'm thrilled. If I didn't have these stents, I wouldn't be golfing."*

Stents apparently work so well that their use has quadrupled across North America. But the sudden rise is bad news for hospital administrators trying to control costs. Their use is being ratcheted down by spending limits and the expensive price of each tube.

"We've had to almost completely stop using stents because of lack of funding, and now ration their use," said the Director of Interventional Cardiology at a metro hospital. *"Our battle is to prove there's a long-term financial benefit to using stents."*

By cutting the number of angioplasty cases requiring further operations, it is likely that using stents saves the system money. Research on cost-effectiveness is underway. Until the funding issue is resolved, doctors have to make frustrating decisions that sometimes force them to withhold stents from some patients who could benefit from them.

This illustrates just one of the dilemmas for a health system pushed by both rapid medical progress and limited budgets—somehow more funds need to be found to assure access to stent surgery for patients with occluded coronary arteries. Yet, it begs the question of how we set limits to funding new medical interventions. How high can a nation's health care expenditures rise before a revolt occurs due to the siphoning of funds from other areas, such as education and social services?

The dilemma over stents raises the question of whether we need a fundamental change in our approach that would emphasize the prevention of heart disease. For example, did this 52-year-old man engage in risk behavior (e.g., smoking, elevated cholesterol, high-fat diet) and live under adverse social conditions that could have been modified earlier and thus have reduced the probability of atherosclerotic vascular disease?

Table 2.1   Ten Great Achievements in Public Health:
Adding 25 Years to Life Expectancy in the 20th Century

	Examples
1. Vaccination	Eradication of small pox; elimination of poliomyelitis; control of measles, rubella, tetanus, diphtheria, *Haemophilus influenzae* type b
2. Motor-Vehicle Safety	Engineering efforts making vehicles and highways safer; personal behavior change (e.g., using seat belts, child safety seats, motorcycle helmets, decreased drinking and driving)
3. Safer Workplaces	Control of environments: e.g., reducing coal workers' pneumoconiosis (black lung) and silicosis; reduction in severe injuries and death related to mining, construction, manufacturing and transportation industries
4. Control of Infectious Diseases	Resulting from clean water and improved sanitation. Typhoid and cholera transmitted by contaminated water reduced dramatically; discovery of antimicrobial therapy to control tuberculosis and sexually transmitted diseases
5. Prevention of Heart Disease and Stroke	Risk factor modification such as smoking cessation and blood pressure control combined with improved access to early detection and better treatment
6. Safer and Healthier Foods	Decreases in microbial contamination and increases in nutritional content; establishing food-fortification programs to eliminate diseases such as rickets, goiter, and pellagra
7. Healthier Mothers and Babies	Resulting from better hygiene and nutrition, availability of antibiotics, greater access to health care, and technologic advances in maternal and neonatal medicine
8. Family Planning	Access to family planning and contraceptive services has altered social and economic roles of women; smaller family size and longer interval between birth of children; fewer infant, child and maternal deaths; using contraceptives to prevent pregnancy and transmission of HIV and other STDs
9. Fluoridation of Drinking Water	Safely and inexpensively benefits children and adults by effectively preventing tooth decay, regardless of socioeconomic status or access to care
10. Tobacco Prevention	Recognition of tobacco as a health hazard and subsequent public health anti-smoking campaigns changed social norms to prevent initiation of tobacco use, promote cessation and reduce exposure to environmental tobacco smoke. Since the 1964 Surgeon General's Report on the health risks of smoking, smoking among adults has decreased substantially and millions of smoking related deaths have been prevented.

Source: U.S. Centers for Disease Control and Prevention, *Morbidity and Mortality Weekly Report,* 1999 issues. Available on CDC website at: *www.cdc.gov/epo/mmwr/*

Rather than waiting for the problem and 'fixing' it once it occurs (e.g., occluded coronary arteries), practitioners and health organizations are increasingly called upon to take a central role in prevention and health promotion. This change is supported by evidence that over half of premature deaths in North America are preventable (McGinnis & Foege, 1993; Wigle et al., 1990). Yet, we continue to allocate over 95% of health expenditures to medical care and less than 5% to prevention and community health. For instance, U.S. federal, state and local health agencies spent an estimated $14.4 billion on core public health functions in 1993. This represented only 1–2% of the almost one trillion ($903 billion) in total health care expenditures (U.S. Centers for Disease Control and Prevention, 1999a).

Are we getting the best value from the current balance of expenditures? Major improvements in life expectancy in the 20th century came primarily from public health initiatives and only to a minor extent from medical care. The U.S. Centers for Disease Control and Prevention (1999a), estimate that 25 years are added to life expectancy of people in the United States due to the Ten Great Achievements of Public Health (Table 2.1). Since 1900, the life expectancy of Americans has improved by more than 30 years, with most (25 years) attributable to advances in public health (Bunker et al., 1994). However, people in the lowest income households have poorer health status and on average die 3 to 7 years younger.

These imperatives underscore the need for health care reform. We are spending more and more on medical care, while neglecting to realize the real potential of public health. Practitioners and health care organizations are caught in a maelstrom of unmet expectations, cost containment and discontent. *"That's not the way I want to practice."*

Understanding the Forces of Change

Various factors driving the need for health care reform are given in Figure 2.1. Decter (2000) likens these forces to 'four strong winds': 1) powerful new ideas about the broader determinants of health and system organization; 2) public expectations about quality, speed and appropriateness; 3) technology; and 4) the big squeeze due to fiscal constraints. Understanding and responding successfully to these forces requires a fundamental shift in how health organizations work to achieve the dual goals:

- promoting health and reducing risk behavior of individuals (patients), while …
- enhancing the health status of the population served by the organization.

To achieve these goals, a new alliance is needed between clinical and public health perspectives within integrated delivery systems.

In the United States, there is growing concern that the health care system needs change (Lurie, 2000). Even the much-heralded national system

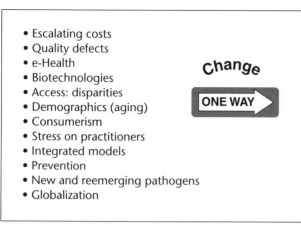

- Escalating costs
- Quality defects
- e-Health
- Biotechnologies
- Access: disparities
- Demographics (aging)
- Consumerism
- Stress on practitioners
- Integrated models
- Prevention
- New and reemerging pathogens
- Globalization

Change

ONE WAY

Figure 2.1. Twelve major factors influencing health care.

in Canada is being questioned. A survey by PriceWaterhouseCoopers (1999b) found the following:

- Although 95% of Canadians support the Canadian Health Act and its five tenets (universality, accessibility, portability, comprehensiveness, publicly funded), half reported having extended or private health insurance.

- Only four out of 10 Canadians agreed that the health care system was currently able to meet the needs of the aging population. In addition, many did not believe this would improve significantly in the future.

- More than 60% of Canadians used complementary therapies in the past year, with vitamins, minerals and herbal remedies being the most popular, in descending order.

What lies at the root of these concerns? The HealthCast 2010 report (PriceWaterhouseCoopers, 1999a) identifies three key forces of change affecting health care: 1) *Empowered Consumers,* some complaining of marked disparities in access, and others, 'impatient' patients, demanding enhanced services; 2) *e-Health,* which is creating a whole new site and model for health care delivery and consumer access to health information (National Research Council, 2000); and 3) *Biotechnology Advances,* particularly genomics, the basis of many new approaches and services such as genetic susceptibility screening and, eventually, designer drugs and gene therapies (Crow, 2000; Keller, 2000; Ridley, 1999). These three forces raise major concerns about access to and financing of these expanding services. Also, these rapid changes are creating ethical dilemmas that challenge our traditional concepts of right and wrong (Somerville, 2000). In particular, there is growing expectation and pressure on the scientific and health care community to engage in public discourse about advances in genetic knowledge (Reilly, 2000).

Health care organizations face difficult choices regarding how they will adapt to these forces. HealthCast 2010 underscores twelve implications arising out of these forces of change (p.3):

1. Health care organizations that are consumer friendly will be winners.
2. Organizations must distinguish themselves through brand-name services or products.
3. Service and speed will be the key to customer satisfaction.
4. New e-business models will emerge and challenge traditional medicine.
5. The race for capital will hinge on the ability to demonstrate quality, efficiency, and customer focus.
6. Resources must be reallocated to retain the work force.
7. Isolated service units in health care organizations must be eliminated and replaced with seamless service.
8. Payers must stress prevention because early detection and intervention will cost more.
9. Consumers will want more and won't want to pay for it.
10. The rate of ethical dilemmas will accelerate for consumers, providers and purchasers.
11. New opportunities for private health insurers outside the United States will expand rapidly.
12. Medical professionals need to work toward global standards of medical treatment.

The Institute for the Future (2000) provides an excellent synopsis of the increasing diversity of the patient population, rise of new consumers, growing gap between 'haves' and 'have-nots', impact of new medical and information technologies, pressure on both public and private sectors for increased funding, and trends in the demand for and supply of health care workers. This report reviews both medical care and public health approaches and underscores the need for an approach integrating both.

New and re-emerging pathogens pose major challenges at the dawn of the new millennium (Brundtland, 2000). Throughout the 20th century the use of antibiotics had a major impact on reducing and controlling once-common infectious diseases (e.g., whooping cough, polio, scarlet fever).

However, the overuse of antibiotics in developed countries and underuse in developing countries has created a huge problem of antimicrobial drug resistance that has potentially catastrophic implications. Formerly curable diseases such as typhoid and gonorrhea are becoming difficult to treat, and major threats are re-emerging from old killers such as tuberculosis and malaria. Globalization, including increased international travel and migration, are exacerbating the prevention and control of infectious disease.

Let's look at some of these forces in more detail.

Quality in Health Care

An analysis by the Institute of Medicine (Kohn et al.,1999) raised critical questions about the quality and safety of the U.S. health care system and, by implication, the quality of health care in other countries. The study estimates that between 44,000 and 98,000 Americans die each year because of adverse events such as medication errors. All of these deaths are preventable.

Substantial opportunities exist for improving quality and reducing costs by focusing on organizational improvement. Berwick (1998) and Chassin et al. (1998) review three types of quality problems or 'defects' in American health care:

1. **Underuse:** failing to identify conditions or offer treatments of known effectiveness (e.g., failure in primary care to diagnose and treat depression in almost half of cases: Wells et al., 1989)

2. **Overuse:** subjecting patients to tests, procedures or medications that are unnecessary or of questionable value on scientific grounds (cf., RAND corporation study, estimated that 30% of acute care is unnecessary: Chassin et al., 1987)

3. **Misuse:** errors (e.g., medication errors) and poorly executed tests and procedures (cf., Harvard Medical Practice Study of hospitalizations found adverse medical events in over 3% of patients: Brennan et al., 1991).

Quality improvement in these three areas requires behavior change in practitioners, patients and health care organizations alike. However, major disparities in access loom as an overshadowing impediment to quality health care and the redirection of resources for promoting health (Ayanian et al., 2000; Eisenberg and Power, 2000).

A subsequent study by the Institute of Medicine (2001) entitled: "Crossing the Quality Chasm: a New Health System for the 21st Century" calls for an urgent reorganization and reform of the health care system to improve quality, access and efficiency. A key component is to apply advances from information technology to address sources of error and continuous system improvement. The report proposes six aims for improvement (p.6):

- **Safe**: avoiding injuries to patients from the care that is intended to help them
- **Effective**: providing services based on scientific knowledge to all who could benefit and refraining from providing services to those not likely to benefit (avoiding underuse and overuse, respectively)
- **Patient-centered**: proving care that is respectful of and responsive to individual patient preferences, needs, and values and ensuring that patient values guide all clinical decisions
- **Timely**: reducing waits and sometimes harmful delays for both those who receive and those who give care
- **Efficient**: avoiding waste of equipment, supplies, ideas and energy
- **Equitable**: providing care that does not vary in quality because of personal characteristics, such as gender, ethnicity, geographical location, and socioeconomic status.

A renewed health care system that makes major gains in these six dimensions would be better for both patients and clinicians, and it would integrate a full array of preventive, acute and chronic services.

At the international level, the World Health Organization (2000) conducted a comprehensive comparison of the performance of health care systems in 191 developed and developing countries. Their analyses concentrated on four vital functions of a health system: delivering services (provision); creating resources (investment and training); financing (collecting, pooling and purchasing); and stewardship (overall management). A number of health status indicators were compared across countries to assess overall performance. Interestingly, countries that spent the most per capita on health did not necessarily have the best health status indicators. Inequalities were noted in life expectancy, inequalities that are strongly associated with socioeconomic class, even in countries with good health status on average. The report makes specific suggestions for improving the four vital functions of a health care system.

Social Determinants

Personal health behavior takes place in a context and is influenced, often powerfully, by proximal (e.g., peer pressure on a teen to smoke) and distal factors (e.g., policy regarding taxation on and thus price of cigarettes). These social, economic, and environmental circumstances are frequently beyond individual control. Wilkinson and Marmot (1998) summarize the evidence and make policy recommendations regarding ten interrelated social determinants of health:

1. **Social gradient:** the poorest and most disadvantaged are especially affected

2. **Stress:** social and psychological environment

3. **Early life:** importance of a good start in life

4. **Unemployment:** job security and satisfaction

5. **Work environment:** impacts on health and risk of disease

6. **Social support:** positive role of friendship and social cohesion

7. **Social exclusion:** impact of social isolation and relative deprivation

8. **Addictions:** effects of tobacco, alcohol and other drugs

9. **Food:** access to nutritious food is a political issue

10. **Transport:** better public transport, reducing driving and encouraging healthier means (walking, cycling)

Their review points out that high standards of health are not shared by all. "Even in the richest countries, the better off live several years longer and have fewer illnesses than the poor" (Wilkinson & Marmot, 1998, p.1).

Social and economic factors influence all levels in a society. The authors draw attention to health disparities in age (children and youth), gender, population groups (e.g., aboriginal people), and socioeconomic conditions including income and education/literacy levels. Economic inequality affects health in three main ways (Raphael, 2000; Wilkinson, 1996):

- Economically unequal societies have greater levels of poverty.

- Economically unequal societies provide fewer social safety nets.

- Economically unequal societies have weaker social cohesion.

This economic disparity is reflected in health status. For example, in southeast Toronto, there is a large gap between two adjacent wards, the poorest ward (Don River: $29,000 average family income) and the wealthiest ward (Rosedale: $74,000 average family income). In comparison with the highest income families, the lowest had 40% more low birth weight infants, 73% more children's hospitalizations for respiratory diseases, and fourfold more adult hospitalizations. Glazier et al. (2000) found that hospital costs were 50% higher for the poorest neighborhoods than for the wealthiest, and one-third higher than neighborhoods with average family income.

Socioeconomic status also affects access to care. Alter et al. (1999) examined how access to invasive cardiac procedures influences mortality after acute myocardial infarction. They found a strong inverse relationship between income and mortality at one year. Each $10,000 increase in the neighborhood median income is associated with a 10% reduction in the risk of death within one year.

Similarly, socioeconomic status affects access to prevention services and health promotion. O'Loughlin et al. (1999) evaluated a Healthy Heart program in a low income community and found that prevention programs do not benefit the poor. People in this community were more concerned with day-to-day challenges of living than with developing a chronic disease. The Healthy Heart program faced virtually insurmountable obstacles: high illiteracy rates, overburdened community groups, and low participation rates (2%). The situation is clearly illustrated by one person's decision:

> The winner of a smoking cessation contest was offered a choice between a $2,000 vacation or $300 cash. The winner took the cash needed for living expenses.

Health disparities within a nation regarding access to quality services and resources for health, as well as disparities between nations (e.g., access to medical treatments for HIV/AIDS in developed versus developing countries) will undoubtedly create major political challenges. Indeed, Michaud, Murray and Bloom (2001) argue that the major challenge in the 21st century is allocation of resources to reduce the burden of disease globally and to reduce disparities in population health between poor and affluent countries.

Shifting Demographic Profile

The changing demographic profile is creating new pressures. The health care system is under increasing demands to address diversity, such as women's health and ethnoracial background. The aging population in most developed countries, and especially in North America, is challenging our ability to control heart disease and cancer if we are to decrease disability in the 21st century.

Boult et al. (1996) evaluated the effects of reducing six fatal and non-fatal conditions (i.e., coronary artery disease, stroke, cancer, diabetes, confusion and arthritis) on the number of functionally limited older Americans. If the prevalence of these six conditions remains unchanged, then the increase in functionally limited older Americans will be at least 311% by the year 2049. The greatest potential for reducing functional limitation lies in lowering the prevalence of arthritis. Assuming a 1% biennial reduction in the six conditions between 2001 and 2049, a decrease in arthritis would yield a reduction in functional limitation of 4 million person-years, compared with 0.9 million person-years for cancer and 0.1 million person-years for coronary artery disease. In this context, the unit person-years refers to the time spent in disability (e.g. five years) multiplied by the number of persons affected. These data underscore the need for redefining goals and priorities in health research for a rapidly aging population.

Spending Trap

Over the past thirty years, we have generally followed a policy of 'spending our way' toward health through increasing expenditures on treating acute illness (Evans & Stoddart, 1990; Rachlis & Kushner, 1994). This is particularly the case in the United States. Health care expenditures in 1997 in the Organization for Economic Cooperation and Development (OECD) countries ranged from 4.0% of the Gross Domestic Product in Korea and Turkey to 13.5% in the U.S. (Anderson & Poullier, 1999). Even when limited to high-income countries, the range is still wide: 6.7% (the United Kingdom) to 13.5% (U.S.). When health expenditures are measured per capita in U.S. dollars, the gap is even wider. In 1997, per capita health expenditures, adjusted for differences in purchasing power, were nearly three times greater in the U.S. (US$ 3,925) than in the United Kingdom (US$ 1,347).

Over the past thirty years, health costs have risen faster than income in the U.S., and projections to the year 2030 indicate that health costs will greatly exceed per capita income (Figure 2.2) if corrective action is not taken. Many of the Fortune 500 companies are seeing their net profits overtaken by rising health care costs. This has led to a "revolt of the payer".

Have certain countries overdeveloped their medical capacity? For instance, the United States has invested a high level of resources to perform medical procedures. In the case of magnetic resonance imaging, Orange

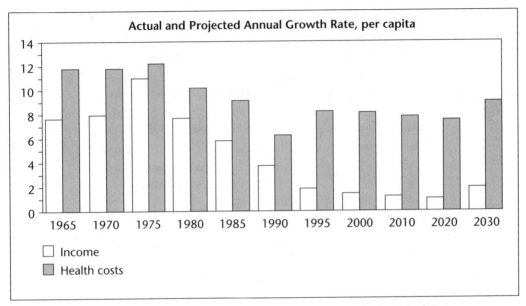

Figure 2.2. Health care costs versus per capita income in the United States over a 65 year period.

County (California) has more imaging machines for its 2.4 million people than all of Canada has for its 30 million people. High rates of utilization and expenditure exist across a wide spectrum of treatments, such as coronary artery catheterization and bypass surgery (Robert Wood Johnson Foundation, 1994). Funds spent on expensive diagnostic and treatment services take away from opportunities to provide essential and cost-effective public health and clinical services, such as immunization, prenatal care and screening, and treatment of hypertension and diabetes. The 'spending trap' for the three leading causes of death in the United States is illustrated in Table 2.2 (McGinnis, 1994). A substantial number (over 50%) of premature deaths could be prevented through control of risk factors via clinical prevention and public health programs.

Critics of U.S. medical expenditures estimate that compared with administrative costs in other countries with national health care systems, the U.S. spends significantly more. They estimate that excess administrative costs in the U.S. account for at least 10% of the $1 trillion national expenditures (Robert Wood Johnson Foundation, 1994). Trimming the administrative 'surplus' (10%) could yield some $100 billion. This would be enough to provide health insurance coverage for every American who is currently

Table 2.2   Risk Factors and Cost of Treatment for
Three Leading Causes of Death in the United States

Cause of Death	Preventable Risk Factors	Cost of Treatment per Patient
1. Heart Disease	Smoking Obesity Inactivity Elevated Blood Pressure Elevated Cholesterol	$30,000 for coronary bypass surgery
2. Cancer	Smoking Diet (improper) Alcohol Environmental Exposures	$29,000 for lung cancer
3. Injuries	Safety Belt (nonuse) Alcohol/Drug Abuse Home Hazards	$40,000 for hip fracture treatment $570,000 for quadriplegia treatment and rehabilitation (lifetime)

Source: McGinnis (1994).

uninsured. By 2000, the U.S. Census Bureau estimates that more than 44 million people, or about one out of every six non-elderly Americans, will lack health insurance, with about a million more Americans losing their coverage every year. The time to take action is now.

Will we be healthier if we increase spending on health care services? Although there is a common belief that *treating illness* will improve health, the evidence points us in a very different direction. For instance, Figure 2.3 summarizes the 1992 per capita spending for eight developed countries. United States per capita spending is well ahead of rates for Canada and substantially above the United Kingdom. Is the U.S. population healthier? Infant mortality rates and life expectancy rates are common indicators of the overall health of a population. Interestingly, countries which spend far less per capita on medical care, such as Japan and Sweden, have better population health indicators, lower infant mortality rates and longer life expectancies. Data such as these have stimulated a resurgence of interest in population health perspectives (Evans et al., 1994).

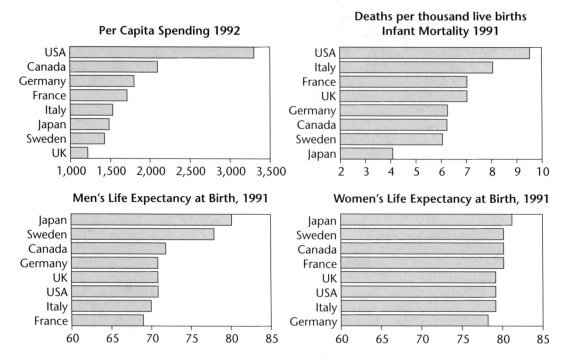

Figure 2.3. National comparison of health care spending with population health status indicators.

'Hidden' Health Care System

The health care system is typically thought of as encompassing only professional assistance: that is, primary care and the various medical subspecialties. This image misses the fact that much health care is achieved by individuals and families either between visits to professionals and hospitals or without any professional care. Indeed, up to 80% of individuals resolve their health issues without seeking professional care (Kemper et al., 1993; Sobel, 1995; Vickery et al., 1983; Vickery & Fries, 1993). Levin and Idler (1982) call this much larger system of lay support and assistance the 'hidden health care system'. Professional care is just the tip of the iceberg (Figure 2.4). This is especially true given the rising consumerism and access to health information afforded by technology (e.g., Internet). We provide a closer look at online self-help and mutual support groups in Chapters 15 and 18.

Borkman (1999) describes the evolution of self-help and mutual aid, and models for understanding the dynamics of how they work. Kyrouz and Humphreys (2000) review studies of the effectiveness of self-help and

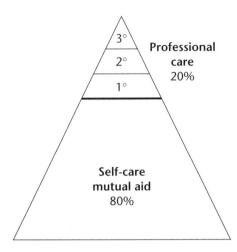

Figure 2.4. Relative magnitude of the professional and self-care (hidden) systems. 1°= primary care (family or general practice), 2°= secondary care, 3°= tertiary care (specialized medical clinics)

mutual support groups. They examine a range of topics: mental health, weight loss, addictions, bereavement, diabetes, caregivers, elderly, cancer, and chronic illness. Their report and updates are available at *http://www.mentalhelp.net/articles/selfres.html.* They conclude that most studies have found important benefits when comparing participants with non-participants (controls) and when data are collected on multiple occasions (longitudinal studies).

Sobel (1995, p.238) summarizes the potential and broad impact of self-care and mutual aid:

> *People are not just consumers of health care, they are the true primary care providers in the health care system. Increasing the confidence and skills of these primary care providers can make health and economic sense.*

Complementary and Alternative Medicine

An important element of both rising consumerism and the 'hidden' health care system is the growth over the past decade of complementary and alternative medicine (CAM). In North America, more than 40% of the public use alternative medicine, although estimates are even higher depending on the breadth of the definition used (Eskinazi, 1998; Kelner and Wellman, 2000). Of particular relevance to mainstream medical care is that approximately two-thirds of patients do not tell their physician about their use of CAM. On the other hand, do health practitioners routinely inquire of their patients about such practices? Use of CAM is higher in specific populations, such as patients with breast cancer or HIV infection (Boon and Verhoef,

2001; Eisenberg et al., 1998). There are major questions regarding the standards of alternative medical care, the quality of products, and the supporting scientific evidence (Jonas, 1998). There are certainly risks to the conventionalization of alternative medicine, but there are also risks and costs to a health care system that avoids this issue. The controversy and complexity surrounding CAM will continue as a major force affecting health care services in the 21st century.

Risk Behavior Costs

Risk behaviors cost money to society. In the U.S., smoking, alcohol and drug abuse are estimated to cost over $250 billion due to lost productivity (illness, premature death), medical care, and other factors such as crime and law enforcement (Robert Wood Johnson Foundation, 1994). The lifetime medical costs of cigarette smokers are approximately one-third higher than nonsmokers (U.S. Department of Health and Human Services, 1991). A study in Canada (Single et al., 1996) estimates the total cost of substance abuse at $18 billion. This equals $649 for every Canadian. To help put these costs in perspective, the economic cost of tobacco use ($3.7 billion) is equivalent to one-half of hospital operating expenses for the province of Ontario, Canada.

Keeler et al. (1989) analyzed U.S. population data regarding the external costs of a sedentary lifestyle. They estimate that the lifetime cost to society (lost production, health care expenses) is $1,900 per sedentary individual. Manning et al. (1991) in a comprehensive study of the costs imposed on others by poor health habits reach the following conclusions:

1. Lifetime per capita cost of smoking is $1,000 per smoker.

2. Lifetime per capita cost of excessive drinking is $19,000 per heavy drinker.

3. Lifetime per capita cost for inactivity is $1,650 per sedentary person.

Prevention Can Pay Off

Would a redirection of resources to fund essential clinical and public health services improve population health status? Results from the World Bank analysis indicate that highly cost-effective gains could be achieved. Bobadilla et al. (1994) estimated that a minimum package of public health and essential clinical services for the entire population cost about U.S. $12 per capita per year for low-income countries and $22 per capita per year for middle-income countries. This package of essential services could eliminate the burden of premature mortality and disability in children under 15 years by 21 to 38%, and in adults by 10 to 18%.

The CDC (U.S. Centers for Disease Control and Prevention, 1999m) conducted an analysis of 19 prevention strategies and the expected returns on investment. Some childhood vaccines are estimated to save up to $29 in direct medical costs for each dollar spent. Other strategies, such as mammograms, have a net cost, yet are assessed to be cost-effective because they achieve considerable return in value.

Bartlett (1995) considered cost-benefit studies in managed care and other settings of patient education for a range of conditions such as minor illnesses, prenatal care, asthma, psychosomatic complaints, diabetes, arthritis and chronic pain. Results indicated that patient education reduced visits for minor illnesses by 35% and resulted in fewer preterm births and three-fold lower use of emergency room visits. On average, for every dollar invested in patient education $3–4 dollars were saved. None of the 12 studies reviewed found that the cost of the patient education initiative was more than it saved.

Tengs et al. (1995) estimate the cost effectiveness of 500 diverse life-saving interventions in the United States. Overall, the median intervention costs $42,000 per life-year saved. Considering medical interventions alone, Tengs et al. (1995) found that primary prevention programs are more cost-effective than secondary or tertiary programs:

- Primary Prevention: $5,000 life/year saved
- Secondary Prevention: $23,000 life/year saved
- Tertiary Prevention: $22,000 life/year saved

Miller and Galbraith (1995) estimate that pediatrician counselling as part of TIPP (The Injury Prevention Program) would achieve an annual cost saving in the U.S. of $880 per child (age 0–4 years). Annual medical cost savings would be in the order of $230 million and injury costs would decline by $3.4 billion if all children ages 0–4 years completed TIPP. Each dollar spent on TIPP would return nearly $13 in cost reductions. Similarly, immunization programs for measles, mumps and rubella can save approximately $14 for every dollar spent (U.S. Preventive Services Task Force, 1989). Programs aimed at bicycle safety in the U.S. would result in estimated net savings of $200 million per year (Newhouse, 1993). Mammogram screening every two years for women 50 to 70 years old would cost $4,050 per year of life saved (Newhouse, 1993).

In a corporate setting, Sokolov (1992a, 1992b) found that employees with three or more risk factors (smoking, obesity, hypertension, hypercholesterolemia, diabetes) have twice the health claims of those with no risk factors. Shepard (1994) estimates that 44 exercise interventions would yield annual savings of $61 to $450 per employee per year and coronary heart disease cost reductions ranging from $75 to $300 per employee annually. Pelletier (1993) comprehensively reviewed 28 studies of health promotion in the workplace and concluded that the savings (reduced health care utilization and absenteeism) are three or more times greater than the program costs. Recently, Pelletier (1996) updated his analysis to cover 1993–1995.

Over the past 20 years, researchers have directed their efforts to evaluating the effectiveness of brief advice by health practitioners to help patients quit smoking (Kottke et al., 1988). In an analysis of 188 randomized controlled trials, Law and Tang (1995) estimate that 2% of smokers (above the control condition) quit and do not relapse (at one year) as a direct result of physician advice. Although this effect is modest, Law and Tang (1995) argue that the cumulative impact is quite cost-effective. They estimate a cost of $1,500 (US) for saving a life through routine 5-minute advice to all smokers to stop: *"Few procedures in medicine carry so small a cost of saving a life"* (p.1938).

Although compelling arguments can be made for increasing the emphasis on prevention, data from cost-effectiveness studies are incomplete and in certain places controversial (Russell, 1993). These estimates provide only one perspective on the cost of health risk behavior to society. Prevention and health promotion can have a broad impact that goes well beyond any economic analysis (e.g., enhanced wellness and quality of life).

Integrating Medical Care and Public Health

In a curious way, escalating costs in health care are stimulating a realignment and even an integration of two broad traditions that split apart at the beginning of the 20th century (Robbins & Freeman, 1999; Roemer, 1984; Starfield, 1996). The first tradition, *medical care*, has focused on the diagnosis and treatment of diseases and the rehabilitation of individual patients. The second tradition, *public health*, has focused on the prevention of disease and the promotion of health mainly at the community and population levels. These traditions have remained two solitudes for most of this century. Thus, it is interesting to observe the advent of managed care approaches (Kongstvedt, 1995) that provide individual patient care within a context that emphasizes maintaining good health for the population served. Community-based, integrated health systems (Decter, 2000; Leatt et al., 1996; McBeth & Schweer, 2000) are advocated as a model for balancing the twin goals of promoting health and treating illness. Some organizations, such as the Group Health Cooperative of Puget Sound (see Chapter 5), Kaiser-Permanente organization of California, and Health Insurance Plan of New York have made important strides in population health improvement and accountability to their consumers.

Health care reform is rolling across most developed countries. In the United States, this is exemplified by the shift away from a fragmented 'cottage industry' of practitioners (predominantly specialists) to an integrated systems approach governed by managed care. Practitioners are under increasing stress as they see a reduction in their professional autonomy and income, deal with more skeptical patients, and endure increasing litigation. Although efforts are being made to shift health care away from hospitals to ambulatory and community-based centers, access to services remains a challenge (e.g., none or inadequate insurance coverage, geographic isolation).

The emphasis on health care reform that began in the 1990s is part of a broader evolution from medical care to primary health care (Starfield, 1992) and a population health perspective (Evans et al., 1994). Essential features of this paradigm shift are summarized in Table 2.3. This new focus encompasses medical care, yet fundamentally extends the boundaries to include different levels of analysis and intervention (individual, community, population-based), emphasis on prevention and health promotion, integrated delivery systems, interdisciplinary collaboration, and active involvement of individuals (patient, family) in decision-making.

Robbins and Freeman (1999, p.121) describe five essential tasks that are facilitated by delivery systems that integrate clinical and public health perspectives:

1. **Disease/Injury Surveillance:** monitor disease, injury, disability and death in the whole population: when, where, and in whom are they occurring?

2. **Environmental Monitoring:** monitor the environment for exposures that may cause disease, injury, disability, or death. Who is exposed to what? How much of it? When? Where? And for how long?

Table 2.3   From Medical Care to Population Health Improvement

	Medical Care	**Population Health Approach**
Focus	Individual	Individual and Population
	Illness/Disease	Health and Illness
	Cure	Prevention and Cure
Content	Treatment	Health Promotion
	Episodic Care	Continuous Care
	Specific Problems	Comprehensive Care
Organization	Specialists	General Practitioners/Specialists
	Physicians	Interdisciplinary Teams
	Single-handed Practice	Integrated Systems
Responsibility	Health Sector Alone	Intersectorial Collaboration
	Professional Dominance	Community Participation
	Passive Role by Patients	Active Role by Patients

Adapted with permission from Vouri (1984). *Community Medicine* (now *Journal of Public Health Medicine*), 6: 221–231.

3. **Population Interventions:** intervene socially and institutionally to protect the public (e.g., remove hazards from the environment, add iodine to salt, ventilate workplaces).

4. **Individual Interventions:** intervene in individual behaviors for population-wide results (e.g., vaccination of all individuals in a community, smoking cessation program delivered to a population using information technology).

5. **Evaluation:** examine all interventions designed to reduce injury and disease and promote health (e.g., evidence-based approaches at clinical and population levels, health services/systems research, quality improvement).

Rising health care expenditures have not resulted in advances in population health indicators, such as the infant mortality rate or life expectancy. Considerable debate has occurred among providers and funders about which strategy (prevention or managed care) will be most effective in reducing the burden of illness and the demand for health care services (Fries, Koop et al., 1993). Regarding the two leading causes of death in North America, a striking decline has been achieved in mortality from coronary heart disease due to both risk factor reduction (prevention) and treatment (Hunink et al., 1997). In contrast, there has been only limited success in reducing cancer mortality (Harvard School of Public Health, 1996). Using a computer-simulation model, Hunink et al. (1997), estimate that primary and secondary risk factor reduction explains more than half of the striking decline in mortality from coronary heart disease in the United States during 1980–1990: 25% of the decline is explained by primary prevention, 29% by secondary prevention of risk factors in patients with coronary disease, and 43% by improvements in treatment of coronary patients. These data underscore the value of both public health (prevention) and medical treatment approaches to the leading cause of death in developed countries.

The impact of medical care and clinical preventive services on U.S. population life expectancy has been analyzed by Bunker, Frazier and Mosteller (1994). They estimate that clinical curative services result in a gain in population life expectancy of approximately 3.5–4 years, and have the potential to extend life by an additional 18 months. The major gains are due to advances in treating ischemic heart disease and diabetes. In comparison, they estimate that clinical prevention services yield a gain in U.S. population life expectancy of approximately 18 months, with the potential of another eight months. Taken together, medical care and clinical prevention yield a gain in population life expectancy of approximately five years, with a potential gain of another two years.

What about the potential gains from primary prevention at community and population levels? McGinnis and Foege (1993) examine factors underlying the major causes of death in the United States. They estimate that *half* of the total premature deaths are attributable to behavioral and social factors, notably, cigarette smoking, improper diet and inactivity, and excessive alcohol use. These risk factors are preventable through individual-, community- and population-based interventions.

Starfield (1994) notes that "much primary care practice is focused on problems that are not, and may never be, resolved to definite diagnosis (p.1129)" Up to 50% of these poorly-defined conditions for which patients seek professional assistance, generally arise from family, social and environmental stresses (Donaldson et al., 1994). In caring for such patients, behavioral medicine and psychosocial interventions are as important as the usual medical response (Rosser, 1996.) Indeed, Sobel (1995) argues that use of clinical behavioral medicine interventions can result in a significant reduction in the frequency of medical treatments:

−17%	Total ambulatory care visits
−35%	Visits for minor illnesses
−25%	Pediatric acute illness visits
−49%	Office visits for acute asthma
−40%	Office visits by arthritis patients
−1.5 days	Average length of hospital stay for surgical patients

An Integrative Approach

Let's further explore the advantages of moving beyond a case-finding approach for high-risk patients to a population-based approach that encompasses health behaviors ranging from low to high risk. For example, let's survey the different interventions for a range of smoking behaviors, from occasional smokers to two-pack-per-day smokers. Lichtenstein and Glasgow (1992) summarize the contrasting elements of a clinical versus public health approach to smoking cessation in Table 2.4. The public health approach has a key advantage; it targets a whole population of smokers and prospective (at risk) smokers using a variety of individual, community and policy interventions (Lichtenstein and Glasgow, 1992).

Abrams and colleagues (1996) analyze conceptualizations of optimal delivery systems for preventive services and behavioral health care, and they estimate the needs for such systems. Using the example of smoking prevention and cessation, they describe a model that integrates illness management, health management, and public health management perspectives. A step-care approach is used to link major intervention domains (primary, secondary and tertiary) for maintaining and improving the health status of the population. Prevention and clinical services are allocated in this step-care approach according to their cost and impact:

- Step 1 represents minimal intensity public health interventions that can be widely disseminated.

- Step 2 represents moderate intensity interventions that are focused on individuals or groups already at risk.

- Step 3 interventions are more specialized and expensive and are targeted at high risk individuals already manifesting major signs or symptoms of disease.

Table 2.4   Clinical Versus Public Health Perspectives on Smoking Cessation

Characteristics	Clinical Perspective	Public Health Perspective
Problem definition	Individual, lifestyle	Community, public policy, environment
Target	Self-referred or recruited samples	Populations and/or high-risk groups
Setting	Medical/specialized clinics	Community environments (work, schools, primary care, home)
Provider	Trained professionals	Professionals, lay, automated (Internet, 1-800 service)
Intervention	Brief counseling or intensive, multisession	Brief, low-cost, self-change focus
Outcome	Higher quit rates (20-30% over 1 year)	Lower quit rates (5-15% over 1 year)
Population of smokers reached	Small percentage	Large percentage
Cost-effectiveness	Lower	Higher

Adapted with permission from Lichtenstein, E., and Glasgow, R.E. (1992). *Journal of Consulting and Clinical Psychology,* 60: 518–527.

Abrams et al. (1996) describe a model that combines individual and population perspectives for smoking cessation. This model emphasizes proactive recruitment of all smokers in the defined population, including those who have little or no motivation to quit. Macrolevel recruitment strategies target subgroups of smokers who vary in their readiness or stage of change. Then, microlevel matching is used at the individual level where the type and intensity of intervention is tailored to the individual's level of nicotine dependence and co-morbidity.

To illustrate the potential cost-effectiveness of this comprehensive approach, Abrams et al (1996) estimate the cost per quality adjusted life-years saved by nicotine dependence treatment (Table 2.5). Because of the relatively low cost and broad reach of Step 1, self-help care, this approach yields the greatest estimated benefits: $100–500 per quality adjusted life-year saved. In comparison, the estimated benefits from Step 2, brief physician counselling and intensive intervention, were $1,000–3,000; and Step 3, behavioral specialty clinic, were $3,000–6,000 per quality adjusted life-year saved. The value from such a multilevel intervention approach is under-scored by smokers' excess cost to the health care system in the United States:

- 14% higher for health care utilization
- $650–1200 more per year to worksites for each smoker

Table 2.5   Cost in Dollars ($) Per Quality Adjusted Life-Year Saved for Smoking and Other Medical Strategies

Step 1. Smoking cessation: self-help	$100–500
Step 1. Smoking cessation: brief physician counselling	$1,000–3,000
Step 1. Smoking cessation: behavioral specialty clinic	$3,000–6,000
Common disease prevention	$7,500–15,000
Hypertension management	$11,000–23,000
Hyperlipidemia treatment	$20,000–100,000
Palliative medicine: tertiary care/rehabilitation	$20,000–150,000+

Adapted with permission from Abrams, et al. (1996). *Annals of Behavioral Medicine,* 18: 290–304.

- Pregnant smokers who quit in first trimester save $22–56 million due to prevention of low birth weight infants

A similar analysis by Orford et al. (1998) examined the trade-offs among clinical, targeted and universal interventions for lowering the burden of suffering from child psychiatric disorders. The authors concluded by recommending a stepped approach: (1) have effective universal programs in place, followed by (2) targeted programs for those not helped sufficiently, followed by (3) clinical services for those unaffected by targeted initiatives.

First Order or Second Order Change?

The previous sections looked at major forces converging on health care and various options for reform. We now look at the level of change needed to provide an effective response. It is instructive to distinguish between two levels of change. First order change involves alterations *IN the system* ('doing it right') to meet a set goal (Watzlawick et al., 1974; Argyris et al., 1985). For example, a thermostat senses when the temperature falls below or above a certain point, and then turns on the furnace or air conditioning. In health care, first order change is exemplified by investing in improving curative care, such as the development of clinical guidelines aimed at improving quality of care and outcome effectiveness. One is working within an established system ('doing it right') that is currently dominated by treating illness through diagnosis, treatment and rehabilitation at the individual patient level. In our thermostat analogy, a first order change could involve installing a computer system that uses sensors to detect when humans are in a room and adjusts the temperature accordingly.

In contrast, second order change entails a radical shift that results in a transformation *OF the system* ('doing the right thing'). New sets of standards, frames, or paradigms are evoked that signal a fundamental shift away from business as usual. In the health field, this transformation could involve a substantial redirection of focus and resources 'upstream' to population-based programs for disease prevention and health promotion. In the thermostat analogy, this could entail a major shift in the expectations and behavior of occupants with respect to their temperature comfort zone along with a structural change to the building (solar panels, special insulation) that substantially reduces the need for fuel.

The distinction between first and second order change is illustrated by our approach to cancer control and treatment. Currently, most cancer-related expenditures are devoted to treatment rather than preventive activities. Would a fundamental redirection of expenditures—'the right mix' of health promotion, early detection and treatment—result in better progress?

The answer is clear if one looks at the major causes of cancer (Harvard Center for Cancer Prevention, 1996). Only a small percentage of cancer is purely hereditary (family history). The major determinants of cancer are behavioral, social and environmental factors. Tobacco is by far the leading cause and is estimated to account for approximately 25% of all fatal cancers and at least eight out of every ten cases of lung cancer. While there is still debate about the specific culprits, diet and nutrition, including excessive drinking, are major determinants. Other important elements include environmental exposure to sunlight, as well as workplace exposure to chemicals and radiation. The Harvard Center for Cancer Prevention (1996) concludes that nearly two-thirds of cancer deaths in the U.S. are linked to preventable risk behaviors:

- smoking (30%)
- adult diet and obesity (30%)
- physical activity level (5%)

In Canada, a cancer prevention blueprint produced by Cancer Care Ontario (2000) estimates that cancer death rates in Ontario could be reduced by at least 20% by implementing four strategies: reducing smoking to equal the lowest level in North America; improving diet and physical activity to match the best in North America; screening 350,000 women annually for breast cancer; and screening for cervical and colorectal cancers.

Yet, there is immense pressure fuelled by public expectations to keep "hacking at the branches" by improving medical treatment. Do we have the resolve to also strike "at the root" determinants of cancer through prevention and public health?

Adapting to the Winds of Change

Health care reform is flailing about on the rising seas of change. Most of the fleet are struggling to hold their course. We decide to downsize with smaller sails; everything is secured or 'ratcheted down'; and sail trim is adjusted again and again (first order change). Some skippers question whether this course will result in the landfall of cost containment and quality care. Meanwhile, a few ships have headed off on a very different tack toward preventive, population-based approaches (second order change). This course offers much promise, yet the chart indicates many barriers, navigation hazards, contrary currents and adverse weather systems. Inwardly, some skippers are unsure that they have sufficient resources, skills and time to reach the new landfall.

There is a pressing need for change in health care. Options exist, but the right choices are difficult to discern.

> There are a thousand hacking at the branches of evil to one who is striking at the roots.
>
> —Henry David Thoreau

Moving On

In the next chapter we look at evolving concepts of health promotion and the importance of behavioral factors as determinants of health and illness. Practitioner and patient perspectives on behavior change are compared. Then, the role of practitioners is described regarding brief advice, motivation enhancement and prevention counselling.

CHAPTER 3

Beyond Clinical Care

*The nation needs stronger education and incentives
targeted to behavioral factors that shape personal
health prospects and to strengthen the state and local
public health infrastructures that are important to
protecting the health of entire populations.*

McGinnis and Lee (1995)

Overview

Health behavior is complexly determined and maintained. This chapter
reviews key concepts and evidence that links behavior with the health status of individuals and populations. Emphasis is placed on four important
aspects:

1. relationship between personal behavior (lifestyle) and health

2. understanding the broader social, economic and environmental determinants of health that influence individuals and communities

3. practitioner and patient perspectives on health behavior change

4. evolving role of health practitioners in providing brief advice interventions, motivation enhancement, and counselling regarding preventive
services

The World Health Organization conceptualizes health promotion largely on
a community and population level; we supplement this approach by focusing on personal and organizational skills of behavior change that impact
both individual and population health. Our person-centered health promotion model brings the motto, *"think globally, act locally"*, to behavior change
at the individual practitioner and patient, the health care organization, and
the community levels.

Why Is Health Behavior Important?

Most people accept that personal behavior has an important influence on health and illness. Indeed, we are constantly bombarded with such messages. Try reading a magazine or watching a talk show without being assailed by the latest strategies for losing weight, getting fit ('washboard abs' and 'buns of steel'), quitting smoking, having safer sex, cutting down on drinking, reducing stress and, above all, enjoying life more! For some, 'good' health is not a goal, but an obsession. Yet, in spite of this knowledge and mass marketing, we engage in risk behaviors.

In North America, an emphasis on personal behavior was given considerable impetus by the Lalonde report, A New Perspective on the Health of Canadians (1974), which identified four major health determinants: 1) lifestyle (personal behavior); 2) human biology; 3) environment; and 4) health care system. The Lalonde Report stimulated much interest internationally. In the United States, the Surgeon General's 1979 report estimated that the major causes of death could be attributed accordingly:

- 50% to health risk behavior (lifestyle)
- 20% to environmental factors
- 20% to human biological factors
- 10% to inadequacies in health care

During the 1980s, there was a major decline in mortality rates for three of the leading causes of death among Americans: heart disease, stroke, and unintentional injuries (U.S. Department of Health and Human Services, 1991). Much of this progress was due to a reduction in social and behavioral risk factors, such as a decline in cigarette smoking. At the same time, there was no progress in other areas (e.g., cancer death rates went up 7% between 1975 and 1990). The emergence of HIV infection and rising rates of other sexually transmitted diseases (e.g., syphilis) became major public health problems, and there was growing concern over environmental pollution.

A study by McGinnis and Foege (1993) underscored the significance of behavior as the major (nongenetic) factor contributing to death in the United States (Table 3.1). Almost half, (1,060,000) of the 2,148,000 total deaths in 1990 could be attributed to cigarette smoking, diet and physical activity pattern, excessive alcohol use, firearms, risky sexual behaviors, motor vehicle accidents and illicit use of drugs. These data offer considerable guidance for shaping health policy priorities. The three leading factors,

Table 3.1   Risk Factors Contributing to Death in USA: 1990

Risk Factor	NUMBER	%
Smoking	400,000	19
Diet/Exercise	300,000	14
Alcohol	100,000	5
Microbial	90,000	4
Toxic	60,000	3
Firearms	35,000	2
STDs	25,000	1
Motor Vehicle	20,000	1
Illicit Drugs	20,000	1
TOTAL	1,060,000	50

Adapted with permission from McGinnis and Foege (1993). *JAMA*, 270: 2207–2212.

tobacco, diet and activity patterns, and alcohol can be modified by individual change strategies and a supportive social environment. Nevertheless, the preponderance of health care expenditures is directed to medical treatment and rehabilitation. Only a small fraction (less than 5%) is directed toward prevention.

In Canada, a study of premature deaths emphasizes the importance of behavioral factors relative to medical care (Figure 3.1). Wigle et al. (1990) found that over 50% of almost 100,000 premature deaths (before age 75) are attributable to personal behaviors or preventable conditions: cigarette smoking, hypertension (obesity/diet/exercise), serum cholesterol (obesity/

Over 50% of premature deaths annually in Canada due to

Smoking: 26,000 deaths

Hypertension: 13,000 deaths
(obesity, diet, exercise)

Cholesterol: 10,000 deaths
(obesity, diet, exercise)

Diabetes: 6,000 deaths
(obesity, diet, exercise)

Alcohol: 5,000 deaths

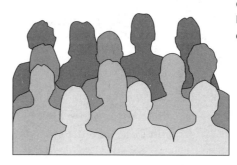

Figure 3.1 Behavioral and social factors underlying premature deaths in Canada. Data taken from Wigle et al. (1990).

diet/exercise), adult-onset diabetes (obesity/diet/exercise), and excessive drinking. In contrast, the authors estimated that only about 6,000 premature deaths, or 6%, could be avoided through improved medical intervention. Charlton and Velez (1986) draw similar conclusions from an international comparison of premature mortality patterns.

Prospective studies have demonstrated that social and behavioral factors can significantly reduce the risk of disease and mortality. The Alameda County Project (Berkman & Breslow, 1983), a landmark study, found that five common habits were strongly related to mortality over a nine-year follow-up:

1. cigarette smoking
2. alcohol consumption
3. physical activity
4. body weight
5. hours of sleeping

To assess the cumulative impact of these five health behaviors, a Health Practices Index sums risk behaviors for each individual. Men aged 30–49 years who followed high risk practices are over 8 times as likely to die as compared with men the same age who followed low risk practices.

In addition, Berkman and Breslow (1983) studied the relationship of social networks in the form of marriage, contacts with close friends and relatives, church membership, and affiliation with non-church groups. They constructed a Social Network Index, which demonstrates a clear relationship between these networks and risk of mortality. Men in the most isolated group have an age-adjusted mortality rate 2.3 times higher than men who have the strongest social connections. Among women the difference is 2.8 times. Moreover, this relationship is consistent across the socioeconomic gradient. Men and women who have few social contacts have higher mortality rates than those who have many connections. This research is consistent with other considerable work demonstrating that social relationships have a causal impact on health (House, Landis & Umberson, 1988; Wilkinson, 1996).

Research has shown that intense or prolonged stressful events lead to physiological effects, such as reduced immunological activities and cardiovascular changes that cause narrowing of blood vessels; these, in turn, are associated with pathological events such as heart attacks or strokes (Barefoote Schroll, 1996; Kop 1997; Ravaja et al., 2000). Stress is also associated with behavioral changes such as decreased likelihood of seeking medical care, smoking, excessive alcohol use, poor eating habits, and insomnia. Although moderate stress can improve performance, excess and chronic levels have profound biological, psychological and social impact. On the positive side, dealing with stressful situations can increase one's sense of personal control and self-efficacy (Bandura, 1997).

Many behaviors leading to later illness and premature death begin during youth; for example, cigarette smoking, excessive drinking, unprotected sexual activity, improper diet and physical inactivity, and preventable injuries (the greatest cause of death and a major contributor to morbidity in youth). Targeting these six major risk factors in the young is an opportune time for health promotion. In terms of health care costs, a Health Canada study (1998) using 1993 data found that those between the ages of 15 and 34 account for more than 15% of all hospital costs, almost 25% of fee-for-service charges by physicians, more than 15% of mortality costs, more than 10% of drug costs, and more than 65% of short-term disability costs (e.g., injuries).

Broader Determinants of Health

In the 1970s, an emphasis on lifestyle behavior, stimulated by the Lalonde (1974) and the U.S. Surgeon General (1979) reports, ushered in a new era—individual responsibility for health risks. The tenor of the time is perhaps best captured in the following quotation from Joseph Califano, U.S. Surgeon General (1979, p.viii):

We are killing ourselves by our own careless habits. We are killing ourselves by carelessly polluting the environment. We are killing ourselves by permitting harmful social conditions to persist—conditions like poverty, hunger and ignorance—which destroy health, especially for infants and children. You, the individual, can do more for your own health and well being than any doctor, any hospital, any drug, any exotic medical device.

The emphasis on lifestyles led to the proliferation of assessment procedures, such as health risk appraisals (Weiss, 1984; DeFriese and Fielding, 1990). This redirection of attention to lifestyle behavior was extremely important; nonetheless, concerns were raised that the pendulum had swung too far.

Critics argued that individual change was being oversold and, what is more, amounted to 'blaming the victim' (Levin, 1987; Becker, 1992). A rebalancing and a focus on structural determinants of health occurred in the 1980s and 1990s. At the international level, the World Health Organization (1978) proposed a wider concept of health: health is not merely an end in itself; health is a resource for living. This declaration (at Alma Ata) was followed by the commitment to "Health for All." This commitment emphasises primary and community-based health care, appropriate technology, community involvement and multisectoral approaches. See Cottrell, Girvan and McKenzie (1999) for a review of the history and development of health promotion and health education.

Health Promotion

At the First International Conference on Health Promotion, a Charter for Action was adopted for the achievement of health for all by the year 2000 and beyond (World Health Organization, 1986). The Ottawa Charter, as it is called, emphasizes five interdependent actions:

1. Build healthy public policy
2. Create supportive environments
3. Strengthen community action
4. Develop personal skills
5. Reorient health services.

The International Union for Health Promotion and Education (2000) provides a comprehensive review of the effectiveness of these five actions for health promotion.

Prevention and health promotion in health organizations must address relevant aspects of *all five actions*, not just lifestyle or personal behavior change. Our book is primarily aimed at action 5. Little systematic progress has been made in reorienting health services to encompass a broader focus on prevention and population health improvement. The Five-Step Model offers a guide and practical tools for achieving this transformation, especially by supporting practitioners and patients in health behavior change at clinical and community levels.

In the 1990s, there was growing appreciation of the importance of prevention and health promotion in clinical practice. Behavioral assessment and change are an important component of a comprehensive approach to health that includes community action, environmental and public policy domains. This perspective is embodied in the World Health Organization definition of health promotion (1986):

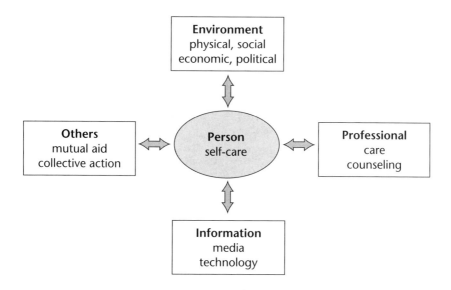

Figure 3.2 Person-centered model for health promotion.
Adapted from Skinner and Bercovitz (1997).

> *... the process of enabling individuals and communities to increase control over the determinants of health and thereby improve their health.*

The development of personal skills through lifelong learning is one of the five central components of the World Health Organization's Charter for Health Promotion (1986). Whereas the other four components conceptualize and promote action at community and population levels, the development of personal skills is located at the individual level. The goal is to enhance life skills and options that will enable individuals to exercise more control over their own health, including their physical, social, and economic environments.

Skinner and Bercovitz (1997) describe a Person-Centered Health Promotion Model (Figure 3.2) as a framework for understanding individual health behavior within a broader systems context. In this model, a person's capacity for self-care and behavior change is influenced by others (mutual aid, family, peer group), by assistance from professionals (care, counselling), by access to information that is timely and pertinent to the individual, as well as by the environment (physical, social, economic, political). Similarly, Raeburn and Rootman (1998) present a comprehensive analysis of the centrality of the individual within community and population health promotion.

Population Health

Parallel to evolving concepts of health promotion, population health and determinants of health perspectives also evolved significantly (Blane et al., 1996; Evans et al., 1994). These perspectives span multiple levels and domains: 1) basic sciences that link biological, developmental and social processes to health and disease expression in populations; 2) social norms and policies, such as regulatory attention to environmental and occupational exposures, that affect populations; and 3) systematic evaluation of interventions, ranging from health behavior change in individuals to environmental regulations, to occupational or community-based initiatives, to health promotion initiatives directed at the entire population, designed to reduce risk and improve health in populations.

The Canadian Federal, Provincial, and Territorial Ministers of Health (1994) adopted population health as a key policy framework. They defined population health as including five categories:

1. **Social and Economic Environment:** income, employment, social status, social support networks, education, and social factors

2. **Physical environment:** physical, chemical, biological, and organizational factors in the workplace, as well as other aspects of the natural and human-built physical environment

3. **Personal Health Practice:** behaviors that mitigate or create risks to health

4. **Individual Capacity and Coping Skills:** personal competence, coping skills, sense of control and mastery, and genetic and biological characteristics

5. **Health Services:** services to promote, maintain and restore health

Similarly, the U.S. Healthy People 2010 initiative incorporates a broad determinants of health framework. The initiative identifies five critical influences that determine the health of individuals and communities: biology; behavior; social environment; physical environment; policies and interventions, including access to quality care and services. These factors are seen as interdependent. For example, violence in the community (social environment) can have a profound effect on personal choice regarding physical activity (behavior); a family history of heart disease (biology) may motivate an individual to avoid smoking (behavior), which in turn may prevent the development of occluded coronary arteries (biology); or a policy regarding low cost public transportation may help achieve cleaner city air (physical environment). The determinants of health framework is used as a basis for identifying health goals and targeting specific action in the Healthy People 2010 initiative discussed next.

Health Goals for the United States

The United States has embarked on an ambitious program of improving public health opportunities. In 1979, the Surgeon General's report, *Healthy People*, provided national goals, and a subsequent report, *Promoting Health/Preventing Disease* (1980), outlined 226 objectives for the next decade. Health goals for the year 2000 are described in *Healthy People* (U.S. Department of Health and Human Services, 1991). They target three broad areas:

1. To increase the span of healthy life for Americans

2. To reduce health disparities among Americans

3. To achieve access to preventive services for all Americans.

McGinnis and Lee (1995) provide a scorecard evaluating the success of meeting specific targets at mid-decade. In the area of **health promotion**, 10 of 17 initiatives are proceeding in the right direction. The greatest concern is prevalence of sedentary lifestyles and the increasing percentage of overweight people. In addition, violence and pregnancies are increasingly problematic for youth. With respect to **health protection**, 8 out of 10 initiatives are progressing in the right direction. Work-related injuries are cited as a major area of increased concern. With respect to **preventive services**, 13 of 19 initiatives are progressing in the right direction. Particular problems are evident for the most vulnerable population: Americans who lack health insurance and have financial barriers to medical care and preventive services.

The Healthy People 2010 initiative furthers these efforts with two overarching goals:

- **Increase quality and years of healthy life:** Help individuals of all ages increase life expectancy and improve their quality of life. Although in the U.S. the average life expectancy at birth is nearly 77 years, at least 18 countries, led by Japan, have better life expectancies.

- **Eliminate health disparities:** Redress disparities among different segments of the population. For example, men have a life expectancy that is six years less than women, infant mortality among African Americans is more than double that of whites, and people in the low-

Table 3.2   Leading Health Indicators: Healthy People 2010

	Example of an Objective
1. *Physical Activity*	Increase proportion of adolescents engaging in vigorous physical activity for 3 or more days per week for 20 or more minutes per occasion
2. *Overweight and Obesity*	Reduce proportion of adults who are obese
3. *Tobacco Use*	Reduce cigarette smoking by adolescents
4. *Substance Abuse*	Reduce proportion of adults engaging in binge drinking of alcoholic beverages in past month
5. *Responsible Sexual Behavior*	Increase proportion of sexually active persons who use condoms
6. *Mental Health*	Increase proportion of adults with recognized depression who receive treatment
7. *Injury and Violence*	Reduce deaths caused by motor vehicle crashes
8. *Environmental Quality*	Reduce proportion of persons exposed to air that does not meet U.S. Environmental Protection Agency's health-based standards for ozone
9. *Immunization*	Increase proportion of young children receiving all vaccines recommended for universal administration for at least the first 5 years of life
10. *Access to Health Care*	Increase the proportion of persons with health insurance

est income households have poorer health status and die three to seven years younger on average.

In achieving these goals, ten leading health indicators were chosen to motivate action (Table 3.2). The Healthy People 2010 website (*www.health.gov/ healthypeople/*) provides a comprehensive description of the prevention agenda, midcourse reviews, progress in meeting specific objectives, and opportunities for getting involved.

New Role of Practitioners in Changing Behavior

Given this increased attention to behavior as a key determinant of health, why are practitioners not routinely using health promotion and behavior change programs in clinical practice? Let's look at both practitioner and patient perspectives on this question.

Practitioners' Perspectives

Practitioners frequently have mixed feelings about their role in prevention and behavioral health care. A study in the 1980s found that nearly three-

Table 3.3   Counselling Practices of Internists

Effective	Counsel Patients	Very Effective	Moderately
Smoking	90%	5%	23%
Alcohol	76%	2%	13%
Exercise	47%	4%	27%
Seat Belt	16%	3%	5%

Source: Lewis et al. (1991)

quarters of primary care physicians feel that they were definitely responsible for educating their patients about behaviors such as cigarette smoking, alcohol use, drug use, stress, exercise and diet (Wechsler et al., 1983). Only about one-quarter (27%) of the practitioners reported that they routinely gathered information about all of these lifestyle behaviors. Moreover, they were generally pessimistic about being able to intervene effectively. For example, only 3–5% report that they were confident about their effectiveness in counselling patients regarding cigarette, alcohol and drug use.

A decade later, a U.S. National Survey found little improvement in the counselling practices of internists (Lewis et al., 1991). Although 90% of physicians report that they counsel all of their patients who smoke cigarettes, 84% report that they never discuss the use of seat belts. Moreover, this study found that physicians' personal health practices are substantially associated with whether or not they counsel patients. For instance, non-smoking practitioners are far more likely to counsel patients who smoke, and physically active physicians are more likely to counsel their patients about exercise. Of particular note is the low number of physicians who believe that they are effective in changing patient behavior (Table 3.3).

In a seven-year prospective study, Scott, Neighbor and Brock (1992) examine physicians' attitudes and intentions to provide 27 preventive services. Respondents are assessed at three career stages: 1) during orientation to medical school; 2) during third year medical school; and 3) at completion of their (three year) residency training. Positive attitudes generally persist, although primary care physicians are more likely than those in medical specialities to view preventive services as important. Residents are most confident in their ability to provide screening and management for hypertension, hyperlipidemia, cancer detection, and immunizations—interventions that conform more closely to traditional medical management protocols. In contrast, attitudes toward and confidence to provide behavioral counselling

Table 3.4   Perceived Importance and Confidence in Preventive Services

	FAIR Confidence	MEDIUM Confidence
VERY IMPORTANT	Smoking cessation	Cancer detection
	Health counselling	Hypertension control
	AIDS education	Hypertension management
	Substance abuse	
IMPORTANT	Exercise/fitness	Immunizations
	HIV screening/management	Hypertension screening
	Weight reduction	Hyperlipidemia screening/management
	Lifestyle modification	Family planning
	Poison control	Health screening physical
	Stress management	STD prevention
	Personal counselling/hygiene	
	Genetic counselling	

Adapted from Scott et al. (1992)

is weak for these health related activities: smoking cessation, exercise and physical fitness, weight reduction, lifestyle modification, substance abuse counselling, nutritional counselling and stress management (Table 3.4).

Patients' Perspective

Patients are often willing to talk about sensitive issues, such as drinking or sexual activities, but they are not likely to do so spontaneously (Murphy, 1980). In a study of patients' perspectives on health behaviors, Wallace and Haines (1984) found that most patients feel that their doctor should be interested in their cigarette smoking, alcohol use, weight control and physical activity. However, less than half of the patients report that their physician had inquired about and seemed comfortable discussing these issues. These findings beg the question, *"who is hiding from whom?"*

In a survey of family practice patients, Skinner (1993) found that over 90% state that it was important that their doctor ask questions and be up-to-date regarding their lifestyle habits. Patients expect their doctor to intervene when appropriate. When asked about what level of help they expect from their doctor regarding potential lifestyle problems (Table 3.5), most patients report that brief advice and support from the doctor are expected

Table 3.5   Level of Involvement Patients Expect from Their Family Physician

Level 1	Level 2	Level 3	Level 4
None	**Refer to a Specialist**	**Advice and Support**	**Counselling/Treatment**
Financial problems	Parenting problems	Poor nutrition	Long-term pain
	Death in family	Nervousness	Drug abuse
	Caffeine use	Drinking problems	
	Social isolation	Weight control	
	Marital separation/	Sleep problems	
	divorce	Depression	
		Family violence	
		Cigarette smoking	
		Exercise	
		Sexual problems	

regarding cigarette smoking, eating habits, excessive drinking, weight control, sexual problems, emotional health and family violence.

What do patients believe is the most effective aspect of the physician's behavior? Insight into this question is provided by a qualitative study by Willms et al. (1991) of a physician-delivered smoking cessation intervention. During open-ended interviews, patients discuss two contrasting roles taken by physicians:

- **Doctor-Centered** (interventionistic), where professional, diagnostic, biomedical and authoritative features are emphasized
- **Patient-Centered** (personalistic), where practitioners are experienced as equals, as supportive, caring, and empowering.

Patients frequently forget the details of the physicians' message but remember the kind of support given ('pat on the back'), positive images used by the physician ('lungs getting clean'), relationship of equality and mutual accountability ("he is doing his best so I need to do mine"). Patients found the personalistic (patient-centered) component of the physician-delivered intervention to be most helpful. This finding reinforces the need for motivational approaches within a patient-centered framework (Stewart et al., 1995).

In review, we find significant differences in the perspectives that practitioners and patients take on health behavior change:

- Practitioners generally believe that they have a responsibility to assess and educate patients about health risk behaviors.

- Most patients believe it is important that their practitioner ask questions and provide assistance (when necessary).

- Patients often are willing to talk about sensitive issues (e.g., excessive drinking, sexual activities), but they are not likely to do so spontaneously.

- Many practitioners do not routinely ask about health risk behaviors.

- Practitioners remain pessimistic about their effectiveness in helping patients change.

These findings underscore a central premise of our book: *if practitioners are to improve their own and their organization's ability to change health related behavior, they need training in both motivational and organizational approaches.* We now turn to an examination of the growing body of research on brief advice interventions and motivational approaches to behavior change. There is a significant gap in professional education in these areas that has contributed to the reluctance of many practitioners to address health behavior with patients.

Brief Advice Interventions

The clinical encounter provides a common meeting ground for the medical care and public health traditions described in Chapter 2. Indeed, Roemer (1984) argues that when patients and their families seek help in hospitals and community health settings we have an ideal opportunity for health promotion and disease prevention. There is a substantial body of research regarding the effectiveness of brief interventions by physicians and other health professionals in helping patients alter health risk behaviors. Comprehensive reviews and meta-analyses of this literature are available: smoking cessation programs by Law and Tang (1995), Ritvo et al. (1997) and Kottke et al. (1988); reduction in problem drinking by Zweben and Fleming (1999), Bien et al. (1993), Babor (1994), Heather (1995) and Kahan et al. (1995); dietary behavior interventions by Brunner et al. (1997); and multiple risk factor interventions by Ashenden et al. (1997) and by Ebrahim and Smith (1997). Also, excellent information sources are available on the Internet, including the evidence cited for the *Clinical Prevention Guidelines* at the Agency for Health Care Policy and Research website (*http://www.ahcpr.gov/guide/*), as well as reviews on the Cochrane Library Website:

United Kingdom: *http://www.cochrane.co.uk*

United States: *http://www.updateusa.com/clibhome/clib.htm*

Canada: *http://hiru.mcmaster.ca/cochrane*

Two reviews of lifestyle behavior change raise concerns about the magnitude of effects achieved by practitioner interventions. Ashenden et al. (1997) examine the impact of general practitioner advice in changing patient behavior in four areas: smoking, alcohol consumption, diet, and exercise. Following an evaluation of 37 randomized controlled trials, they conclude that many brief intervention studies show that practitioner interventions effect small changes, but none show that practitioners produce substantial changes. Similarly, Ebrahim and Smith (1997) review randomized controlled trials of multiple risk factor interventions for preventing coronary heart disease. The six interventions include: stop smoking, increase exercise, dietary advice, weight control, anti-hypertensive drugs, and cholesterol lowering drugs. Interventions using personal or family counselling were effective in changing behavior (e.g., quit smoking) in high-risk hypertensive populations. However, the interventions result in only small changes in risk factors and mortality in the general population. Because of this relatively small impact, the authors of both reviews draw somewhat pessimistic conclusions about the utility of practice-based interventions for altering health risk behaviors among patients. Ashenden et al. (1997) argue for more research on ways to engage a larger number of practitioners in routinely applying practice-based behavior change interventions. However, Ebrahim and Smith (1997) look beyond the clinical setting and recommend greater emphasis on population-based approaches, such as health protection legislation, health policy and fiscal measures.

The potential cumulative impact of brief interventions could be substantial, if health practitioners use them routinely as part of an organizational approach. Russell et al. (1979, p.234) argue that if one could get all general practitioners in the United Kingdom to counsel patients to quit smoking, then "this success rate could not be matched by increasing the number of specialized smoking-withdrawal clinics in England from the present 50 to over 10,000". Similarly, following their demonstration of the effectiveness of practitioners' advice to heavy drinkers to reduce their excessive alcohol consumption, Wallace et al. (1988, p.663) concluded that "if the results of this study are applied to the United Kingdom, intervention by general practitioners could, each year, reduce to moderate levels the alcohol consumption of some 250,000 men and 67,500 women who currently drink to excess." The Five-Step Model described in this book is aimed at the type of organizational change needed to support routine and comprehensive implementation by practitioners of brief advice interventions as well as the motivation enhancement approaches discussed next.

Motivational Interventions

We are in the midst of major advances in understanding motivation and the processes of change (see Chapter 7 for an in-depth presentation). The Transtheoretical Model developed by Prochaska and DiClemente (Prochaska et al.,1992) is particularly fruitful. Their **stages of change** component has broadened and deepened our understanding of health behavior change: it spans a continuum from the early recognition of a health concern to long-term maintenance of behavioral change. Miller and Rollnick (1991) developed another significant component called **motivational interviewing (MI)**. MI concepts and techniques are especially relevant for practitioners in helping patients who are either unsure or not yet ready for change (Rollnick et al., 1999). A third development emphasizes **relapse prevention** and harm reduction stimulated by the work of Marlatt and colleagues (Allen, Lowman & Miller, 1996; Marlatt, 1998; Marlatt and Gordon, 1985). Finally, **self-determination theory** by Ryan and Deci (2000) provides a comprehensive model for understanding the dynamics of motivational approaches. This theory, which emphasizes support of patients' autonomy to make health decisions, is a central element underlying the six-phase negotiation model for practitioners described by Botelho (2001) and Botelho, Skinner et al. (1999).

Stages of change: transtheoretical model. In attempting to understand how people change health behavior, Prochaska, DiClemente and Norcross (1992) describe a progression through five stages:

1. **Precontemplation:** not thinking about change

2. **Contemplation:** unsure or ambivalent about change

3. **Preparation:** ready to initiate change in next four weeks

4. **Action:** taking steps toward the behavioral goal

5. **Maintenance:** trying to maintain change over the long term—at least 6 months

Most people do not progress in a linear fashion through these stages; relapses are common. With respect to cigarette smoking, Prochaska and DiClemente (1986) found that self-changers make at least three serious attempts to quit before they achieve long-term abstinence. Thus, individuals may recycle through the stages several times before achieving a long-term goal.

The stages of change model can help practitioners understand how the patient 'sees' the health issue (concern or problem) and then take appropriate steps based on the patient's readiness for change. Change is most likely to occur if both patient and practitioner focus on the same stage of change and use the appropriate process for that stage.

For example, the PACE project is designed to encourage primary care providers to counsel patients about regular physical activity (Patrick et al., 1994). One of its innovative features is to link specific counselling strategies to the patient's readiness for change. Results from a controlled trial (Calfas et. al., 1996) support this tailored approach. A series of studies described in Chapter 16 demonstrate how the stage-based *Pathways to Change* computer-based system can outperform traditional interventions in a variety of community and health care settings.

Motivational interviewing. Motivational interviewing (MI), developed by Miller and Rollnick (1991), has sparked considerable interest among practitioners and researchers. Motivation is traditionally viewed as a trait of the individual that is difficult to change: *'It is the person's problem ... a reason why the patient did poorly in treatment'*. In contrast, our view is that motivation is a state that is changeable and influenced very much by the practitioner's interviewing style (cf., Miller, 1985). Motivational interviewing is particularly relevant for working with patients who are in the precontemplation or contemplation stages of change. Both patient and practitioner play key roles in fostering a commitment toward changing a health behavior. Although initially developed in the addictions field, MI is being applied to a broad range of behaviors (Miller, 1996). With respect to health care settings, Rollnick et al. (1999) have published a guide for practitioners based on motivational interviewing principles.

Miller and Rollnick (1991) describe five basic principles for enhancing motivation:

1. **Express empathy:** listen rather than tell.
2. **Develop a discrepancy:** distinguish between where a patient is now (i.e., risk behavior) and where he/she wants to be (goal).

3. **Avoid argumentation:** the force of argument alone rarely convinces patients.

4. **Roll with resistance:** avoid meeting patient resistance head-on.

5. **Support self-efficacy:** instill hope and support patients' belief that they can change.

The use of these principles requires health practitioners to take a very different stance (e.g., nonconfrontational) with respect to the patient. The basic goal is to develop a 'shared' understanding of the health issue and to stimulate the patient's commitment to change.

The Motivational Interviewing website gives an updated list of research publications including outcome studies:

http://www.motivationalinterview.org/library/biblio.html.

Relapse prevention. When an individual takes action to change a health behavior, the most likely outcome is not successful maintenance (at least, not on the first attempt), but rather relapse. Our approaches to intervention tend to focus on making initial changes, rather than on maintaining these changes in behavior over time. What often results is a 'revolving door' where patients relapse and return again and again into care, or they simply give up (precontemplation). Relapse prevention was initially developed for the treatment of addictive behaviors, with abstinence as the primary goal. Subsequently, these interventions have been extended to a range of health behaviors and outcome goals consistent with a harm reduction philosophy (Marlatt, 1998; Brownell et al.,1985).

Self-determination theory. Ryan and Deci (2000) developed self-determination theory as a comprehensive approach for understanding human motivation. Its central achievement is a description of how behavior is regulated. Any intentional behavior can be analyzed according to the extent that it is self-regulated (**autonomous**) or regulated by forces (**controlled**) outside the individual.

Autonomous behaviors are regulated by the individual's willingness to engage in a behavior: *"I want to do it of my own choice"*. Since this behavior emanates from the self, Deci and Ryan (1985) consider it self-determined. In contrast, controlled behaviors are regulated by a process of compliance and pressure to behave in a certain way: *"I am taking action because I feel that I should or have to do it"*. Fully autonomous and fully controlled motivation are poles of a continuum. Any action, such as beginning an exercise program, can be located along this continuum by assessing the degree to which it is being freely chosen by the individual.

Self-determination theory also includes dimensions that characterize interpersonal environments. Of particular relevance to health care organizations is whether practitioners support the patient's autonomy or try to control the patient's behavior. Autonomy-supportive practitioners take time to listen to patients, try to understand their perspective on the health issue, and offer choices or options on how to deal with the health issue. This characterization is consistent with motivational interviewing (Rollnick et al., 1999), with the patient-centered approach (Stewart et al. 1995), as well as with the six-step model for becoming a motivational practitioner (Botelho, 2001; Botelho, Skinner et al., 1999).

Williams, Deci and Ryan (1998) summarize research that has applied self-determination theory to health behavior change. Their basic premise is that patients are more likely to achieve long-term success when they take action for autonomous reasons. Their model is guided by two interrelated hypotheses:

- **Practitioners' Approach**: when practitioners use an autonomy-supportive rather than controlling approach, they increase patients' intrinsic motivation, and this produces better outcomes

- **Patients' Autonomy**: personal choice rather than controlled motivation predicts self-care and adherence to treatment protocols (prescriptions, attendance in programs), which in turn enhances the likelihood of positive behavior change and maintenance over time.

Autonomy support is hypothesized to consist of three aspects: 1) a meaningful rationale is given so that patients understand the personal importance of the activity; 2) patient's feelings and perspectives are acknowledged, so they feel understood; and 3) an interpersonal style is adopted that emphasizes choice and minimizes control. When health practitioners try to pressure patients to change using words such as 'should', 'must', or 'have to', patients are likely to feel less autonomous and are more susceptible to relapse. Williams et al. (1998) found that patients' autonomous motivation was a strong, positive predictor of medication adherence, assessed with both self-reports and pill counts.

Preventive Services Guidelines

This final section reviews the role of practitioners in providing preventive services. Comprehensive guidelines on a full range of preventive services have been compiled by three expert panels: the U.S. Preventive Services Task Force (1989; 1996), the American College of Physicians (Hayward et al., 1991; Sox, 1994), and the Canadian Task Force on the Periodic Health Examination (1994). The three panels agree on seven policies for disease prevention in low-risk patients:

1. Blood pressure measurement

2. Breast examination by a physician

3. Serum cholesterol

4. Mammography

5. Cervical cytological screening

6. Vaccination

7. Counselling

With respect to behavioral (lifestyle) issues, the three panels underscore 10 areas of focus for counselling:

1. Tobacco use

2. Alcohol use

3. Nutrition: diet, weight, calcium, and iron levels

4. Physical activity

5. Injury prevention

6. Sexual practices, prevention of unwanted pregnancies

7. Breast and testes self-examination

8. Drug use

9. Dental hygiene

10. Functional assessment

Table 3.6 provides a synopsis of specific recommendations from the expert panels. They all insist on a comprehensive literature search, critical evaluation of the available evidence, clear rationales for their recommendations and external review by experts. The importance of cost and ethical issues (e.g., do the benefits of a given preventive measure outweigh the harm) are also taken into consideration. For up-to-date reviews on achieving specific objectives in clinical preventive services consult the U.S. Healthy People 2010 website *(www.health.gov/healthypeople/)*.

While keeping in mind the weight of these expert task force recommendations, one must remain cognizant that preventive services can have potentially negative effects on individual patients and the health care system in general (Marshall, 1996a, b, c, d). This may be the case for both procedural (e.g., screening) and behavioral (e.g., counselling) interventions.

For example, a 50-year-old woman with a family history of breast cancer is referred by her primary care physician for mammography. Because of time pressure during the clinical encounter, the physician describes the mammography procedure but only superficially explores the patient's concerns. In the time between the referral and the mammogram appointment, she worries about whether the procedure will be painful and about the mammogram results. As the appointment date approaches, she becomes even more anxious about any abnormalities. This affects her ability to function personally, socially and professionally. During the mammogram itself, she suffers some discomfort and breast compression. An abnormal mammogram result leads to further investigations. The woman feels both angry and dejected by the investigative process.

In their book on evaluating prevention effectiveness, Haddix et al. (1996) pose seven basic questions for making decisions that draw upon epidemiology, public health surveillance, intervention studies and economic analyses:

1. What is the magnitude of the problem addressed by the prevention strategy?
2. Can the intervention work (efficacy)?
3. Does the intervention work (effectiveness)?
4. What are its benefits and harms (individual and societal perspectives)?
5. What does the intervention cost?
6. How do the benefits compare with the costs?
7. What additional benefit could be obtained with additional resources?

These questions provide a comprehensive framework for evaluating the impact of prevention policies, programs and practices on health outcomes.

Another excellent framework for evaluating the healthcare system is given by Aday, Begley, Lairson and Slater (1998). They describe a health services research framework for addressing effectiveness, efficiency and equity of health care and health promotion initiatives.

TABLE 3.6   Preventive Counselling Recommendations of Three Task Forces

	Canada	U.S. ACP	U.S. PSTF
Nutritional Counselling	General dietary counselling, advise patients to reduce fat intake, increase fiber intake (fair evidence)	Counsel on balancing diet with reduced fat intake; reduce cholesterol and sodium; increase vegetables, fruits, and grains. For women: advise on folic acid and calcium intake.	Counsel patients to lower fat and cholesterol intake, increase complex carbohydrates and fiber, limit sodium. For women: counsel on iron and calcium intake.
Physical Activity: Encourage regular moderate-intensity physical activity that is appropriate to health status and lifestyle.	(Poor evidence but recommendation made on other grounds)	✔	✔
Dental Health: Counsel on daily oral hygiene.	(Poor evidence but recommendation made on other grounds)	✔	✔
Alcohol Use: Identify problem drinking and offer counselling.	(Fair evidence)	✔	✔
Tobacco Use	Counsel on smoking cessation. May use nicotine replacement as an adjunct (good evidence). Advise young non-smokers not to start (fair evidence).	Advise and assist patients to stop smoking.	Provide tobacco cessation counselling. Nicotine gum may be used as an adjunct. Advise young against smoking initiation.

✔ means agreement among the task forces

Moving On

Stimulated by recognition of the broad determinants of health, there is an increasing call on practitioners to play new and enhanced roles in helping patients change risk behaviors. These roles, which integrate clinical and

TABLE 3.6   Preventive Counselling Recommendations of Three Task Forces

	Canada	U.S. ACP	U.S. PSTF
Intravenous Street Drug Use: Case identification and counselling. Warn users of the risks of sharing needles/using contaminated needles. Provide information on cleaning needles.	Not considered	✔	✔
HIV and Other Sexually Transmitted Diseases: Counsel patients on STD transmission and prevention.	Counselling for adolescents (fair evidence). Counselling for general population (poor evidence but recommendation made on other grounds)	✔	✔
Contraception: Provide counselling on contraception and prevention of unwanted pregnancy.	Specific recommendation made only for adolescents (fair evidence)	✔	✔
Injury Prevention	Counsel parents of young children on home risk factors and poisoning. Counsel on seat belt use and drinking and driving (fair evidence). Counsel on general household and recreational safety (poor evidence but recommendation made on other grounds).	Counsel on safety belt and helmet use, alcohol and driving and/or recreational activities, smoke detectors for the home, proper firearm storage, workplace safety.	Advise patients against engaging in potentially dangerous activities while under the influence of alcohol or other drugs. Provide counselling on household and recreational safety. Counsel on seat belt use and drinking and driving.

✔ means agreement among the task forces
CTF–Canadian Task Force on the Periodic Health Examination
U.S. ACP–American College of Physicians
U.S. PSTF–United States Preventive Services Task Force

population health approaches, require a transformation in how health organizations work and function. The next chapter looks at the dynamics of this type of organizational change.

CHAPTER 4

Improving the Organization

*It's easy to get the players.
Gettin' 'em to play together,
that's the hardest part.*

—Casey Stengel

Overview

Health care organizations often fall short of their potential to promote health, manage chronic disease and increase quality of life. The organization itself, rather than practitioners and patients, is usually at the root of failures to achieve health behavior change.

Practitioners face various problems in changing health behavior: relentless time pressures, inadequate reimbursement, role conflicts (clinical versus prevention), insufficient training in motivation and handling patient resistance. Substantial improvements are needed at the organizational level to address these problems. Various strategies are outlined in this chapter, integrating approaches from 'top-down' quantum change and 'bottom-up' incremental change. We focus on six guiding principles:

1. Foster leadership at all levels

2. Use a systematic protocol

3. Develop office systems

4. Tailor the approach to your organization

5. Work with complexity

6. Use quality improvement knowledge and tools

A final section of the chapter written by Pearl Bader reviews major individuals and events in the history of quality improvement in industry and health care.

Shifting Approaches

As you walk into the clinic, the waiting room is jammed with patients, staff look harried, the intercom pages you—urgent! You can't escape the pressures, ...too many demands, too little time, too few resources.

Increasingly, you are faced with managing patients with chronic disease and unhealthy behaviors. Motivational skills and system supports are essential for helping these patients. The rapid pace of change makes it difficult to develop new initiatives. You address these issues whenever you can fit them in. But you lack the resources to do the job right. You do not even have data on how well you are doing with most patients. You have time only to react to patient needs, give advice and move on to the next patient. You feel trapped!

How do you get out of this trap? This book will give you the tools to rejuvenate your health care organization. First, you need to broaden your perspective.

Patients often resist health education and advice for behavioral change. Such resistance is a clear signal that we must shift our approach with patients to include motivational interventions. However, many practitioners work in time-pressured settings with limited incentives and supports for changing behavior. Resources for prevention continue to lag far behind investments in acute treatment. There is a compelling need to shift our approach to develop organizational resources for prevention and behavioral health care. Even when organizational systems are in place to support practitioners, an additional shift is needed. To have impact on the broad determinants of health, we need to shift our approach to a population perspective that integrates individual, organizational and community health.

Making Health Care Organizations Healthy

Organizational culture powerfully shapes practitioner behavior and vice versa. Practitioners typically lack organizational supports to use motivational approaches with patients. Patients sense this problem (Willms et al., 1991):

> *With the case-loads they've got nowadays, they're just too damn busy;*
> *if you don't really want to quit (smoking), I don't think they're going to*
> *help much.*

Practitioners are under mounting expectations to take a greater role in promoting health, improving quality of life and managing behavioral aspects of chronic disease. These expectations coincide with increasing time pressures and rationalizing of resources. Practitioners struggle with the competing demands of patient care, excessive workloads and behavior change targets that are often too ambitious (Cheung et al., 1997; Frame, 1992; Jaen et al. 1994; Kottke et al., 1993; Walsh & McPhee, 1992).

One asks: How healthy really are health care organizations today? Some problems practitioners face include:

- Inadequate reimbursement
- Drive for productivity—lack of time
- Inadequate training
- Clinical care is given priority over prevention
- Little feedback about results of preventive services (patient and population levels)
- Disorganized medical records
- Patients with multiple practitioners involved
- Preventive services often do not correspond to practitioners' images of their primary work and themselves

Progress has been slow incorporating prevention and behavioral health care into the mainstream of clinical practice. To redress the problem, we must alter our approach in three important ways.

Address organizational barriers and supports. The complexity of training practitioners about behavior change, prevention, and disease management has been underestimated. Skill development in motivational approaches will have limited impact unless one also deals with organizational constraints inherent to a busy clinical practice. We need to nurture leaders who can guide the change process, reduce barriers and enhance supports.

Focus on both individual and organizational levels. We are preoccupied with the individual patient and practitioner; we wrongly take the individual as the major locus for changes (see Figure 1.1, p. 5). Patients and practitioners do make choices about their behavior, but they do so in a social and physical environment that exerts considerable influence (Stokols, 1992). Effective strategies for changing behavior integrate individual, organizational and community health (Wallerstein, 1992).

Emphasize training in motivational skills. We are preoccupied with screening and diagnostic techniques. Relatively little attention is given to providing practitioners with sufficient training in motivational approaches. Screening and case findings must be linked with interventions for lowering patient resistance and enhancing motivation to produce behavior change. Often, clinicians identify a patient's health concern (e.g., excessive drinking or risky sexual practices) yet feel unable to intervene effectively (Lewis et al., 1991; Scott et al., 1992). Far greater attention should be focused on advances in motivational approaches to behavior change, and these advances should be incorporated into professional training and continuing education.

Where to Start, Top or Bottom?

Where are the best leverage opportunities for change in your organization? Quantum leap change requires senior level commitment and leadership ('top-down'). This magnitude of change can result in a complete transformation of the organization's culture and performance. In comparison, microlevel changes ('bottom-up') that operate at specific points can have solid and cumulative impact. These improvements are vulnerable even if the organizational culture is reactive and non-supportive. Both top-down and bottom-up approaches are vital for long-term success. The Five-Step Model described in Chapters 8 to 14 provides a framework and the practical tools for linking macro- and microinitiatives. High performing organizations demonstrate a synergistic interplay among top-down and bottom-up approaches. They weave all levels together through ongoing cycles of renewal.

What can you do when strong leadership is lacking or when the organizational climate is reactive? Concentrate on Step 1: generate momentum for organizational improvement. Various strategies are described in Chapter 9 for using *Your Organizational Prototype* analysis as a way to stimulate interest among senior management and create an imperative for change.

Another strategy is to pick a 'winner' and start momentum from the bottom-up. Begin with one idea for improvement that offers considerable impact yet will be relatively easy to do. Often this idea is readily apparent, if you ask! For example, have a team brainstorm about specific aspects of the organization that most need improvement: "*one specific idea that would make the most difference is ...*" Have team members discuss and agree upon a short list of opportunities that could yield the highest impact or leverage. Then, have the team rate these opportunities according to their ease of implementation (e.g., use the *Payoff Matrix Analysis*, Worksheet 11.5 in Chapter 11). From this list, start with the change opportunity that is easiest to do yet offers high impact.

Deming's 85:15 Rule

How do you identify which opportunities for change will lead to sustained gains in performance? According to Deming's 85:15 Rule (Figure 4.1), approximately 85% of opportunities for improvement lie with system changes such as role assignment, whereas 15% lie with people (Gaucher & Coffey, 1993). Cohen (1983) found that a simple change in the clinic routine had a profound effect on physicians' behavior regarding preventive care of diabetic patients. Whether or not the physician performed a foot examination was largely determined by whether the nurse instructed the patient to remove his/her shoes and socks before being seen by the physician. Physicians were almost five times as likely to examine the feet when patients presented barefoot (70%) than when wearing shoes (15%) (Figure 4.2). Such is the impact of a simple organizational change on practitioner behavior. Consider the cumulative impact on patient outcomes if this process improvement was made routine in primary care settings.

Contrast this organizational improvement approach with one targeted at individual practitioners. Does a continuing medical education (CME) seminar on preventive care with diabetic patients improve practitioner's preventive care? Research on CME effectiveness indicates that this approach by itself is unlikely to produce sustained change in physician behavior (Davis et al., 1999; Greco and Eisenberg, 1993). Would a fee for preventive services change practitioners' behavior? Adding a financial incentive is hardly viable in today's cost containment climate.

Deming's Rule also rings true in a study for identifying patients who smoke (Agency for Health Care Policy and Research, 1996). Based on a meta-analysis of nine randomized controlled trials, the AHCPR panel found that having a smoking status identification process in place resulted in these improvements:

- threefold increase in the likelihood that clinicians would conduct a smoking cessation intervention with patients who smoked
- twofold increase in smoking cessation

Again, these findings illustrate how a simple organizational adjustment leads to significant change in practitioner behavior, which leads to positive change in patients' behavior—i.e., successful modification of the most significant preventable cause of death (cigarette smoking). An update to the AHCPR Tobacco Cessation Guideline is available at their website: *www.surgeongeneral.gov/tobacco/*

Opportunities for Improvement

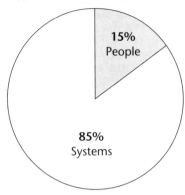

Figure 4.1 Comparison of the relative size of opportunities for organizational improvement—changing individuals versus changing processes in a system, Deming's 85:15 rule.

Diabetic Foot Examination by the Physician

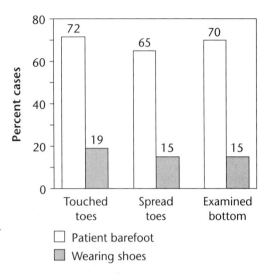

Figure 4.2 Impact upon physician behavior of changing a simple organizational process (asking patients to remove their shoes and socks). Data taken from Cohen (1983).

Guiding Principles for Organizational Change

Here are six keys to unlocking organizational change. They will guide you to the areas where you can have the most impact transforming your organization.

Foster leadership at all levels. At the core of every organization, however big or small, is an individual who can have a profound effect as a champion for change. Consider the accomplishments of Dr. Paul Frame at the Tri-County Family Medicine Service in upstate New York. Together with colleagues, he prepared a series of handouts for helping patients deal with various health issues:

- Injury Prevention for Children
- Screening for Prostate Cancer
- Estrogen for Prevention of Heart Disease and Thin Bones
- Health Is Your Responsibility

Yet, he was frustrated because even he did not routinely give these self-help guides to patients! The problem: The pamphlets were stored in the waiting room near the reception desk. This meant that either the practitioner had to walk out to the reception area to get a guide, or ask the patient to pick one up on the way out.

Frame hit upon a solution: Hot Files. In each examination room a plastic file folder (Hot File) was installed on the wall. A staff member was given the responsibility of keeping the files stacked with pamphlets. This meant that during the clinical consultation the practitioner only had to reach into the Hot File to obtain the appropriate guide. A simple organizational change improved practitioners' behavior in providing patients with advice, health education and self-care guides. Beer et al. (1990) called this strategy 'task alignment'. Task alignment focuses on change in the work itself through a realignment of roles and responsibilities.

When you draw back the curtain from an organization that has been successful in sustaining change, you undoubtedly find the presence of a champion or "bee in the bonnet" (Miller et al., 1998). In Chapter 5, we profile Dr. Robert Thompson, a leader who has successfully put prevention into practice at clinical and population levels in a large health maintenance organization.

Use a systematic protocol. Hahn and Berger (1990) evaluated the impact of introducing a health maintenance protocol systematically to all patients within a multi-site, family medicine practice. Their Systematic Health Maintenance (SHM) Protocol was tested on over 1400 patients over an 18-month period.

Hahn and Berger (1990) found excellent physician compliance (97% of eligible patients were included). The time taken by the physician to introduce the Protocol was less than 4 minutes. Patient acceptance ranged from good (77% for sigmoidoscopy) to excellent (97% for cholesterol screening). Of particular note was the finding that the patients in the SHM group were offered and completed more health maintenance procedures than a control group, the usual care group. The increase was quite dramatic with respect to encouraging seat belt use, skin self-examination, breast self-examination and postmenopausal bleeding. Advice regarding cigarette smoking increased from 60% for usual care patients to 95% for patients receiving SMH. Thus, a practical and effective health maintenance protocol was integrated into routine office care.

Develop office systems. The practice environment is a key source of both problems and solutions for improving quality. It is necessary to understand and focus efforts on the whole system, not just components that may be easiest to implement. Solberg et al. (1997) provide an excellent overview of essential components in a systems approach to delivering clinical prevention services. Anderson, Jaines and Jenkins (1998) conducted a meta-analysis of office-based interventions from 43 studies designed to alter practitioner and patient behavior in the delivery of preventive care. They found positive effects of the systems approach on both practitioners' and patients' adherence to preventive recommendations (e.g., mammography screening).

Allen Dietrich and colleagues from the Cancer Prevention in Community Practice Project have developed and evaluated an office system based on four components (Dietrich et al., 1994):

1. Identifying patients in need of services

2. Monitoring patients' receipt of services over time

3. Reinforcing positive patient behavior

4. Providing feedback to practice members that reinforces use of the system

Emphasizing teamwork and using trained facilitators, the office system was implemented at 50 primary care settings in Vermont, New Hampshire and Maine. Customized flow sheets were used in all practices. The use of other office system tools varied between 32% and 75% across study sites.

When compared with control sites, the office system practices demonstrated a significant increase in preventive services evident throughout the study's 12-month evaluation period (Dietrich et al., 1994). For example, mammography increased 33%, and a 20–25% increase was noted for occult blood-testing, clinical breast examination, breast self-examination and smoking cessation. This study demonstrates that community-based primary care practices can implement and maintain important improvements in preventive activities through an office systems approach.

Moreover, this project developed a practical *Office Systems Workbook* for the Cancer Prevention in Community Practice program and tools for applying this system in a wide variety of practice settings. (Contact: Dr. Allen Dietrich, Primary Care Research Projects, HB 7250, Strasenburgh Apt. A, Dartmouth Medical School, Hanover, NH 03755, USA; Tel. 603-650-1992).

Dietrich et al. (1994) recommend a four-step method termed GAPS:

- **Goals:** Goal-setting regarding preventive care

- **Assessment:** Assessment of existing routines that support preventive care and the current level of attainment of preventive goals

- **Planning:** Planning to modify existing routines that support preventive care

- **Start-Up:** Starting and maintaining the improved preventive care office

Tailor the approach to your organization. One size does not fit all! Put Prevention Into Practice (PPIP) is a state-of-the-art office system program, whose major components have been successfully tested in a clinical trial (Dickey, 1994). This program is designed to address patient, clinician and systems barriers. How well has the PPIP program been incorporated into clinical practice? Stange (1996, p. 358) concludes that "despite the excellent pedigree of PPIP, none of the physicians who had voluntarily ordered the material were actually using it in practice."

A study by McVea et al. (1996) raises serious questions. They examined eight family practice sites in the midwestern U.S. where all eight practices had purchased PPIP kits. Their major finding is startling: the PPIP material was not being used! McVea et al. (1996) identify three practice types according to delivery of preventive services:

Case 1–This practice provides a limited range of preventive services and has difficulties because its office systems are not well organized. Lack of time is identified as a major obstacle to doing a better job in prevention. "We spend so much time putting out fires" (physician 1, p. 364). They simply have no time to consider, let alone implement, preventive practices.

Case 2–This practice does a good job of providing screening and early detection services, such as immunizations and early cancer detection. However, little activity is noted in the way of counselling, especially counselling for behavior change. The physicians in this practice are strong leaders and have developed some good office systems of their own. PPIP was not used because they are already doing it.

Case 3–This practice provides lifestyle counselling as well as screening and early detection services. In addition to having office routines that facilitate preventive services, the physicians in these practices are quite enthusiastic and skilful at counselling patients to change health behaviors. One physician was noted because "he creates" windows of opportunity "to discuss prevention issues during almost all visits." (p. 366).

Table 4.1 summarizes the adoption of preventive services across these three types of practices. Some of the differences are striking.

These practice settings present strong challenges. The first type lacks sufficient organizational capability to begin a serious initiative at incorporating a comprehensive protocol such as the PPIP. Concerted efforts are needed to support a culture of change and quality improvement in this environment. The second practice type is already proficient at delivering preventive services (procedural, advice giving) and has a number of independently developed office systems in place. However, they need to take

Table 4.1   Differential Adoption of Preventive Services
in Family Practice Settings

	Case 1	Case 2	Case 3
Smoking History Taken (eligible patients)	23%	100%	93%
Health Maintenance Visit			
a) Prevention topics raised	4.0	10.1	16.0
b) Counselling	0.5	1.0	5.9
c) Biomedical*	0	1.4	1.6
Acute/Chronic Care Visit			
a) Prevention topics raised	3.4	2.7	3.5
b) Counselling	0.6	0.7	0.9
c) Biomedical*	0.4	0.4	0.2

*Laboratory tests, immunizations, chemoprophylaxis, interventions
Source: McVea et al. (1996).

the next step and actively engage patients in motivational counselling regarding health behavior change. It is noteworthy that the PPIP program does not address the issue of how to develop motivation enhancement skills. The third practice type is already highly proficient at screening, early detection and behavior change counseling. Here the PPIP has little to offer.

In a study of the dissemination of PPIP by the American Academy of Family Physicians, Medder et al. (1997) conducted pre- and postdissemination surveys that included purchase order data. They find that after two years of active promotion, 27% of Academy members had heard about PPIP and 2,004 purchased components, which represented less than 5% of active members. Barriers to using PPIP included too little time to look at the materials, staff are too busy to implement the system, materials are too expensive, and there is too much stuff: "it is overwhelming".

A similar finding was found in a study of tobacco prevention and cessation in Nebraska physicians' offices (McIlvain et al., 1997). None of the 11 practices were using any specific package, such as the PPIP kit, the 4-A (Ask, Advise, Assist, Arrange) National Cancer Institute model, or the American Academy of Family Physicians smoking cessation kit. Considerable variation was observed in the scope and intensity of tobacco control activities. Many provided little prevention. McIlvain et al. (1997, p. 201) conclude that 'prevention packages' need to be tailored to a practice's readiness for change, specific needs and organizational culture:

> *Like patients, practices and physicians are similar but unique and resist being forced into a one-size-fits-all pattern. Like patients, it was not a lack of knowledge or skill that usually defined their "non adherence"; rather it was little things particular to the system, the physicians' beliefs, and the culture of the practice.*

Work with complexity. The provision of behavioral change and disease management programs in primary care is much more complicated than generally acknowledged. This organizational complexity and 'chaos' (Goldberger, 1996; Stacey, 1996; Waldrop, 1992) can stymie efforts at changing practice behavior and improving organizational outcomes.

The multiple dimensions of primary care practice are described by Crabtree et al. (1998). Using qualitative methods in observing 138 family physicians, they identify a set of practitioner and system level variables that are important for understanding how practices are organized (Table 4.2). Three key dimensions emerged for understanding the physicians' component: philosophy (e.g., disease- or patient-focused), style (e.g., efficiency in time management), and doctor-patient continuity (e.g., remembered shared experiences). At the practice and patient population levels, four significant dimensions are identified: organization (e.g., clarity and agreement on roles), office staff (e.g., friendly atmosphere), patient population (e.g., dominant demographic group), and practice continuity (e.g., personnel over time). Crabtree et al. (1998) conclude that success in stimulating meaningful change in preventive service delivery is contingent on a comprehensive approach that addresses the spectrum of variables described in Table 4.2.

Use improvement knowledge. A comprehensive body of knowledge has developed over the past decade regarding the continuous improvement of health organizations and systems (Berwick & Nolan, 1998; Langley et al. 1996). Practitioners are encouraged to improve and perfect their clinical skills through continuous education and to do their best working within the system. However, this training does not prepare practitioners for taking effective roles in redesigning health care practices and organizations to produce better outcomes. Training in organizational improvement needs to be incorporated as an essential 'basic science' in professional education.

Efforts that actually produce results and improve systems have four elements (Berwick & Nolan, 1998):

Table 4.2   Understanding the Organization of Primary Care Practices

Physician-Level Constructs	System-Level Constructs
Physician-Philosophy:	*Practice Organization:*
Problem- or patient-focused	Degree to which role expectations are clear and shared among staff
Scope of clinical information	Degree to which there is clear and shared communication among staff
Approach to preventive service delivery	Efficiency of the office in moving patients through the system
Physician Style:	Presence, clarity and shared use of protocols
Degree of shared power in patient encounters	Volume of patients seen
Degree of affective connection with patients	Sense of being busy
Perception of competing demands	Perception of overwork or burnout of office physicians and staff
Efficiency in time management	Cohesiveness of physicians
Amount of teaching and use of health education materials	
	Office Staff:
Doctor-Patient Continuity:	Degree to which office staff were friendly
Personal knowledge of the patient	Degree to which staff shared knowledge with each other and their families
Longitudinal relationship over time	Staff were involved in the delivery of preventive care
Remembered shared experiences with the patient	
	Patient Population:
	Degree to which the patients identified with the practice
	Level of medical and socioeconomic need of the patient population
	Presence or absence of a dominant demographic group
	Practice Continuity:
	Personnel over time and place

Additional Features
Bee-in-bonnet
Openness

Reproduced with permission from Crabtree et al. (1998). *Journal of Family Practice*, 46: 403–409.

1. **Aim:** Organizational improvement is not an accident; it is the result of a clearly intended aim.

2. **Measurement:** Data collection and feedback are necessary to testing whether a system change has actually resulted in an improvement.

3. **Good Ideas for Change:** Gather good ideas from all available sources, and use them to identify opportunities and alternatives for change.

4. **Testing:** Ideas for change are tested on a small scale, adjustments are made based on test results, and redesigns are tested in an iterative fashion.

Understanding the Roots: A Brief History of Quality Improvement

Pearl Bader

While the subject of quality has a lengthy history, most of it took place in relative obscurity. A massive change then took place late in the twentieth century—quality moved to centre stage, and became a major parameter in human affairs.

—Juran (1996, p.634)

A comprehensive body of knowledge has developed over the past decade regarding the philosophy and practice of continuous improvement of health organizations and systems. This conceptual foundation is generally referred to as 'quality management' or 'quality improvement,' QI. Central to quality improvement is the concept of systematically building knowledge through collecting data, using statistical analysis, and selecting and testing solutions by experiment.

The history of quality improvement has followed two somewhat parallel but separate paths (Figure 4.3). Quality, as a specific approach to organizational change and improvement, began in industry (Juran, 1996). It was not until the mid-1980s that the science of quality improvement received recognition and application in health care (Brennan & Berwick, 1996). However, the history of the pursuit of quality in health care began in the early 1900s with Ernest Codman, who is credited with pioneering outcome measurement in health care. Even earlier concepts of quality can be traced back to Florence Nightingale in the 1860s. By publishing the mortality rates of patients in London hospitals and stressing the importance of data, she established herself as a true innovator in providing information regarding quality of health care. She stated:

> *What is wanted is: not theory nor opinions, but facts and the results of actual experience ... upon a uniform basis, of course; so as to secure uniform data, which can be compared and tabulated.*

A Brief History. . .

Improvement in Health Care	Improvement in Industry
1900 Codman	
1920 Hospital Standardization Program	Shewhart
1930 Lee-Jones Report	
1940 (no significant advances)	
1950 Lembcke	Deming
1960 Health Service Research (White)	Juran
Donabedian	Ishikawa
Williamson	
1970 Health Insurance Experiment	
1980 Medical Outcomes Study	U. S. industries adopt quality improvement

1987 U. S. National Demonstration Project
1988 Institute for Healthcare Improvement
1991 University of Toronto CQI Symposium
1999 Institute of Medicine study: To Err is Human
2001 Institute of Medicine: Crossing the Quality Chasm

Figure 4.3. Significant individuals and events in the history of quality improvement in industry and health care.

Beginnings in Health Care

Ernest Codman is generally recognized as the pioneer of the scientific study of quality in health care. In a seminal paper in 1914, he strongly advised hospitals and physicians to measure and report the outcomes of their work. He believed that consumers both need and have a right to this information to make informed health care choices—a version of the current vogue of hospital report cards. Moreover, he believed this information was critical for enabling practitioners to compare their results in order to improve patient care.

The American College of Surgeons launched the Hospital Standardization program in the early 1900s. This was the most important effort in the first half of the twentieth century to link standard setting and audit with actual day-to-day care. By 1920, surveyors accumulated data on almost 700 hospitals to address various aspects of hospital performance. The findings indicated a dramatic lack of conformity among US hospitals in approaches to clinical care.

In 1930 the Lee-Jones Report, a study of the resource needs of the health care system in the U.S., was published. This study, reviewing the economic aspects of prevention and care of illness, was led by I.S. Falk through the Committee on the Costs of Medical Care (Brennan and Berwick, 1996). A short time later, in the late 1930s and 1940s, there was a hiatus in the study of quality in health care. The reasons for this are not clear.

Paul Lembcke, a surgeon at Johns Hopkins University Medical School, resurrected interest in health care quality in the 1950s and 1960s. Like Codman, his predecessor of fifty years, Lembcke believed in the value of examining outcomes of care. He added to the work of Codman by designing methods for collection and analysis of information regarding variation in clinical practice. Fuelled by his concern regarding the high degrees of variation in utilization rates and patterns of care among surgeons, he began conducting medical audits. His 1956 article, *Medical Auditing by Scientific Methods Illustrated by Major Female Pelvic Surgery*, was a significant contribution to the history of medical quality (Brennan and Berwick, 1996). He managed to increase the appropriateness of pelvic surgery from thirty to eighty percent, through a simple system of audit and feedback.

In the early 1960s, Kerr White, Chair of Medicine at Johns Hopkins University, provided leadership for the development of the field of health services research. Quantitative methods of studying quality of care were used. Building on this evaluation work and the works of Lembcke and the Lee-Jones Report, was Donabedian, a Lebanese physician who came to the U.S. in the 1950s. His 1966 article, *Evaluating the Quality of Medical Care*, is considered a hallmark in the field of health care quality (Brennan and Berwick, 1996). Of particular importance and relevance even today, is his identification of structure, process, and outcome of care as the three main entities of study in quality.

Also in the 1960s, John Williamson was interested in understanding the processes of adult learning and knowledge acquisition in physicians. He emphasized the importance of focusing on physicians 'thinking' processes as integral to improving quality. His views are consistent with current wisdom in quality improvement, which links measurement and feedback to processes of learning.

The RAND Corporations's Health Insurance Experiment and Medical Outcomes Study in the 1970s and 1980s are landmark projects in measuring results of health care. Hulk, Newhouse, Ware, and Brook are some of the leaders at the forefront of these initiatives. The Health Insurance Experiment assessed how variations in patients' share of health costs affected their utilization of health services, satisfaction with care, quality of care and health status (Taylor et al., 1987). As part of the Medical Outcomes Study, numerous instruments were developed for assessing both the processes and outcomes of care. Multiple dimensions of quality were identified, including functional health status, emotional health, appropriateness of care and patient satisfaction. This was the first time patients' self-reports were recognized as an important and reliable source of information regarding their own functional status and satisfaction. As well, robust measures of system cost and efficiency were designed.

Beginnings in Industry

While health care was involved mainly with assessing and measuring outcomes of care, the manufacturing industry was developing and implementing methods regarding the processes of care leading to the outcomes (Juran, 1995). The goal was to understand the causes of the results. Industrial quality improvement techniques have gained increasing prominence in health care today. The concepts, techniques and tools borrowed from industry offer great promise in improving health care.

Shewhart, Deming, Juran, and Ishikawa are considered the founders of quality improvement (Hackman and Wageman, 1995). Our current wisdom of quality improvement draws almost exclusively on the works of these leaders. Walter Shewhart is considered the 'father' of scientific methods of quality management. He began his work as a statistician and physicist at the Bell Telephone Laboratories in the U.S. He was convinced that improving processes in complex systems of production was key to improving quality. This was a departure from the prevailing practice of standardization and control as being central to quality. His ideas were largely ignored for the next thirty years, almost the same time that there was no movement in the study of the health care side of quality. In the early 1950s, his ideas were resurrected in Japan as part of American activities in postwar reconstruction of the deteriorating Japanese economy.

Following World War II, Japanese manufacturers changed over from military production to civilian products. They encountered major difficulties on the international market because of a reputation for poor quality goods. The Japanese became convinced of the need to improve their quality reputation (Juran, 1995). Ishikawa, chairman of the Union of Japanese

Scientists and Engineers (JUSE), helped translate statistical and engineering principles of quality improvement into a series of tools and approaches that everyone in an organization, at all levels, could use in their daily work (Brennan and Berwick, 1996). Ishikawa invited Deming and Juran to Japan to help teach quality concepts to their manufacturers. The U.S. government supported them in this endeavour.

W. Edwards Deming was a physics instructor and later a mathematical physicist for the U.S. Department of Agriculture. Joseph Juran began his career at the Western Electric Company in 1924. He began work in the inspection branch and eventually became quality manager in 1934. Both Deming and Juran were students of Shewhart, and built on Shewhart's principles to implement a framework for redesigning Japanese industry. Deming and Juran were instrumental in helping the Japanese achieve a position of global market dominance by offering products of superior quality and value.

Despite Japanese dominance on world markets, American companies were slow to accept the need for quality improvement. Deming and Juran did not achieve any impact in North America until many years later. The 1980 NBC television documentary, *If Japan Can, Why Can't We*, helped put quality improvement on the agenda of American industry.

Recent Events in Health Care Quality

The first major application of modern industrial quality management methods to health care occurred in 1987 with the National Demonstration Project on Quality Improvement in Health Care (Brennan and Berwick, 1996). Donald Berwick, then Vice-President of the Harvard Community Health Plan, and Blanton Godfrey, then head of Quality Systems and Theory Division at AT&T Bell Laboratories, submitted a proposal for a trial of applications of modern quality improvement methods in health care settings. Twenty experts from industry quality management and twenty-one health care organizations participated in the project. Some issues addressed included: access and waiting times, clinical and financial data management, human resources issues and patient satisfaction (Brennan and Berwick, 1996). In 1988 the Institute for Healthcare Improvement (IHI) was established in the United States, with Berwick as the current Chief Executive Officer. IHI has quickly established itself as a premier force, initially in the U.S. and now internationally, for leadership and dissemination of QI concepts and tools.

A decade later, the Institute of Medicine (Kohn et al., 1999) published the first of a series of reports by the Quality of Health Care in America project. The main results, described more fully in Chapter 2, estimated that up to 98,000 preventable deaths occur per year as a result of medical errors. Total national costs (lost income, productivity, disability) of preventable adverse events were estimated to be between $17 billion and $29 billion, with health care costs representing over half. This hard hitting report called for a comprehensive approach to improving health care safety, with a national goal of 50% reduction in errors over 5 years.

Quality improvement in health care in Canada has a much shorter history. In 1991, Ross Baker and Peggy Leatt, of the University of Toronto, organized a symposium on Continuous Quality Improvement (CQI) in Health Care. Speakers at the symposium included Don Berwick and Maureen Bisognano from the Institute for Health Care Improvement, Don Sherman from Alberta, and Phil Hasson from London. There was an enthusiastic response with 250 people in attendance. Following this symposium, the University of Toronto sponsored the formation of the Ontario CQI Network with five Toronto teaching hospitals and St. Joseph's Hospital in London as initial members. Currently, the CQI network is sponsored by its more than 65 members in Ontario (*www.thecqinetwork.com*).

A challenge for quality improvement in health care is to maintain the momentum it has generated. Quality improvement practices must be integrated into every facet of the organization. It must become incorporated into the fabric of the organization, driving values, behavior, and organizational learning. When this occurs, quality improvement will be integral to all aspects of the organization's performance.

While formal application of quality improvement to health care has a relatively short history, achievement of quality has always been an aspiration of human effort. According to Juran (1996, p. x), in his monumental work, *A History of Managing for Quality*, "our archaeological sites, ancient cities, and modern museums provide convincing evidence that 'invention' of managing for quality has been a continuing process over the millennia." Indeed, we can trace our roots in the pursuit of quality improvement to the wisdom of Aristotle (Clemmer, 1992, p. 220):

> *The way to achieve success is first to have a definite, clear practical idea–a goal, an objective. Second, have the necessary means to achieve your ends–wisdom, money, materials and methods. Third, adjust all your means to that end ... Quality is not an act. It is a habit.*

Moving On

Despite the many challenges to improving health organizations, certain organizations have paved the way in demonstrating that a proactive, population-based approach to health care is possible. The next chapter profiles one such organization, the Group Health Cooperative of Puget Sound.

CHAPTER 5

Putting Prevention into Practice

Quality is not an act. It is a habit.

—Aristotle

Overview

This chapter describes a success story in organizational improvement by the Group Health Cooperative of Puget Sound. Experiences are reviewed in the development, implementation and evaluation of preventive services. Five organizational factors are deemed essential to this success:

1. A population-based epidemiological viewpoint coupled with specific evidence-based criteria,

2. Involvement of all stakeholders in the process, including patients, practitioners, managers and the community,

3. A systems approach to implementation that focuses on predisposing and enabling factors both in the organization and in the community,

4. Feedback on program outcomes,

5. Use of clinical information systems.

The Group Health Cooperative reported some impressive results: a 38% decrease in late-stage breast cancer, a 90% immunization rate for two-year-old children, a decrease in adult smokers from 25% to 15%, and an increase in bicycle safety helmet use among children from 4% to 48% which resulted in a 67% decrease in bicycle-related head injuries.

Creating a Health-Promoting Organization

The Group Health Cooperative of Puget Sound (GHC), located in Seattle, Washington, is a consumer-governed Health Maintenance Organization (HMO) with almost 500,000 members residing in the greater Puget Sound area and approximately 675,000 members overall in Washington and Idaho. The GHC employs approximately 1000 physicians (40% in primary care). The population served by the GHC is similar to that in the surrounding area in terms of age, race, gender distribution and income. What sets GHC apart from other HMOs in the region (and in the country) is its approach to primary and secondary prevention. Indeed, this focus has been evident since the GHC's inception in 1947; the original bylaws decree:

> *The Cooperative shall endeavor to develop some of the most outstanding hospitals and medical centers to be found anywhere, with special attention to preventive medicine.*

The GHC organizes its clinical practices to facilitate the delivery of preventive services. It has successfully developed and implemented a number of preventive initiatives: immunizations, breast cancer screening, colon cancer screening, cholesterol screening, and smoking cessation. In addition, the Cooperative has developed and disseminated a number of preventive care guidelines for clinical practice. Successful outcomes from these clinical prevention programs are described by McAfee et al. (1995), Rivara et al. (1994), Thompson (1996) and Thompson et al. (1995a; 1995b).

Four Examples

Key results from four initiatives are highlighted in Figure 5.1. Each initiative demonstrates the differential use of clinical, organizational and community-based strategies.

Breast cancer screening. One of GHC's first successes was the breast cancer screening program developed between 1981 and 1983 and implemented between 1985 and 1986. A computer database was used to identify eligible women (70,000 women aged 40 years or older) and to manage correspondence regarding screening (i.e., automated information and reminder system). Periodic reports on the screening status of women in the practice panel were generated and fed back to practitioners. The overall impact was a 38% decrease in age-adjusted incidence of late-stage breast cancer.

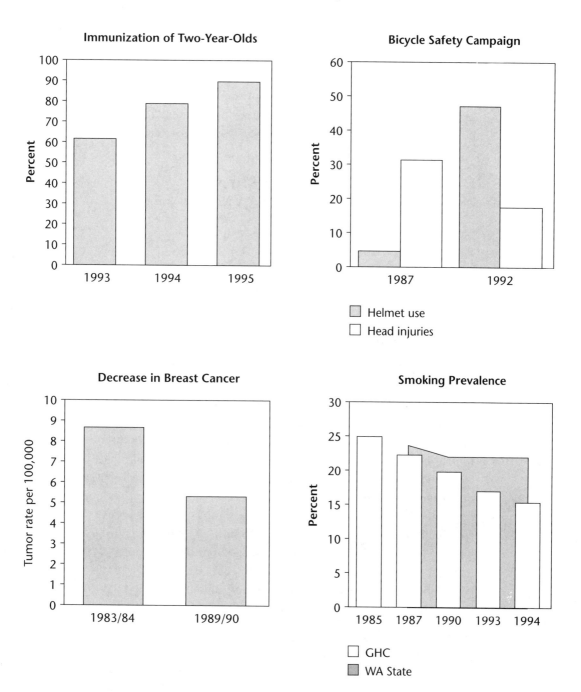

Figure 5.1 Key results from putting prevention into practice at the Group Health Cooperative of Puget Sound. Source: Thompson (1995a, 1995b).

Tobacco use. The GHC banned smoking from its clinical facilities in 1982, and has devoted considerable efforts to the development of a cessation program, Free and Clear (Orleans et al., 1991). In 1991 a task group was formed to devise a 'Tobacco Roadmap' to focus efforts on smoking cessation. The program used both a quality improvement and a population-based framework (McAfee et al., 1995). Its key initiatives:

- improved access to tobacco cessation services
- global measurement systems and feedback
- provision of clinical guidelines and implementation tools
- population-based education
- staff support.

By 1994, the prevalence of tobacco use among GHC adult patients dropped to 15.5%. Relative to the rate of decline of adult smokers in the state of Washington over the same period, GHC achieved a more significant reduction in tobacco use (Figure 5.1).

Bicycle safety. This program uses research on barriers to, and effectiveness of, bicycle helmet use and relies on broad-based community participation to achieve its positive outcomes. GHC was one of 18 community groups participating in this campaign, which included extensive media coverage and discount coupons for helmets. Participation by primary care physicians in distributing the discount coupons was a significant component. Between 1987 and 1992, a 67% decrease was found in the rate of GHC emergency department attendee head injuries due to bicycling in the target population of children aged 5 to 14 years. During the same period, helmet use in school aged children in the general Seattle community increased from 5.5% to 40.2%. The GHC thus served as a mini-population laboratory to assess the effects of the broader community campaign. Helmet usage rates in GHC emergency department attending children increased from 4.3% to 48.0% during this campaign (Figure 5.1).

Immunizations. An automated recording and tracking system for immunizations was developed in 1991. The system generates reports for practitioners about the immunization status of every child. Records are reviewed and deficiencies are flagged for action. As a result, complete immunization levels for two-year-olds have increased from 63% in the first quarter of 1993 to 90% in the first quarter of 1995 (Figure 5.1) and continued in excess of 90% through 1997.

The Essentials of GHC's Success

The health practitioners at GHC really know what works when it comes to putting prevention into practice. Here are five valuable lessons GHC has learned from its years of developing and implementing clinical preventive systems.

Lesson 1. Clear vision and direction are essential to a preventive care provision system. GHC began in 1947 with a mission statement that emphasized prevention—quite unique at the time. Guided by its mission, GHC determined exactly what it needed to constitute an ideal or 'gold standard' system for preventive care (see Table 5.1 adapted from Thompson et al., 1995b). Clearly articulating the details of a prevention system ensures organizational cohesiveness, sets the direction of efforts (Tables 5.1 and 5.2), plans the route (Table 5.3), and establishes the criteria by which an organization tests its interventions (Table 5.4).

Lesson 2. Leadership and an organizational focus are key. Because a wide variety of GHC departments and individuals are involved in preventive care, effective leadership and good communication is critical to ensure that prevention remains a priority and that preventive efforts are effectively coordinated. The work of a Preventive Care Task Force in 1973 led to the establishment of the Department of Preventive Care. The Department undertook the following initiatives:

- **Committee on Prevention:** a broad-based committee that develops and facilitates implementation of guidelines and provides implementation oversight
- **Center for Health Studies:** conducts epidemiological and health services research, established by Dr. Edward Wagner and now lead by Dr. Susan Curry
- **Center for Health Promotion:** the principal planning and implementation partner.

The Department of Preventive Care is responsible for "bringing an epidemiological perspective to priority setting and analysis of issues" (Thompson et al., 1995b), whereas the Committee on Prevention (COP) is responsible for examining prevention issues and developing guidelines and programs for clinical practice. The COP includes staff representatives from various areas: medicine, nursing, health education, research, information

Table 5.1   Elements of an Ideal Preventive Care System

- A population-based, multilevel planning approach is used.
- Direct your efforts at major causes of morbidity and mortality as determined by epidemiological research. Consider both the epidemiology of "needs" (diseases and risks) and the epidemiology of "wants" (desires of patients and practitioners).
- Evidence for intervention effectiveness is available, or will be generated by well designed program evaluations.
- Functions linked at multiple levels of care: one-to-one, infrastructural, organizational, community.
- Use prospective and automated programs to the maximum extent feasible.
- Health is the result of shared decision-making between practitioners and patients. Informed consent encourages shared planning and input from patients.

Adapted with permission from Thompson et al. (1995b). *JAMA*, 273: 1130–1135.

systems, GHC's quarterly publication, quality improvement, government relations and communications, and marketing. In addition, the COP consults specialists on an ad hoc basis for input on specific issues. Members of the COP are required to work on at least one priority area each year and to keep their respective departments informed of the Committee's activities. The circulation of committee minutes to all staff ensures dissemination of information. In recent years, all clinical guidelines and many patient education items have been made available on clinical computer workstations in doctor's office and in clinical practice areas.

Lesson 3. Criteria used to examine primary and secondary prevention must be explicit and must reflect an evidence-based approach. At the heart of GHC's work on preventive care are the six-point criteria given in Table 5.2. The Committee on Prevention uses these, time and again, as a basis for critically reviewing the literature and developing evidence-based guidelines. Once an issue has been examined using the six criteria, the COP provides a framework for practice guidelines and development. The guidelines are, for the most part, written by the practitioners themselves with technical assistance from the various departments of the organization.

Lesson 4. Take a systems approach to address individual, organizational and community levels. GHC found that a systems approach is necessary to enable, develop and smoothly integrate clinical preventive services (Table 5.3). In practical terms, this involves the use of Green and Kreuter's (1991) PRECEDE/PROCEED and other systems approaches (Dever, 1997) as frameworks for the implementation of prevention pro-

Table 5.2 Criteria Used to Evaluate Prevention Issues

1. The condition (disease/risk factor) is important to the individual and society. What is the burden of suffering due to the condition (individual, community, population perspectives)?

2. The risk factor or disease has a recognizable pre-symptomatic stage. The natural history of the disease is known.

3. Reliable methods for detecting the risk factor or disease exist. Consider screening test validity: sensitivity, specificity, and predictive values.

4. Intervention effectiveness is considered. Modification of the risk factor or intervention at the pre-symptomatic stage reduces morbidity and mortality more than intervention after symptoms appear.

5. Facilities or capacity to address the identified risk factor or condition exist.

6. The cost/harms and potential benefits of implementing a state of the art approach have been considered.

Adapted with permission from Thompson et al. (1995b). *JAMA*, 273: 1130–1135.

grams. According to the PRECEDE/PROCEED model, strategies to bring about behavior change (in this case, implementation of specific prevention protocols) are most effective when targeting predisposing, enabling and reinforcing factors of the behavior in question.

a) Predisposing factors: Factors that predispose a health professional to change his or her clinical practices include a sense of self-efficacy; acquisition or possession of the skills necessary to perform the new behavior; and the health care provider's knowledge, attitudes and beliefs towards the new behavior. Specific interventions directed at identifying barriers and increasing provider predisposing factors include focus groups, surveys of GHC staff, and direct practitioner involvement in planning and training activities (e.g., workshops and role-playing exercises). Similarly, focus groups with GHC members and surveys are useful in designing prevention programs that are acceptable and relevant to populations served by GHC.

b) Enabling factors: Enabling factors are those in the practice, organizational and community environments that make change possible. At the level of individual practice, program elements such as clear guidelines with summaries of the evidence and protocols, prompts and reminders for clinicians, and an organized system for follow-up activities are instrumental to the successful implementation of preventive services. At an organizational level, factors such as explicit support from the top brass, continuing education programs for GHC staff on topics such as patient behavior change, staff involvement in research projects on clinical prevention, the use of computer

Table 5.3   Systems Approach to Clinical Prevention Services

PREDISPOSING FACTORS

1. Barrier identification
2. Practitioner involvement in planning
3. Training for practice integration (workshops, role playing and videos). Focus on skill acquisition and practitioner self-efficacy

ENABLING FACTORS

1. Practice Level
   - Clear guidelines
   - Reminders
   - Chart stickers/flags
   - Health questionnaires with behavioral risk factor information
   - Patient flow planning
   - Organized follow-up

2. Organizational Level
   - Chief executive officer/medical director commitment
   - Organizational focus for clinical prevention services development and implementation planning
   - Postgraduate educational programs directed to physician skill development, practice, integration, and patient behavior change
   - Staff involvement in research and evaluation projects of clinical prevention services
   - Automated clinical information systems

3. Community Level
   - Community coalitions
   - Collaboration with university-based researchers and/or public health agencies
   - Community policy development

REINFORCING FACTORS

1. Personalized feedback
2. Newsletters
3. Awards

Adapted with permission from Thompson et al. (1995b). *JAMA,* 273: 1130–1135.

Table 5.4   Program Evaluation Criteria

- **Capacity Enhancement/Barrier Reduction:** measures of attitudes, knowledge, beliefs and skills of practitioners and patients.
- **Process of Care:** measures of screening tests performed, identification of risks, counseling directed to behavior change, and medical care utilization.
- **Health Outcomes:** For disease screening this may include decreased disease incidence, decreased morbidity, decreased mortality. Other outcomes include reductions in risk behavior, enhanced health status, increases in the readiness for change.

Adapted with permission from Thompson (1996). *The Millbank Quarterly*, 74: 469–509.

technology to facilitate the delivery of services, and patient-centered communications (verbal and written) stressing preventive health care are invaluable to the success of preventive efforts. Finally, at a community level, GHC actively participates in community coalitions, collaborates with university research groups, and works with public health agencies on policy development issues.

c) Reinforcing factors: Reinforcing factors such as peer support, timely feedback of results, and recognition of preventive efforts help to ensure the adoption and maintenance of preventive protocols by GHC staff.

Lesson 5. Assess outcomes at various points in the system, and incorporate this feedback in cycles of improvement. The final component of the comprehensive population-based approach is to define measurable criteria (Table 5.4) for evaluating a preventive program at multiple levels (individual, organizational, population) and at various points throughout the system—e.g., at the point of barriers or bottlenecks, throughout program implementation (process), and at health outcomes.

The Group Health Cooperative has been a trail-blazer in achieving comprehensive population-based programs in disease prevention and health promotion. Results from specific initiatives are impressive. At the same time, GHC has generated a wealth of knowledge on 'how to get there', how to get through the difficult terrain of organizational and community change to success in disease prevention and health promotion. Despite its leadership, indeed, despite its gold-standard role in prevention, the GHC is challenged to maintain its commitment to prevention at a time of fiscal restraint and mounting competition in the marketplace. The following interview with Robert Thompson provides fascinating insights into the value of sustained leadership, the value of a champion for organizational transformation.

A Conversation with Dr. Robert 'Tommy' Thompson

"After reading your papers which describe some impressive progress that GHC has made in putting prevention into practice, I am curious about the following question: How did you really do it, what's the story behind the story?" His eyes widened and a smile came to his face—we were off on a fascinating 90-minute conversation.

For someone who has taken a leadership role in preventive medicine, it is interesting to note that Dr. Thompson's initial interest while a medical student at Johns Hopkins University was in basic science and bench research. He decided to focus his clinical interests in the fields of pediatrics and infectious diseases. Then, a turning point occurred in his career that would have longstanding ramifications.

Halfway through his pediatric specialty training, he was called into military service and elected to spend his time in public health. The military sent him to train at the Centers for Disease Control, Atlanta, and he got a glimpse of a whole new world: *the public health perspective*. His two years spent in public health as an epidemic intelligence officer for CDC left a lasting impression that stimulated his vision of merging clinical medicine and public health perspectives.

He came to the Group Health Cooperative in 1972 as a pediatrician but soon began lobbying for time to spend on preventive medicine. By 1975, he was allowed to spend half his time on preventive activities (but with no other resources), and the Department of Preventive Care was initiated. At that time, there was little opportunity to discuss system-wide primary and secondary prevention. Dr. Thompson advocated for and initiated the Committee on Prevention in 1978. This Committee became instrumental in the development and implementation of preventive guidelines.

During these formative years, Dr. Thompson quipped that he was in "serious negative numbers". In stimulating organizational change, he had become both an advocate and a pain. One thing that he found extraordinarily helpful was specifying six criteria (Table 5.2) as an evidence-based approach to identifying prevention initiatives that helped him establish credibility with his colleagues; as well, it provided a tool for arbitrating between competing recommendations ... and fiefdoms! He found that while various factions could 'run' from the evidence, they could not 'hide' from it forever.

Another critical factor was the charge he gave members of the Committee on Prevention. Every member was required to select one preventive issue and work it through the criteria each year. This participatory approach stimulated broader ownership of the preventive initiatives.

By the early 1980s, Dr. Thompson reported that he had achieved "positive numbers" for the organization with the first major success, cost-effective breast cancer screening. In 1983, a new CEO provided resources for strengthening internal research. As a result, Dr. Edward Wagner from the University of North Carolina was recruited to spearhead epidemiological studies and health services research. Since the early 1980s, Drs. Thompson and Wagner have recruited an exceptional cadre of clinical and basic researchers: Today, the Center for Health Studies has over 20 investigators and a staff of approximately 200.

"What kept you going during the early years when you encountered so many obstacles?" Dr. Thompson attributed his success to three factors:

1. **Vision and Direction:** He came to GHC in 1972 with a vision of merging clinical and public health perspectives. He never wavered from this vision. Related to this was his specification of the six criteria to identify prevention initiatives and to help to arbitrate conflicts.

2. **Initial Success:** The breast cancer screening program developed between 1981 and 1983 and implemented in 1985 and 1996 proved that a system-wide preventive care initiative could be cost-effective. This screening program established the credibility of such initiatives.

3. **Critical Mass:** With the backing of senior management, Dr. Edward Wagner was recruited in 1983. He proved to be a key partner, who quickly established an excellent research department.

In addition to vision and determination, Dr. Thompson exhibits a knack for understanding the dynamics of organizational change. In a rather low-key manner, his aim initially was to get a specific preventive activity 'on the table' for consideration by the Committee on Prevention and then to have the preventive activity implemented without it getting in the way of the doctor-patient relationship. This approach is participatory, flexible and practical. He continually looks for opportunities for organizational change, often in areas where the organization is preoccupied with other issues. Dr. Thompson characterizes his philosophy as: a little vision and some evidence coupled with "riding the wave of apathy to victory".

Moving On

The next chapter reviews physicians' perspectives on organizational change. It focuses on their stresses and pressures and considers proactive approaches physicians can take to improve the quality of health care, prevention, and health promotion.

CHAPTER 6

Physicians' Perspectives on Organizational Change

MARTIN SOMMERFELD

It is not only going backward that the plain practical workman is liable to, if he will not look up and look around; he may go forward to ends he little dreams of.

—Oliver Wendell Holmes

Overview

This chapter gives voice to physicians' perspectives on organizational change. It does not demand this or that change; it seeks to stimulate discussion around problems and values. The chapter reviews the broad forces of change, the troubles physicians presently feel, and the responses of individuals and medical organizations. How should physicians respond? What sort of change should they make? The chapter ends with a case study that can be used to stimulate discussion, to help physicians think about their problems and values and their potential responses to the ongoing changes to the health care system.

This book has a good deal to say about change: what motivates individuals and organizations to change, how change is facilitated, achieved, and maintained. In describing the Five-Step Model, the authors insist that it is vital to have a clear start. Step 1 requires developing motivation and building momentum and capacity. This chapter focuses on Step 1, that is, on the experiential process: on questions of resistance, problems, values, capacities and direction—the physician's perspective.

Forces of Change

The recent and ongoing changes to the health care system affect all health care practitioners. Physicians, because of their traditional role and position as the primary coordinators of health care, feel the most pressure to change. Calls for change come mainly from economic and political quarters. Initially, these calls were quite strident, accusing physicians of organizing medical care as a guild or craft union that benefited largely their own economic and social self-interests (Freidson, 1970; Freidson, 1994; Starr, 1982), Since the public backlash against managed care organizations (MCO) in the U.S. (Anonymous, 1999) and government rationing of health care resources in Canada, these calls are more conciliatory. Both corporate medicine and public medicine need the good will of physicians (Anonymous, 1999; Mechanic, 2000; K. White, 1991).

Nonetheless, the calls for economic and political accountability persist. From the economic side, they ask doctors to change their traditional compact, to assure customers and the market that doctors are accountable (Silversin & Kornacki, 2000) From the political side, they ask doctors to change their traditional covenant, to assure not only individual patients but also the community, population, and society that doctors are accountable.

Physicians are indeed participating in this unprecedented economic and political reorganization of health care systems. Many are participating with reluctance and resistance. They complain of lost autonomy, increased stress and workload, decreased income, and decreased ability to provide quality patient care.

In the U.S., physicians are increasingly involved in some form of managed care. "Managed Care On-Line" estimates that Health Maintenance Organizations (HMOs) and Preferred Provider Organizations (PPOs) have enrolled some 165.4 million Americans. A Commonwealth Fund survey found that 87% of physicians have at least one managed care patient and contract with at least one plan. An American Medical Association (AMA) survey estimates that, on average, contracts with managed care organizations comprise 45% of physician revenues (Collins et al., 2001; Scheffler, 1999).

U.S. physicians are increasingly joining labor unions. The American Medical Association estimates that 45,000 doctors belong to unions, up 250% from 1997 (Albert, 2000). U.S. physicians have also formed their own not-for-profit HMOs or joined large physician-groups to aggressively negotiate contracts with MCOs (Bodenheimer, 2000; Ginzberg & Ostow, 1997; Greenberg, 1998; Grumbach et al., 1998). In Canada, physicians are increasingly involved in government rationing of health care resources. Recently, they are participating in pilot projects to reform primary care through even more fundamental changes to funding, payment, delivery, and access (Coburn et al., 1997; Graham, 1996).

Certainly these economic and political perspectives capture public attention. They have been met and often opposed by a 'professionalism perspective', physicians' retrenchment to the values and goals of the physician-patient relationship (Emanuel & Emanuel, 1996). The authors of *Promoting Health* offer a broadly conceived public health perspective: health promotion, disease prevention, population health, and behavioral medicine. This approach, through the Five-Step Model, offers a means to integrate professional and organizational-economic perspectives. It offers a means for practitioners to provide appropriate, effective, and cost efficient care.

Will clinicians respond to and integrate these other approaches? Clinicians are not health economists, politicians, or public health academics. The profession of medicine is none of these; it has a unique perspective, expertise and professionalism. This chapter is about the clear and valued medical perspective and about its present diffraction in the face of massive organizational changes. In the language of the transtheoretical model (Prochaska et al., 1992) described in Chapter 3 and elaborated in Chapter 7, many frontline clinicians either directly oppose changes, are resistant to changes, or are not yet contemplating the issues. How can physicians prepare themselves for an active response, that is, a thoughtful and innovative response on the organizational-change front?

Doctors' Troubles

Doctors are well aware of the changes in the content and context of medical practice—changes in the art and science of practice and its organization and financing. Doctors are vocal critics of these changes, and they express their personal and professional concerns and troubles. This section focuses on their expression of troubles, in particular, time and money.

Time

Again and again one hears doctors talk about the amount and quality of their time. For some, one hopes a very few, their offices and careers have become prisons that they yearn to escape (Canadian Medical Association, editors, 2000a). For many others who are seeing more patients over longer

days, the office has become a place of constant stress and urgent demands
(Sheehy, 2000; editors, 2000). Many doctors have little time and energy to
do more than react to these demands. In a recent survey by the Canadian
Medical Association Journal, of the almost three thousand doctors surveyed, over half believe their workloads have increased over the past 12
months; almost two-thirds have a workload they consider too heavy
(Ontario College of Family Physicians, 2000). Doctors feel that such medical practice undermines their ability to provide sensitive and compassionate care, indeed to provide quality care in general (Sheehy, 2000).

An international survey of physicians from five countries conducted by
the Harvard School of Public Health, the Commonwealth Fund, and Harris
Interactive Inc. found that more than half of all physicians surveyed in the
United States and Canada, and a large percentage of those in three other
countries, Australia, New Zealand, and the United Kingdom, believe that
over the past five years their ability to provide quality health care to
patients has deteriorated. Overall, 41% report a decline in time spent with
patients in the past three years. Doctors feel that spending more time with
patients would improve quality, but extra time is often unavailable (Collins
et al., 2001).

Nor are academic physicians insulated from time troubles. In a survey
of U.S. physicians' attitudes to managed care, Simon et al. (1999) found
63.1% of faculty, directors of residency programs, and department chairs
believe that managed care has decreased their time for research, and 58.9%
believe it has reduced teaching time.

New medical inductees, medical students, interns and residents, have
long complained about the maniacal rush from patient to patient, the vital-
ity-sapping workloads, and the insensitivity and callousness of their supe-
riors (DeCastro, 2000; Haddock, 2001). Most disturbing, recent surveys
indicate an undiminished rate of abuse of students and residents; almost
40% report at least one episode of abuse, mainly humiliation and belittle-
ment, during their education and training (Cook et al., 1996; Daugherty,
1998; Kasebaum & Cutler, 1998). What is worse, students describe their
accommodation to these apparently accepted pressures and practices
(Friedly, 2000).

Money

Do physicians feel they have money troubles? In Ontario, Canada, 60% of
doctors surveyed report an increase in expenses, and about 75% believe

their incomes have decreased (32.1%) or stayed about the same (44.9%) during the past 12 months (Canadian Medical Association, 2000b). New medical graduates in Ontario may feel even less financially secure. The Ontario provincial government recently deregulated medical school tuition fees; Ontario universities responded with steep tuition increases, doubling and even tripling fees over the past three years (Duffin, 2001). Some young doctors certainly feel the financial burden; despite hard-working practices, they still carry significant debts years after graduating (Keegan, 2000). Things are no better in the U.S. After graduation and on average, the U.S. doctor owes about US$93,000 (Korcok, 2001).

Doctors feel they are working much harder and being paid less; they have less time with their patients, and they believe they are less able to provide quality patient care. They are stressed, demoralized, and increasingly fed-up. How have doctors responded to these experiences?

Doctors' Responses

Individual Responses

Most doctors it seems are muddling through. They complain to their family, friends, and colleagues, and they squeeze in a bit more time and another patient. Some have decreased the services they provide and cut back on hospital committee and education duties (Kassirer, 1998). A mere decade ago in Canada, many physicians billed their provincial medicare plans more aggressively to shore-up flat or declining incomes (Shortt, 1999). Since 1993 in Ontario, after the introduction of a definitive cap to physicians' incomes, physicians are taking 'reduced activity days'. A few are taking early retirement. And an unprecedented number of a typically stoic profession are making disability claims and quitting on the income therefrom (Kassirer, 1998; Pincus, 1995).

An increasing minority of physicians, perhaps a prescient minority, are actively taking up the tools of managed (U.S.) or integrated (Canada) care. In the U.S., physicians' organizations are aggressively negotiating contracts and fees with the multiple insurers of the American managed care environment. They are learning to use the tools of business and population health, and they are joining hospitals and academic medical centers and establishing not-for-profit HMOs. These American physicians hope thereby to practice good medicine, maintain their medical decision-making autonomy, and provide quality service at a much lower cost (Greenberg, 1998;

Kassirer, 1998). By taking up the tools of their adversaries, physicians have not been entirely successful in avoiding trouble. The recent financial collapse of two large physician-practice-management companies left thousands of physicians with a total of more than $100 million in unpaid bills (Bodenheimer, 2000; Scheffler, 1999).

In Canada, hundreds of physicians are participating in pilot projects whose object is reform of the health care delivery system. For example, in Ontario, 200 family physicians are participating in a primary care reform project conducted by the Ontario Medical Association and the Provincial Ministry of Health. These physicians hope that the project's unique interlocking of a modified fee-for-service payment method with a capitation funding system, an information technology (IT) infrastructure to share and integrate information, the use of clinical practice guidelines, and the assistance of nurse practitioners will lead to better medical practice; that is, "a balance between reasonable working conditions for physicians and sustainable access to high-quality care for patients" (Graham, 1996; Graham, 1999; O'Reilly, 1998).

Responses of Medical Organizations

How have medical organizations responded to recent changes? The troubles of medical organizations relate to and differ from the troubles of doctors in clinics, offices and wards. Doctors discuss their relationships with patients; they discuss their own experiences, and the local context in which these occur. Medical organizations and their spokespersons talk about stakeholders: physicians, patients, and governments. This section deals with organizational responses to change under two broad categories, value for money and value for value.

Value for money. Certainly the most talked about changes and responses to changes involve money. In Canada over the past decade, public opinion, and the translation of public opinion into legislation, has produced cuts to federal-provincial transfer payments for social welfare programs (health and education). In 1999, federal funding was only two-thirds of 1995/96 levels (Canadian Medical Association, 2001). Provincial governments responded with cuts to hospitals, health and social programs, and claw backs in payments to physicians. A study sponsored by the Ontario Hospital Association (OHA) called the resulting hospital mergers, closings, reorganizations, and continued funding cuts "the largest public sector restructuring ever undertaken in North America" (Richard Ivey School of Business, 1997).

The OHA sponsors of the above study concluded in a way typical of medical organizations. The latter have produced hundreds of guidelines and parameters, commissioned reports, written policies and position papers, and conducted studies, many of which intend to show stakeholders that their members are increasingly providing appropriate and effective health care, and that they are doing it cost-effectively (Shortt, 1999). I discuss these responses under three headings: improved value, rationalization, and alternatives.

Improved value. Organizational efforts in this direction intend to assure or reassure stakeholders that physicians are of the highest value, that they are eminently qualified to provide the value for money stakeholders seek. Both the College of Family Physicians of Canada (CFPC) and the Royal College of Physicians and Surgeons of Canada (RCPSC), the bodies that accredit postgraduate medical education programs and examine candidates for certification, have recently revised their accreditation and certification standards (College of Family Physicians of Canada, 2000; Royal College of Physicians and Surgeons of Canada, 2000).

The CFPC examines candidates for certification in relation to four principles of family medicine: 1) the family physician is a skilled clinician; 2) family medicine is community-based; 3) the family physician is a resource and advocate for both individual and community health; and 4) the patient/physician relationship is paramount. The first and most traditional principle prescribes clinical skill and competence. The RCPSC, in a similar vein, prescribes seven "essential roles and key competencies of specialist physicians" (Royal College of Physicians and Surgeons of Canada, 2000). The physician's central role is medical expert and clinical decision-maker (College of Family Physicians of Canada, 2000; Royal College of Physicians and Surgeons of Canada, 2000). Contributory to the success of the physician expert are the other traditional roles: scholar, communicator and professional. Both colleges have developed roles that they recognize are increasingly valued by their public and academic stakeholders: the physician as health advocate, manager, and collaborator. Both colleges explicitly affirm their stakeholders' interests in broadening physicians' responsibilities. Physicians traditionally see themselves as clinical experts, medical scholars, and professionals, who provide the highest quality care to their individual patients. The RCPSC and CFPC in addition see their physician members as stewards of scarce health resources, collaborators with patients and participants in multidisciplinary health-care teams, and promoters of population health. Undergraduate medical curricula and continuing medical education programs in Canada and the U.S. also increasingly reflect this role expansion.

If stakeholders' demands for increased collaboration, health promotion, and judicious use of resources are legitimate demands, and physicians can best meet them, then medical organizations argue that we need such physicians, and that we may need more of them (Canadian Medical Association, 2000c Ontario College of Family Physicians, 2000).

Rationalization: standardized and predictable outcomes. Can physicians' organizations assure that the health care their members provide is of a high and consistent standard, that the standard is continuously maintained and improved, and that it is achieved cost-effectively? The structures, practices, and evaluation tools of medical education are designed to ensure certification of doctors of a consistently high standard. There is, however, a disjunction between the educational laboratory and the real world, the world of apprenticeship and the clinic and ward. For most of the last century, medical teachers could only hope that the physician would actively respond to the challenges of the real world and continue the educative process, that the doctor would be a lifelong learner.

Medical organizations primarily use two means to assure their stakeholders that their members provide consistent and efficient care: 1) peer review and audit, and 2) clinical practice guidelines. In the U.S. the Agency for Health Care Research and Quality sponsors and conducts research that "provides evidence-based information on health care outcomes; quality and cost; use and access" (Agency for Healthcare Research and Quality, 2001). As of early 2001 their researchers have published and made available in partnership with the AMA and the American Association of Health Plans approximately 1500 clinical practice guidelines. Canadian and Provincial Medical Associations enthusiastically endorse the use of clinical guidelines and make these readily available to members.

Peer Review Organizations have existed in the U.S. as a legislated part of Medicare since 1982. The College of Physicians and Surgeons of Ontario (CPSO) established an ongoing peer review process in 1981. Since 1999 the CPSO has been investigating ways to expand its review, and to make its audit more effective and efficient. The College's Peer Assessment Committee plans to be in a position to audit all Ontario physicians every five years. In addition to revoking the licenses of those unable or unwilling to improve substandard practices, the CPSO wants to play a larger role in education, in improving the good practices of the majority of physicians.

Alternatives. Medical organizations have responded to their stakeholders' movements for change by offering alternatives. Calls for fundamental changes to the health care system have, not surprisingly given the different organization and financing of their systems, produced distinct responses from American and Canadian medical organizations. The AMA and CMA do share some broad values and approaches. Both believe that their respective systems have served their nations very well. Both argue that fee-for-service payment is better for all stakeholders than any other method. Both call for gradual and incremental changes based on reform of what are presently good health care systems (American Medical Association, 2001a; Graham, 1996).

United States. The AMA believes that a pluralistic health care system open to market competition will provide the best and most efficient health care with maximum freedom of choice for both providers and patients. Single payer systems like Canada's unfairly concentrate the market power of payers. The AMA is opposed to the encroachment of government in the practice of medicine (American Medical Association, 2001a, 2001b).

Both the AMA's earlier *Health Access America* and its present proposals call for reform of the health insurance market (AMA 2001a, AMA 2001b; Todd et al., 1991). In its present proposal, the AMA details the unfair protection of employment-based insurance coverage from competition, and it proposes legislative reforms that would shift the contracting of health insurance from employers to employees. A capped, refundable tax credit inversely proportional to income would, the AMA argues, encourage the majority of America's working poor, the majority of those now uninsured, to purchase health insurance. Reform of tax and insurance laws, the AMA argues, would increase competition and keep premiums affordable. Loosening the requirements on basic sets of insured services and encouraging voluntary risk pools and 'Medical Savings Accounts' would further reduce premiums while maintaining adequate coverage. The unemployed poor and the uninsurable would be covered through government established or subsidized high-risk pools and further reforms to Medicare. The AMA calculates that its proposal would provide approximately 93% of Americans with health insurance coverage. It estimates that the federal government would have to provide between $39 and $65 billion in new funding to insure approximately 56% of those presently uninsured. This would leave 18–20 million Americans uninsured.

Canada. The Canadian and provincial medical associations believe in a plurality of payment methods "each tailored to the needs of the population and the considerations of providers, and designed to ensure the most efficient and effective provision of service within a variety of practice environments" (British Columbia Medical Association, 1995). Surveys of their members make it clear that they prefer fee-for-service, and for some of the same reasons the AMA gives: it provides the greatest choice for both physician (clinical autonomy) and patients (choice of provider); it rewards those who are efficient and hard-working; and it favors completeness of care. Canadians add that it produces a record of service as a by-product of the payment for service and thus generates detailed information useful to quality measures and population-based analyses (British Columbia Medical Association, 1995; Graham, 1996).

Despite these traditional commitments, there is a sense among Canadian medical organizations that "maintaining the status quo is untenable in view of the prevailing political and economic climate" (Graham, 1996). Two reports commissioned by government in the early and mid-1990s suggested that the Provincial Ministers of Health were moving toward a system of wholesale capitation payments for physicians (British Columbia Medical Association, 1995). This suggested the ministers were moving from a fee-for-service payment system to a system based on a flat rate per rostered patient. This has not happened, but governments continue to push for reform of the primary care system. The College of Family Physicians of Canada was the first medical organization to respond with an alternative, *Managing Change: The Family Medicine Group Practice Model*. Both the CFPC in its follow-up document, *Primary Care and Family Medicine in Canada: A Prescription for Renewal*, and the Ontario Medical Association (OMA) in its *Primary Care Reform: A Strategy for Stability* recommend some form of integrated group and multidisciplinary practice and a mixed payment system. The first strategy is designed to ensure both supply of the full complement of primary care services and patient access to services 24 hours per day, 7 days per week. The payment recommendations hope to balance predictability and control of costs with autonomy and service incentives. Both strategies attempt to balance communitarian values in health insurance with individual autonomy—fiscal with clinical accountability (Graham, 1996).

The OMA in conjunction with the Ministry of Health is conducting a pilot project of the OMA's plan at seven sites throughout the province. The Primary Care Reform (PCR) pilot project involves approximately 200 family physicians and 300,000 or more rostered Ontarians. A 1997 survey of Ontario physicians indicated general support for the OMA's approach (PCR survey):

- 60% believe doctors will be able to provide better preventive care under PCR

- 70% agree PCR will allow information technologies to better manage care

- 74% believe rostering will help eliminate waste in the health care system

- 80% believe PCR will confirm the role of doctors as the primary coordinators of health care (Jenkins, 1997)

Value for value. The categories 'value for money' and 'value for value' suggest some traditional value distinctions: means and ends, extrinsic and intrinsic value, self-interest and altruism. Earlier medical educators talked to students and colleagues about the dual nature of medicine: on the one hand, medicine is a means to make a living; on the other, it is the art and science of healing. They cautioned their listeners to avoid making the former the primary business of medicine (Gregory, 1772; Osler, 1930).

If those who paid no heed to the old docs ran medical businesses, they were private businesses. The resources they took in and profited from were private resources. For most nations today medical care is a public business. Even in the U.S., medicine is the public's business and takes in public resources that are measured in percentages of gross domestic product (GDP). Although U.S. insurance companies are not public businesses, they are certainly population businesses; insurance premiums are still determined and insurance profits projected in relation to population risks.

The duality of values with which doctors and indeed patients struggle today is not that described by Drs. Gregory and Osler. Today, on the one hand, medicine is steward of certain public resources and, on the other hand, is the art and science of healing. The latter implies both physician and patient autonomy. The former is not the value of prudent self-interest; it is a community and economic value—wise management of community resources. The duality has changed. Has the caution changed as well? Must doctors avoid making the stewardship of public resources the primary business of medicine?

Medical organizations recognize troubles generated by this dual responsibility. They have responded by revitalizing and sometimes expanding the core values of the profession. The American Board of Internal Medicine (ABIM) recently undertook Project Professionalism. ABIM affirms the core value of the medical profession, altruism; the medical professional upholds

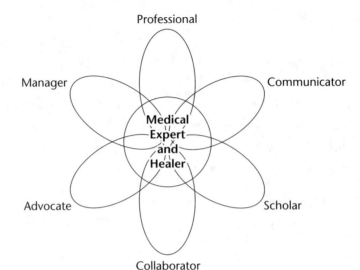

Figure 6.1 Seven key roles for physicians. Adapted from the Canadian Medical Association's Futures Project (Canadian Medical Association, 2000c)

the patient's interests above his or her own. The project conceptualizes professionalism and offers vignettes to stimulate discussion and aid doctors to further develop professional attitudes and behaviors. Professionalism stands beside clinical competence as essential to specialty certification. Project Professionalism is a response, ABIM says, to "changes in the health care environment … that can negatively affect the professional behavior of physicians. This concern is sharpened as physician reimbursement is changing and health care is provided in a competitive environment of managed and prepaid care, threatening to reduce the status of patients to commodities rather than people with an affliction" (American Board of Internal Medicine, 1998).

The Canadian Medical Association's Futures Project seeks to develop a vision and core values for the medical profession and an action plan to achieve these values. These core values, the CMA says, "must be upheld in whatever health system emerges." The first core value: medicine is a health profession, dedicated to serving *humanity*. The cornerstone of this value is the "relationship of trust between the patient and the physician." In addition, the CMA says, the medical profession should "encourage the development of healthy communities and of practices and policies that promote the well-being of the public" (Canadian Medical Association, 2000c).

The Royal College of Physicians and Surgeons of Canada in its *Skills for the New Millennium: Report of the Societal Needs Working Group* developed

Table 6.1   Key Physician Roles

Medical Expert & Healer

Physicians have always been recognized for their role as medical experts and healers; it is the defining nature of their practice, and derives from the broad knowledge base of medical practice – an interlocking of art and science. Medical expert and healer is the foundation for continuing physician leadership in the provision of health care.

Professional

Physicians must reaffirm the principles of the medical profession, including upholding its unique knowledge and skills; maintenance of high standards of practice; and commitment to its underlying values of caring, service, and compassion. The medical profession of the future must continue to develop standards of care and ongoing assessments of competency, and it will continue as a valued, self-regulated profession worthy of public trust and respect.

Communicator

Physicians will emphasize their ability to gather and communicate medical information in a compassionate and caring fashion, to enter into partnership with patients when organizing care plans, and to provide education and counseling bearing on the promotion of health. As always, the patient–physician relationship remains paramount, with its essential features of compassion, confidentiality, honesty and respect.

Scholar

Medical scholarship contains three essential parts: creation of new knowledge (research); delivery of rational and high quality care (clinical practice); and induction of novices into the culture of scholarship, of life-long learning (education). It is the interchange between these essential parts of medical scholarship that continue to renew medical expertise and professionalism.

Collaborator

Interdisciplinary teams increasingly provide health care services throughout the continuum of care. As collaborators, physicians recognize the essential and valued functions of all health care workers, and they contribute their unique values and expertise to patient-centered health care delivery.

Advocate

As health care becomes increasingly complex and integrated with other societal values and endeavors, it is essential for physicians to increase and expand their roles as health advocates. Physicians have excellent opportunities to advocate for the resources and social conditions that promote improved individual, family, and community health.

Manager

Providing quality care requires that physicians must now be effective resource managers at the individual practice level, at the health care facility level and as part of the wider health care system.

Adapted from the Canadian Medical Association's Futures Project (Canadian Medical Association, 2000c) seven essential roles (Figure 6.1) and their corresponding competencies as a framework for specialty training and certification in Canada (Table 6.1). In addition to the traditional roles of expert clinician, scholar, and professional, the RCPSC includes advocate, manager, and collaborator. The RCPSC emphasizes the profession's responsibilities to society. The overall goal of the project is "to ensure that postgraduate specialty training programs are fully responsive to societal needs"; indeed, "[m]edicine has a solemn covenant to serve society." The RCPSC authors are responding to a particular imbalance of interests, which the project should remedy: the project intends to change "the focus of specialty training from the interests and abilities of providers (supply) to the needs of society (demand)." This stated, the authors further describe medicine's covenant: specialty training programs are "to consider the needs of individual patients in context of the population at large" (Royal College of Physicians and Surgeons of Canada, 2000).

Looking Around & Going Forward

Many authoritative commentators on health care and health care systems remark on the fact of change: "Change is the order of the day!" (K. White, 1991). They call on doctors to perceive the disjunction between their traditional practices, their traditional professionalism, and the changed environment (Mechanic, 2000). They imply and sometimes demand that doctors change themselves, or be changed (K. White, 1991).

Disjunction between one's goals and the environment, that is, between intentions and the real world, can be a most valuable stimulus to change. To wield the environment as something fixed, however, is to take it as something necessary to which one submits, either by conforming oneself to this necessary environment or being conformed by it. Environmental necessity then provides the ends and standards of change. Whether these necessary standards are utilitarian, the greatest health for the greatest number, or whether they are economic, the best value for the health customer, doctors are asked to change or be changed. Both demand static adjustments, mere conformity to fixed ends.

By contrast, physicians can begin from their unique perspectives and capacities to assess their values and their problems, and thus mount an active response to the present environment. Rather than submitting to a pre-given environment or pre-set standards, physicians can receive and respond to the environment by thoughts and initiatives that apply their capacities to new and valued aims. Physicians will thereby add their unique values and skills to the ongoing structuring of the new health-care environment at the same time that they are developing new capacities as physicians.

Case Study: Elsewhereville

Use the following case study to stimulate discussion and raise questions around the problems, values, capacities and goals of the practicing physician: the physician's perspective. You may find it useful to refer to Table 6.1 on the physician's roles.

Elsewhereville, Part 1

Dr. H. and his partner are the only doctors for a town of 3500 and for a First Nations, or aboriginal, community of 1000. The town's major employer is a lumber and sawmill company. Dr. H. came here shortly after family medicine residency; he started as a three-month locum, a temporary replacement for the previous doctor, and now he and his partner own the practice. He has been here three years, his partner two. They have tried to attract another doctor; six have come and gone. No one stays, and Dr. H. well understands why; the pace of practice is grueling. Dr. H. works 10–12 hour days, often seeing 30–40 patients in the office. Every second day and weekend on call, the small emergency in their 10-bed hospital keeps them hopping. They see one major trauma a week, either a vehicle or industrial accident or the violent results of alcohol use.

He is glad that he did an extra six months in ob-gyn, even though he is still paying back his university debts. He and his partner do five or six deliveries a month. He likes it here; he would have to be crazy if he didn't. Because of the isolation and difficulties of getting patients in to specialists, Dr. H. and his partner carry many interesting cases; it keeps them in the top of their form. What is more, his patients like him, and he feels he is making a valuable contribution.

The truth is, he is getting worn out. It isn't simply the workload; he is used to that. His wife is unhappy and wants them to move on. He has not been much company for her; when he is not at the office or hospital, he practices the flute; it helps him relax. Unfortunately, he is usually too tired to do even that. Last week a friend invited him to join their three-doctor practice in the city. Perhaps he should. He has heard rumors that the hospital may close, and if that happened, he doesn't know how he and his partner could continue.

Questions for Discussion

1. *What should Dr. H. do? What values could inform Dr. H's possible decisions?*

2. *Who has a stake in his decision?*

3. *What capacities does Dr. H. need to build to change and improve his practice? Refer to the seven key roles of a physician (Table 6.1) as an aid to thinking about capacity building.*

Elsewhereville, Part 2

A week later, Dr. H. attends a weekend Advanced Trauma Life Support course in the city. His city-friend is there, as is a physician and clinical epidemiologist, Dr. C., a guest of one of the instructors. Over lunch Dr. H. shares some of his practice problems with Dr. C. He didn't expect a city doc to understand, but he and Dr. C. have many common interests. Dr. C. works part-time at an inner-city clinic in the capital, where he also teaches clinical epidemiology at the medical school. He is in town to give a special lecture on child poverty and health.

The lecture moves Dr. H.; it puts words to something he has always known: much of the illness in his community is due to environmental, social, and economic factors. This illness should be preventable. He realizes too why he has not given this much thought; he feels completely helpless to do anything about it. He has little enough time or energy to fully meet today's demands let alone engage in prevention and health promotion. This weekend's conversations with Dr. C. help him realize that if he were to try and change his practice, he cannot do it alone. He makes a start by talking to the four docs from Nextville. Perhaps, despite the distance, they could share on call duties and resources.

Questions for Discussion

1. *Who else might Dr. H. talk to? Who are the other health professionals in his community?*

2. *What resources and capacities might the community, the regional medical association, the University, the Public Health Department contribute?*

Elsewhereville Six Months Later, Part 3

Sharing call with the Nextville doctors was unworkable. Dr. H. did succeed in attracting an assistant on a three month contract, in part through the medical school's rural medicine training program. He was instrumental in helping the public health nurse attract an experienced midwife to the community, and he has a good working relationship with her. His regional medical association helped with guidelines. He has also become involved in a joint medical association and government pilot project to test the integration of nurse practitioners.

Despite these successes his workload has not noticeably eased, and the rumors of hospital closure are now real. He realizes that despite working daily in the hospital, he hardly talks to the hospital director. And although he feels the need more acutely, he has been unable to find time to expand his efforts at disease prevention and health promotion. He gives Dr. C. a call, who puts him in touch with a colleague, Dr. A.

Dr. A. has expertise in health systems management and is particularly interested in aiding health professionals to succeed in providing cost-effective primary care. Dr. H. is skeptical, but they agree to meet. Dr. H. is impressed with Dr. A.'s advice, in particular, the potential benefits of using information technologies and e-Health applications. They arrange a one-day workshop involving Dr. H., his partner and locum; the hospital staff and administration; and the community health personnel.

This is the first time all the health professionals in the community have met together. Many are interested in improving the community's efforts at health promotion and disease prevention, but it becomes difficult to keep this in mind when the hospital director takes this opportunity to announce that the hospital is merging with Nextville's. Dr. A. leads the group through many of the practices in this book; and using several of the worksheets from *Promoting Health*, in particular the *Decision Balance* (Worksheet 9.2) and the *Building Motivation* guide (Worksheet 9.3), the group becomes clearer on its values and goals. Health promotion and disease prevention become an explicit priority. Even the merger may have its benefits: the integration of acute care services in Nextville will make shared call workable, and the old hospital may be home to obstetrical and home care services. The health-care team arranges a future workshop to discuss strategic directions.

Worksheet Practice

1. Complete and discuss Worksheets 9.2 and 9.3 regarding motivation for change (instructions in Chapter 9).

2. Take a look at Worksheets 11.1, 11.2, and 11.3 on stakeholder analysis, environmental scanning, and strategic directions (Chapter 11). How

could these be used to clarify action steps for physicians regarding organizational improvement?

Conclusion

This chapter will have succeeded if it helps the reader actively think about and openly discuss the values of the medical profession. Medical organizations have strongly renewed traditional values and developed new values that address the profession's present problems and challenges. The profession's traditional challenges remain providing appropriate and effective patient care within a compassionate and increasingly collaborative patient-physician relationship. Physicians have always taken this professional accountability as paramount. With the development of new values and capacities based on their traditional responsibilities, I have no doubt that they will become increasingly accountable, economically and politically, to their communities.

It is well within their values and capacities to embrace a public health approach, indeed it is a traditional medical approach (K. White, 1991). If it has been set aside during the past century, that is due also to broader social and political forces. To shift our communities toward health promotion and disease prevention, doctors will need the help of those broader forces. This book hopes to make its small contribution to that effort.

Moving On

The next chapter reviews several theories on motivation. It describes the dynamics of both resistance and motivation, and discusses why and how people change. The insights from these theories are integrated in a ten step index, and presented as a worksheet that aids analysis of an individual's likelihood to change.

CHAPTER 7

What Motivates People to Change

A cigarette is the perfect pleasure. It is exquisite, and it leaves one unsatisfied. What more can one want?

—Oscar Wilde (late 1800s)

Overview

This chapter reviews concepts that are important for understanding the forces for changing individual behavior. In particular this chapter reviews the following: Health Belief Model, Theory of Reasoned Action/Planned Behavior, Social Learning/Social Cognitive Theory, Self-Determination Theory, Transtheoretical Model (stages of change), motivational interviewing, and relapse prevention. These concepts are integrated into a ten-step Likelihood of Action Index, which provides a practical guide for analyzing when an individual is more or less likely to change a behavior. This heuristic method can be used to guide intervention approaches at both individual and organizational levels. For example, organizational improvement initiatives often encounter individual-level resistance from key stakeholders, such as physicians or clinical unit staff. Understanding what underlies this resistance and what approaches you can take to build motivation is pivotal to effect changes needed for organizational improvement. Sooner or later, it all comes down to addressing the root causes of resistance and motivation of individuals by shifting their give-get balance in the organizational context.

Dynamics of Motivation and Resistance

Human motivation is rather curious. Consider our actions in buying lottery tickets. British statisticians have determined that anyone who buys a

National Lottery ticket on Monday is 2500 times more likely to die before the draw on Saturday than to win the jackpot. Yet, the lottery business is booming! Given the huge profit margin, one can readily understand why governments and other organizations run lotteries. But, with minuscule odds of winning, why do so many people continue to buy tickets, week in and week out?

This illustrates the human tendency to accentuate the benefits of a behavior (e.g., winning the lottery) and downplay its risks (e.g., losing money). These tensions regarding the pros and cons of behavior are at the core of understanding motivation.

Both individual- and systems-level forces influence the likelihood of behavior change. This is embodied in the concept of Reciprocal Determinism, that is, the dynamic and simultaneous interaction between a person, the behavior of that person, and the environment (system or organization) in which the behavior is performed (Bandura, 1986). These components are constantly interacting and influencing each other, which is a central tenet of systems theory (Miller, 1978; Prigogine and Stengers, 1984; Stacey, 1996). The likelihood of behavior change in health organizations is

- **Increased** by approaches that enhance individual motivation and build organizational (system) supports,
- **Decreased** by approaches that stimulate individual resistance and create organizational (systems) barriers.

Our aim in this chapter is to help you understand the dynamics of motivation and change at the individual level. This understanding is critical for increasing your effectiveness in changing health organizations using the Five-Step Model described in Chapters 8–14. Even if you are focusing on a macro-level change in the organization, sooner or later you will be sitting across the table trying to influence another person such as your boss, another department head, or an external partner or funder. Understanding why people resist advice and what motivates action will help you in these situations.

Understanding Resistance

Someone may resist your advice about behavior change for a variety of reasons. In this section, we examine four dynamics that underlie resistance: 1) your communication style, 2) mismatches in readiness for change, 3) differing perspectives on how a 'problem' is defined, and 4) alternative values about the pros and cons of change (give-get balance). By under-standing these perspectives, you open the door to more effective ways in negotiating change. Botelho et al. (1999) give practical strategies for work-ing with, not against, resistance in the context of primary care patients with alcohol problems.

Your communication style. How often have you found yourself in the sit-uation where the harder you try to persuade someone to change, the more the individual digs in his or her heels regarding the prospect of change? A classic example is a parent (or teacher) arguing with a teen about a risk behavior, such as wearing protective gear while skateboarding or inline blading. Both parties are pushing with increasing intensity on the gate—but from opposite directions!

We have all experienced this: people frequently act counter to pressure put on them. Reactance theory, articulated by Brehm and Brehm (1981), provides a useful way of understanding this form of resistance. This theory emphasizes the importance that individuals place on having control or free-dom. Any threat results in the individual attempting to restore the freedom in question. This helps explain why individuals may cling to a 'problem' or risk behavior, in the face of increasing evidence and pressure to change. Ironically, the attractiveness of a risk behavior can be increased, if the per-son feels that his or her freedom (right of choice) is being threatened. A principle of this theory is that the amount of reactance will increase as a direct function of the number of freedoms threatened. In other words, the more one tries to persuade (push) an individual to change on an issue where they feel threatened, the more likely the individual will react by dig-ging in their heels (pushing back).

Resistance and reactance can be demonstrated in controlled studies. Patterson and Forgatch (1985) had therapists switch back and forth between either 1) a directive-confrontational style and 2) a supportive-reflective style in a study of family therapy. Every 12 minutes, the therapist switched from one style to the other, back and forth. Interestingly, clients' behavior mirrored the therapists' approach. When the therapist adopted a directive-confrontational style, client resistance increased. Conversely, when the therapist used a supportive-reflective style, behaviors reflecting client resistance decreased.

Similarly, Miller, Benefield and Tonigan (1993) compared two therapist styles in a study with problem drinkers. Patients were randomly assigned to three conditions: 1) directive-confrontational counselling, 2) client-centered counselling, or 3) waiting-list control. The directive-confrontational style yielded significantly more resistance from clients, such as arguing, interrupting and diverging from the focus of therapy. In comparison, problem drinkers who received client-centered counselling were more likely to exhibit positive behavior. Thus, the clients' behavior was strongly correlated with the therapist's style: the more the therapist confronted, the more likely the client would argue. Similarly, at the organizational level, a highly controlling leadership style can evoke resistance among staff.

Mismatches in readiness for change. Another area for the generation of resistant behavior stems from differing perspectives regarding stages or readiness for change (Prochaska et al., 1992). The stages of change model is depicted in Figure 7.1 (also see the Readiness for Change Analysis Worksheet 9.1 in Chapter 9). Often, you may be far out in front of the other person, working on the assumption that the individual is ready to take action.

For example, research on cigarette smokers and related health behavior indicates that only approximately 10–20% are at the point where they are ready or prepared to take action (Prochaska et al., 1992). More likely, smokers are either ambivalent or unsure about change (are in a contemplation stage), or they are not engaged or even thinking about change (are in a precontemplation stage) (Velicer et al., 1995).

As the degree of mismatch increases between yourself and the other person in readiness for change, the likelihood of resistance increases proportionately. A key task is to explore and reach a shared understanding

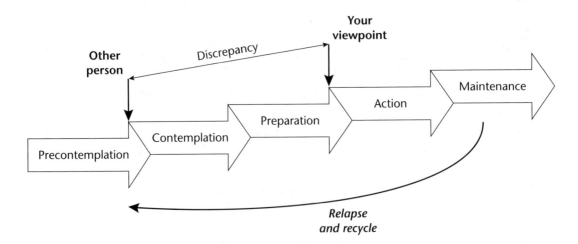

Figure 7.1 Differing viewpoints on readiness for change.

about where you both are on readiness for change, and then adapt by taking the appropriate problem-solving and negotiation approach.

Who defines the 'problem'? Another way for understanding resistance is to consider the level of agreement between yourself and another person about defining an issue as a problem. For instance, health care professionals may assess the risk from a given behavior (e.g., physical inactivity) to be higher than the patient's estimate. In an organizational context, you may falsely assume that others share your evaluation about the need to respond to substance abuse patients missing routine follow-up appointments. Also, there is a tendency to minimize personal susceptibility to a risk behavior (e.g., getting an STD from unprotected sex) due to an 'optimism bias' (Olson, 1992, Weinstein, 1987). *"I am less vulnerable to the health consequence; it is more likely to happen to someone else than to me."*

For these reasons, you may be at a quite different point than the other person in their assessment of whether the issue is a 'problem' that warrants action. Resistance is a function of this degree of separation.

Differing views on the pros and cons of change. Another area where significant mismatches can occur lies in different values placed on the benefits and costs of change. Ambivalence and resistance result when individuals experience competition on both sides of a decision (pros and cons of change). Silversin and Kornacki (2000) describe this dynamic as the 'give' and 'get' members expect from an organization. The term **compact** refers to this implicit or explicit contract between an organization and its members. The Decision Balance Worksheet 9.2 in Chapter 9 is a useful heuristic tool for helping you become more aware of the benefits (actual or perceived) that the individual gains from not changing, as well as concerns if they were to change.

Typically, health practitioners and patients are focusing upon different aspects. Practitioners are more likely to emphasize the benefits (pros) of behavior change and the costs or harms (cons) to the patient of maintaining the risk behavior. Alternatively, patients are more likely to value how a risk behavior may function (pros) for them (e.g., smoking a cigarette to relax) and, conversely, be quite concerned about the costs (cons) of change. Similarly, the chief information officer in a health care organization may place great value on implementing a computerized patient record and management system, whereas practitioners see this change as more complication and an intrusion on their time and professional autonomy.

The flip side of resistance is motivation. Let's look at the dynamics of individual motivation.

Understanding Motivation

Motivation addresses why one takes action (or not) in a given situation. From a lay perspective, motivation is viewed as the reason why humans feel and behave as they do. Individuals are deemed to accomplish significant acts because they are 'motivated'. This student achieved an A+ in the course because of her high level of motivation and academic drive. Conversely, individuals are frequently labelled 'unmotivated' when they fail to achieve a certain standard of behavior, such as maintaining abstinence following alcoholism treatment, or failing to alter a risk behavior such as quitting cigarette use. Motivation is seen to stem from forces within the individual (e.g., needs, drives), as well as factors in the environment (e.g., incentives, barriers).

Deci and Ryan (1985, 2000) distinguish between two fundamental aspects of motivation: 1) energy and 2) direction. Consider a ski jumper depicted in Figure 7.2. The goal is to land as far as possible down the hill but still within the 'sweet spot' (K point). If the jumper has too little momentum (energy), he will land too close up on the steep pitch of the hill. Conversely, if the jumper has too much momentum, he will land too far down the hill on the flat pitch. In either case, the jumper risks serious injury. In addition, the jumper must adjust his body lean and backswept arms to fine tune his directional stability so that he lands in the middle of the hill.

Energy results from needs that are either innate to the organism or are acquired through interactions with the environment. Energy can also result from the degree of discrepancy between an individual's current state (e.g., poor physical fitness level following an injury) and a highly valued goal (e.g.,

Figure 7.2 Two essential components of motivation.

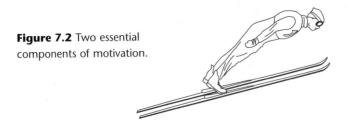

Energy plus direction

winning a 10-K running race). **Direction** is given by structures and processes that relate needs to behavior. For instance, weighing the pros and cons (decision balance) of adopting a new training program, along with the prospect of training with several highly competitive athletes (social rewards), may compel a runner to join an elite track club. In brief, direction determines toward what, and away from what, an individual will move.

A number of theories and integrative models have been proposed to help explain whether an individual will engage in a health behavior. From a review of the health education, medical and behavioral science literature published during 1992–1994, Glanz et al. (1997) found that the five most commonly used theories and models were, respectively:

- Health Belief Model
- Social Learning Theory/Social Cognitive Theory
- Theory of Reasoned Action/Planned Behavior
- Transtheoretical Model (Stages of Change)
- Community Organization

One concept that has attracted considerable attention is self-efficacy (Bandura, 1995; 1997). Although this concept evolved out of Social Cognitive Theory, self-efficacy is now incorporated in both the Health Belief Model and the Transtheoretical Model.

The first three theories/models address health behavior acquisition and maintenance. These models, along with Self-Determination Theory (Deci & Ryan, 1985), will be examined in more detail below. Basically, they address the question of **why one acts**. The Transtheoretical Model, on the other hand, focuses more on the question of **how people change**. The final section of this chapter reviews research on the increasingly popular Transtheoretical Model, especially the Stages of Change component. Also, see the discussion about practitioner interventions in Chapter 3 using the principles of motivational interviewing and relapse prevention.

Why One Acts: A Primer

The diversity of concepts and theories for understanding health behavior can be quite bewildering. In Table 7.1, a succinct integration of concepts is given in the form of a Likelihood of Action Index, initially formulated by Skinner and Bercovitz (1997). Specifically, the likelihood (probability) of

Table 7.1   Likelihood of Action Index*

"A Person Is More Likely To Act If ..."	Concepts
Sees the health risk as serious and is personally concerned	Severity,[1] Encodings,[3] Precontemplation[5]
Feels personally susceptible to the health risk	Susceptibility[1]
Believes the recommended change to be effective in reducing risk	Outcome Expectations,[3] Beliefs[1,2,3]
Assesses that expected benefits (pros) are greater than (cons) of change	Decision Balance,[1,5] Expectancies,[3] the costs Values,[3] Contemplation[5]
Believes that significant others (family, friends, practitioner) think the behavior should be changed	Normative Belief[2]
Is motivated to comply with the other person's desire	Compliance[2]
Is in a context (environment) that is supportive of the action	Environment,[3] Situation[3,4]
Has the knowledge, skills and emotional coping responses to change successfully	Capability,[3] Affects (emotions),[3] Self-regulation[3,4]
Feels capable of carrying out the action successfully	Self-efficacy[1,3,5]
Wants to engage in the action because of personal choice	Self-determination,[4] Preparation,[5] Perceived Control[2]

*The likelihood (probability) of an individual taking action increases
as a function of the number of factors present (range 0–10).

[1]Health Belief Model
[2]Theory of Reasoned Action/Planned Behavior
[3]Social Cognitive Theory
[4]Self Determination Theory
[5]Transtheoretical Model

behavior change increases as a function of both the presence and intensity of ten factors. The greater the number of factors, the more likely the person is to act.

A person is more likely to take action when the potential health risk is seen as not only serious, but also of personal concern to the individual. For instance, a woman may view having unprotected sex as a significant health risk for STDs and HIV. However, the woman is not personally concerned nor feels susceptible to the risk because she is in a long-term relationship with the same partner whose sexual history she is fairly confident about.

In weighing of pros and cons of change (decision balance), an individual is more likely to act when the expected benefits are assessed to be greater than the costs (barriers) of change. Note: the decision-weighing process is a central feature of most theories/models of intentional behavior. It incorporates not only a cognitive component (i.e., the rational decision-maker), but also affective/emotional processes (e.g., anxiety or fear reduction), perceptions about the expected benefits and barriers, and the importance (value) placed on a desired outcome. For these reasons, the Decision Balance Worksheet 9.1 is discussed in Chapter 9 as a key tool for understanding differing perspectives and building motivation for organizational change.

The next three factors involve the extent of social and environmental influence. Specifically, a person is more likely to act if he or she believes that significant others support the behavior change, and this person cares about complying with the desire of the other persons (friend, family, practitioner). Also, the likelihood of action can be powerfully influenced by the broader social and physical context, which either supports or oppresses the action. For instance, a middle-aged man is more likely to increase physical activity and keep a low-fat diet if family members also stress low-fat food in the home and when eating out, he takes out a membership at a health club where some friends also exercise, and he lives in a safe community that encourages its members to walk/cycle to work (e.g., special bike paths).

A person is more likely to act when she or he has the relevant capabilities, including knowledge, skills and emotional responses. Yet, knowledge and skills are often not enough to produce behavior change. Someone may feel susceptible to a health risk, believe it to be severe, have the capabilities to change and believe that the benefits of change (including social recognition) outweigh the costs. However, whether or not a person takes action is highly correlated with the sense that *"I can do it"* (self-efficacy). Indeed, a person's confidence in performing a particular behavior such as quitting smoking is generally the most important predictor of success.

A final element for increasing the likelihood of change is the person's sense of personal choice or freedom to engage in the action; that is, *"I want to do it"* (self-determination). Two individuals can have the same level of capabilities and strong confidence (self-efficacy) that they can cut down on their drinking. Yet, one may feel pressured by family members and resist change, whereas the other feels little pressure and decides to cut down due to personal choice.

Note: the last two factors (self-efficacy—'can do it'; self-determination —'choose to do it') are generally determined by or are derivative of the other components in Table 7.1. For this reason, self-efficacy and self-determination are often good predictors of behavioral intention and actual behavior change (Bandura, 1997; Ryan & Deci, 2000).

Likelihood of Action Analysis (Worksheet 7.1) is designed to help you put the likelihood of action index into practice. You can use it with a person such as a friend, family member, coworker or even yourself, who may consider changing a health behavior.

Exercise 1: Self Analysis

Think about a behavior that you might change. You may have made attempts in the past or it may simply be an item on your personal 'to consider' list. Write your target behavior on Worksheet 7.1. Before you go further, rate the likelihood that you will successfully take action using the following ten-point scale:

not at all: 0   1   2   3   4   5   6   7   8   9   10: definitely

Carefully review each of the ten factors regarding the prospects of your taking action to change this behavior. If you have difficulty or insufficient information, then try talking to someone you know and trust about it. Check off your self-assessment for each factor (1 = yes, 0.5 = somewhat, 0 = no) on Worksheet 7.1. Give specific reasons for each rating in the Rationale section. Finally, sum up your ratings on the ten factors to give your overall Index Score.

Now, work through the following Guiding Questions:

1. *How did the self-assessment Index Score compare with your initial rating?*

2. *Which factor is your greatest strength? Which is your most concern?*

3. *In what ways did completing Worksheet 7.1 help you think about where to concentrate your efforts in changing this behavior?*

Case Study

Louise, a 23-year-old woman, is having unprotected sex. She is in a stable relationship with the same partner whose sexual history she feels fairly confident about. Her boyfriend, Jim, does not use condoms. Their sexual behavior is a risk factor for STDs and HIV.

Recently, Louise contracted a sexually transmitted disease (chlamydia infection), but feels that she is not susceptible to contracting the AIDS virus. She has not had an HIV test. However, after learning that a girlfriend had contracted HIV, Louise is thinking about having the test. She now insists that her boyfriend start using a condom. However, Jim hates the use of condoms. Also, he is terrified of AIDS and refuses to have the blood test.

Use Worksheet 7.1 to analyze the likelihood that Louise and Jim will take the following actions. Then, compare your assessment of their overall index scores, as well as which factors are most salient for them:

1. *What is the likelihood that Louise will have the HIV test?*
2. *What is the likelihood that Jim will start using a condom?*

The Likelihood of Action Index is meant to serve as both a heuristic and assessment tool for understanding what motivates people to take action in a particular context. How did these two exercises increase your understanding of the range of factors that influence why people act?

We now turn to a more detailed examination of four theories/models.

Why People Engage in Health Behavior

Health Belief Model

The Health Belief Model (HBM) was developed in the early 1950s in an attempt to understand why people fail to take part in screening tests and disease prevention services (Rosenstock, 1974). This model draws upon psychological and behavioral theory that hypothesizes that behavior depends upon: 1) the value placed by an individual on a particular goal (e.g., good health), and 2) the individual's estimate of the likelihood that a given action will achieve that goal (e.g., regular physical activity). The central concepts of the Health Belief Model are depicted in Figure 7.3. The energizing component of motivation results from the perceived magnitude of a threat to the individual's health. This entails a belief in personal susceptibility and anticipated severity of the health consequence (disease). The direction component of motivation results from the individual's assessment that the advised action will reduce risk as well as alleviate barriers such as negative side effects.

The HBM also incorporates various modifying factors such as demographic characteristics and socioeconomic status, which are known to influence health behavior. Another class of modifying factors, Cues to Action, are included in the Model as triggers of action (e.g., mass media campaign), even though there has been limited research on this component. More

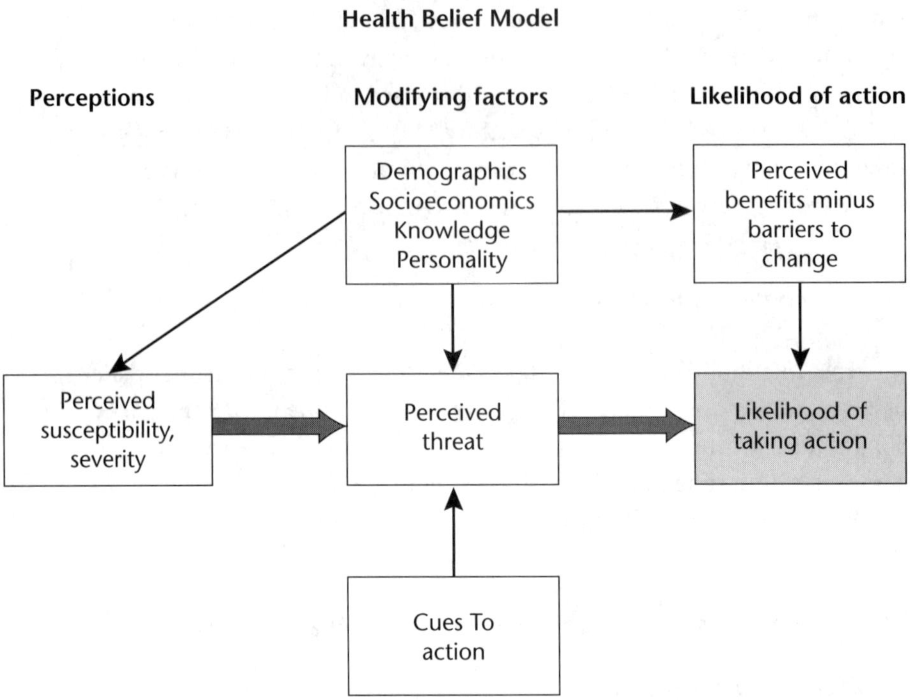

Health Belief Model

Figure 7.3 Overview of concepts in the Health Belief Model. Reproduced with permission from Strecher and Rosenstock (1997). The health belief model. In: Karen Glanz, Frances M. Lewis and Barbara K. Rimer (Eds.), *Health Behavior and Health Education: Theory, Research, and Practice,* 2nd ed. San Francisco: Jossey-Bass Publishers.

recently, the concept of self-efficacy (Bandura, 1986, 1997) has been added to the Health Belief Model in order to increase its explanatory power (Rosenstock et al., 1988). Lack of self-efficacy is viewed as a perceived barrier to taking a recommended health action.

Strecher and Rosenstock (1997) provide an overview of evidence for and against this model. The Perceived Barriers component has been found to be the most powerful single predictor of action among the Health Belief Model dimensions across studies and behaviors.

Theory of Reasoned Action/Theory of Planned Behavior

These two related theories developed by Fishbein and Ajzen add several important pieces to the puzzle of understanding why one acts (Ajzen, 1991; Ajzen & Fishbein, 1980; Fishbein, 1967; Fishbein & Ajzen, 1975). First, the theories emphasize measures of attitude and social perceptions regarding an action. The intention to perform a behavior is determined by

- Attitudes and beliefs about a specific action and the value attached to the outcome,

- The person's belief about likely social reactions (approval or disapproval) from certain individuals or groups regarding the behavior, and the person's motivation to comply or not with what others think.

Second, the theories propose that the most immediate determinant of behavior is a person's **behavioral intention**. The causal relationship is depicted in Figure 7.4. Third, these theories distinguish between an attitude toward an object (e.g., breast cancer) and an attitude toward a behavior

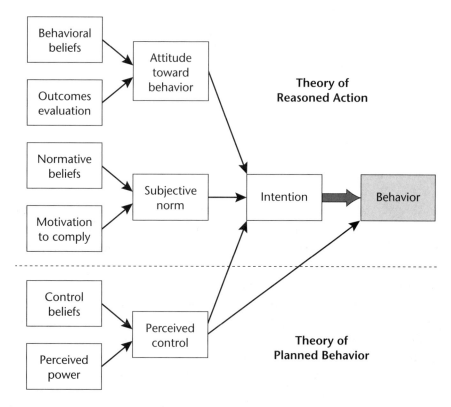

Figure 7.4 Overview of concepts in the Theories of Reasoned Action and Planned Behavior. Reproduced with permission from Montano, Kasprzyk, and Taplin. The health belief model. In: Karen Glanz, Frances M. Lewis and Barbara K. Rimer (Eds.), *Health Behavior and Health Education: Theory, Research, and Practice,* 2nd ed. San Francisco: Jossey-Bass Publishers.

with respect to that object (e.g., seeking mammography screening). Fishbein and Ajzen (1975) have found that an attitude toward a behavior is a better predictor than an attitude toward the target to which the behavior is directed. For example, a woman's behavior in seeking mammography screening will be more closely linked to the woman's attitude toward mammography screening than her attitude toward breast cancer.

The Theory of Planned Behavior extends the Theory of Reasoned Action by adding the component of perceived control (Figure 7.4). Intention can only predict a person's attempt. Whether or not the individual actually performs the behavior may be due to factors beyond the person's control that can interfere with completion of the intention. For this reason, Ajzen (1991) added the concept of perceived behavioral control as a means of accounting for factors outside of a person's control. Performance is a function of the person's attempt as well as the degree of control over that behavior. In this way, the theory incorporates external factors (e.g., unsafe neighborhood) that can influence behavior (e.g., physical activity such as walking alone).

Social Learning Theory/Social Cognitive Theory

This framework, dating back to the 1940s, considers both the acquisition of behavior as well as behavioral change. Of particular relevance is the work of Albert Bandura beginning in the 1960s, in which he demonstrated that children could watch other children and learn a new behavior while not being rewarded directly (i.e., vicarious reinforcement). Bandura continued with a major rethinking of Social Learning Theory, which led to the concept of self-efficacy (Bandura, 1977) and, more recently, to a comprehensive framework termed 'Social Cognitive Theory' (Bandura, 1986, 1997). The key elements of Social Cognitive Theory are summarized in Table 7.2. A related stream of theoretical development has evolved from the work of Walter Mischel (1973; Mischel & Shoda, 1995), who has emphasized cognitive constructs. Miller, Shoda and Hurley (1996) have applied Mischel's framework to the study of breast self-examination in cancer screening (Table 7.3).

Social Cognitive Theory links the individual with salient attributes of the environment (Baranowski et al., 1997). The pivotal concept is reciprocal determinism, which emphasizes the dynamic interplay between the person and the environment. Behavior is seen to result from the continual interaction among three components: 1) characteristics of a person; 2) behavior of that person; and 3) the environment in which a behavior is performed. In

Table 7.2   Major Concepts in Social Cognitive Theory

Behavioral Capability	Knowledge and skill to perform a given behavior
Expectations	Anticipated outcomes of a behavior
Expectancies	Value that the person places on a given outcome (incentives)
Self-control	Personal regulation of a goal-directed behavior (e.g., self-monitoring)
Reinforcement: Rewards/Incentives	Responses to a person's behavior that increase or decrease the likelihood of recurrence
Emotional Coping	Strategies used by a person to deal with emotional stimuli/situations (stress management)
Self-efficacy	The person's confidence in performing a given behavior ("*I can do it*")
Environment	Factors that are physically external to the person
Situation	Person's perception of the environment
Reciprocal Determinism	Dynamic interaction of the person, the person's behavior and the environment

Adapted with permission from Baranowski, Perry and Parcel (1997). In: Karen Glanz, Frances M. Lewis and Barbara K. Rimer (Eds.), *Health Behavior and Health Education: Theory, Research, and Practice,* 2nd ed. San Francisco: Jossey-Bass Publishers.

Table 7.3   Applying Social Cognitive Theory to Breast Cancer

Health Relevant Encodings: constructs for encoding of self and situations regarding wellness, health risks and illness. Includes attentional strategies for selecting and processing health threats (e.g., avoiding information about personal vulnerability to breast cancer).

Health Beliefs and Expectancies: Specific belief and expectations activated in health information processing. Includes expectancies about outcomes (e.g., likelihood of developing breast cancer based on one's family history) and self-efficacy (e.g., can successfully perform breast self-examination).

Affects: emotional states activated in health information processing, such as: anxiety, depression, hopefulness, fear, irritability, anger, self-depreciation (e.g., fear and anxiety over personal susceptibility to breast cancer causes an individual to avoid health information on cancer prevention).

Health Goals and Values: desired health outcomes and their subjective importance (e.g., it is critical to have healthy breasts), and goals for life projects (e.g., dieting and regular exercise).

Self-Regulatory Competencies and Skills: knowledge and strategies for dealing with specific barriers to health-protective behavior (e.g., skills required for proficient breast self-examination), and for maintaining health-protective behavior (e.g., self-rewards and stress management).

Adapted with permission from Miller, Shoda and Hurley (1996). *Psychological Bulletin,* 119: 70–94 this book, we expand the principle of reciprocal determinism to incorporate characteristics and behavior of *both* the practitioner and patient as well as the environment (practice setting, community) in which the clinical encounters take place (also see Baranowski, 1990).

Of particular relevance for our purposes is the distinction between environment and situation. The concept of environment includes physical (e.g., size of clinical room) and social components (e.g., family members present). Both practitioner and patient can share the same environment, such as the clinical examination room. The term 'situation' describes how an individual perceives the environment, including real, distorted or imagined factors. Thus, patient and practitioner can see the situation quite differently. To the practitioner, the examination room is a familiar, comfortable room. To the patient, the examination room can be perceived as quite unfamiliar and frightening.

Social Cognitive Theory incorporates the need for knowledge and skill development in order for an individual to perform a given behavior. This includes availability of strategies to deal with emotional situations (e.g., manage anxiety), as well as the ability to monitor and regulate actions toward achieving a behavioral goal. Behavioral acquisition is governed by principles of learning (reward/incentives that increase or decrease the likelihood of occurrence) and also includes observational learning, where a new behavior is acquired by watching others.

Of the various concepts in Social Cognitive Theory, **self-efficacy** currently attracts most attention. Indeed, Bandura (1997) now proposes self-efficacy as the preeminent construct that underlies social change. Bandura has extended the concept from the individual level, to include larger units of analysis, such as group self-efficacy (e.g., a football team's feeling that they are capable of winning this year's Super Bowl), organizational self-efficacy and community self-efficacy. Self-efficacy is an expression of confidence that a person has the necessary capability to overcome difficulties inherent in achieving a behavioral goal. This should be distinguished from an outcome expectation, which is the individual's belief about a particular outcome (e.g., winning a race) resulting from a given behavior (e.g., rigorous training). Self-efficacy concerns a belief in one's capability to actually produce the behavior. Maibach and Murphy (1995) provide an in-depth analysis of the concepts and measurement of self-efficacy.

In the practitioner-patient encounter, it is not always recognized that both parties bring efficacy expectations. While it is important to assess and

Table 7.4   Types of Self-Efficacy in Addictive Behavior

Prevention

- **Resistance Self-Efficacy** (before initiation of behavior):   one's perceived ability to resist pressure to start smoking, drinking or drug use
- **Risk-Reduction Self-Efficacy** (once behavior is initiated): one's perceived ability to minimize risk or harm by limiting the frequency and amount of use (cigarettes, alcohol, drugs) or stopping use altogether

Stages of Change

- **Action Self-Efficacy** (contemplation ± action): one's perceived ability to go beyond just thinking and initiate change, such as seeking professional assistance or going to a self-help group
- **Coping Self-Efficacy** (action ± maintenance): one's perceived ability to deal success- fully with high-risk situations and maintain a behavioral goal
- **Recovery Self-Efficacy** (maintenance ± relapse): one's perceived ability to reinstate control and maintain a behavioral goal, should a relapse occur

Source: Marlatt, Baer & Quigley (1995)

understand the degree of confidence a patient has in being able to change a health behavior (e.g., wear a seat belt), of equal importance is the efficacy expectation that a practitioner brings to the clinical encounter. As reviewed in Chapter 3 (see Tables 3.3 and 3.4), most practitioners do not feel that they are effective in counselling their patients to change behaviors such as quitting smoking, reducing heavy drinking, starting an exercise program or wearing a seat belt in a moving vehicle (Lewis et al., 1991).

Within the field of addictive behavior, Marlatt, Baer and Quigley (1995) distinguish among several types of self-efficacy (Table 7.4). The first two types deal with behavior acquisition and are particularly important for pre- vention initiatives, especially with adolescents and young adults. Resistance self-efficacy is relevant before a behavior is initiated and concerns the indi- vidual's perception of the ability to resist pressure to start a health risk behavior, such as cigarette smoking, drinking or other drug use. Once a behavior is initiated, risk-reduction self-efficacy concerns the individual's ability to minimize harm by limiting the health risk behavior (e.g., never having more than two standard drinks on a given occasion). Three other types of self-efficacy in Table 7.4 are relevant to the stages of change dis- cussed below.

The central importance of self-efficacy to behavior acquisition, maintenance and change is underscored by Bandura (1991, p. 258):

Perceived efficacy can affect every phase of personal change – whether people even consider changing their health habits, whether they can enlist the motivation and perseverance needed to succeed should they choose to do so, and whether they adequately maintain the changes they have achieved.

Self-Determination Theory

Deci and Ryan (1985, 1990; Ryan & Deci, 2000) provide a comprehensive theory for understanding human motivation. In essence, Self-Determination Theory introduces a continuum (Figure 7.5) that distinguishes controlled behavior (taking action because you 'should' or 'have to') from autonomous behavior that is self-determined (*"I want to do it of my own choice"*). A central concept is how behavior is regulated. According to Self-Determination Theory, any intentional behavior can be analyzed according to the extent that it is self-regulated versus regulated by forces outside the self.

Self-Determination Theory incorporates the concept of autonomy (self-determination) as an integral part. This distinguishes Self-Determination Theory from other theories and models of behavior acquisition and maintenance. For instance, the concept of self-efficacy from Social Cognitive Theory denotes an expectation by the individual that *"I can do it"* (Table 7.2). An individual can have high self-efficacy, yet be driven toward an action, like a pawn, either by external forces or introjected pressures. The sense of personal freedom of choice is absent. By emphasizing personal autonomy (human agency), Self-Determination Theory argues that a person is most likely to take action when *"I want to do it of my own choice"*. An

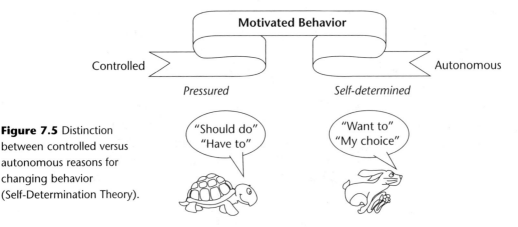

Figure 7.5 Distinction between controlled versus autonomous reasons for changing behavior (Self-Determination Theory).

individual may have a high efficacy expectation regarding a health behavior, such as starting a physical exercise program, yet remain inactive out of choice: *"I don't want to do it"*.

Self-Determination Theory is particularly relevant for understanding the dynamics of the practitioner-patient interaction. Practitioners frequently take an action-oriented role where they are directive and at times confrontational in providing advice to patients that they should change a health behavior. The practitioner takes the 'one up' position relative to the patient: *"I'm the expert and you should follow my advice"*. In these types of interactions, patients often feel pressured or even coerced. They may attempt or even change a health behavior, but do so because of perceived demand from the practitioner. Patients feel controlled—they have to change the health behavior in order to feel better about themselves.

Behavior regulation under this highly controlled condition is labelled External (Figure 7.6). That is, whether a patient changes a health behavior or not is largely regulated by contingencies that are external to the individual. For example, a patient may comply with taking his anti-hypertensive medication because he feels pressured and does not want to get his doctor upset. He feels that the locus of initiation of the behavior (taking medication) is external to one's self. In this instance, the patient feels that he has very little choice (autonomy).

At the other end of the continuum (Figure 7.6), individuals experience a true sense of volition or choice about whether they will change a health behavior. The individual believes that the initiation and regulation of behavior change is largely within her/himself (internal). This sense of personal control that the behavior is emanating from oneself is more likely to result when the practitioner takes a motivational role (see Chapter 3), where the patient's right to choose (autonomy) is respected and supported. For example, a practitioner might spend a session exploring what this patient sees as both the benefits and concerns regarding changing a health behavior (Worksheet 9.2). Following the discussion, the patient may have a better sense of his/her personal balance sheet regarding the pros and cons of change and subsequently choose to look into joining a health and fitness club (self-determined). Deci and Ryan (1990) describe this condition as Integrated regulation, where the patient has identified the underlying value of the behavior and chooses to do it.

A third type of regulation characterizes the central region of the continuum in Figure 7.6. Introjected regulation appears to be 'autonomous' to

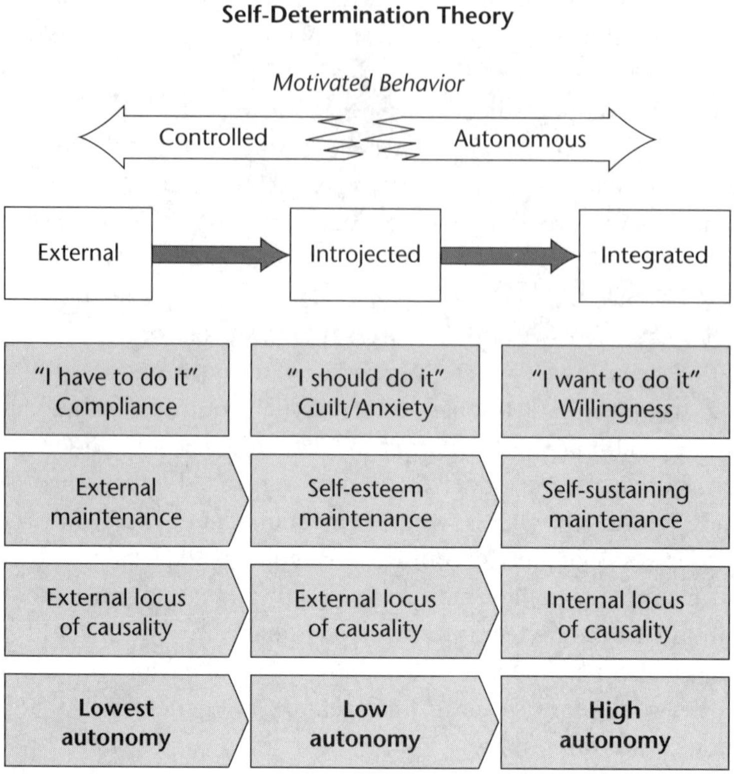

Self-Determination Theory

Figure 7.6 Comparison of external, introjected and integrated forms of behavior regulation (Self-Determination Theory).

an outsider. Yet, the individual takes action more out of a sense of guilt or anxiety that he/she has to change the behavior in order to feel a worthy person. An individual feels that he/she should do it. Deci and Ryan (1985; 1990) point out that when behavior regulation has been introjected, it appears to be internal to the person, since there are no external prods or prompts. However, the individual is not choosing to take action out of choice but rather by inner conflict and tension. For instance, an individual may attempt to lose weight because of an internalized (introjected) image promoted in the popular media regarding an 'ideal' body weight. The person's self-esteem is contingent on achieving the desired weight loss.

A working hypothesis of Self-Determination Theory is that patients are more likely to achieve long-term success in behavior change when they take action for autonomous reasons (Williams et al., 1998). Externally regulated behavior (e.g., losing weight in order to make the class limit for wrestling) is less likely to be maintained when the external contingency is not present (e.g., the college wrestling season is over). Introjected regulation can also be associated with less persistence in maintaining behavior change, since it is driven by internal conflicts. Deci and Ryan (1985; 1990; Ryan & Deci, 2000) have found that autonomous-determined decisions (integrated regulation) are more robust against relapse than controlled behavior change. In the practitioner-patient interaction, this is most likely to occur when the practitioner supports the patient's autonomy.

For example, Harackiewicz et al. (1987) found that smokers who were randomly assigned to an autonomy-supporting self-help condition remained abstinent longer than those in two more controlling conditions and in the reference condition. Similarly, Curry, Wagner and Grotaus (1991) found that an autonomy-supportive approach yielded the best abstinence record at 12-month follow-up for cigarette smokers. Ockene et al. (1991) had physicians vary their style of counselling with patients. At six-month follow-up, patients in the more autonomy-supportive (patient-centered) style achieved greater abstinence rates. Patients also liked the autonomy-supportive style better than when physicians took a directive style.

Ryan and colleagues applied Self-Determination Theory for understanding intrinsic motivation and adherence to physical exercise and alcohol treatment. Ryan and Frederick (1997) found that extrinsic motives, such as fitness and appearance improvement, were important determinants of the initiation of an exercise program. However, intrinsic motivation (enjoyment, competence) was the critical factor for sustaining physical activity (adherence). In a study of outpatient alcoholism treatment, Ryan, Plant and O'Malley (1995) found that patients reporting a greater internalized motivation at the start of the program demonstrated greater involvement (adherence) and retention in treatment, as well as better outcomes at eight weeks.

Although Self-Determination Theory is anchored at the individual level, it incorporates the broader social and environmental context. According to Deci and Ryan (1990, p. 280):

> *Our theory ... affords people their human essence, while also accounting for the processes through which they appear to be controlled. It places the active organism in a social context that can either support or impair its natural development and self-determination.*

How People Change

Several recent developments have renewed a focus on understanding the dynamics of change summarized in Figure 7.7 (also see Chapter 3). Some milestones include the emphasis on maintaining change by concentrating on what happens to an individual following treatment. This has been stimulated by work on relapse prevention by Alan Marlatt (Marlatt & Gordon, 1985) and colleagues (Brownell et al., 1986). A second important development is the Transtheoretical Model (Prochaska & DiClemente, 1983; Prochaska, DiClemente & Norcross, 1992; Prochaska, Redding & Evers, 1997) which considers 1) stages of change; 2) decision balance; 3) self-efficacy; and 4) processes that produce change. The stages of change component, in particular, has extended our focus of attention to the broad continuum which includes the recognition or admission of a health concern, ambivalence about change, taking action and maintenance components. A third significant development by Miller and Rollnick (1991) is interviewing strategies to enhance motivation for behavior change, termed **'motivational interviewing'** (MI). Practical strategies are described for building motivation and strengthening commitment to change.

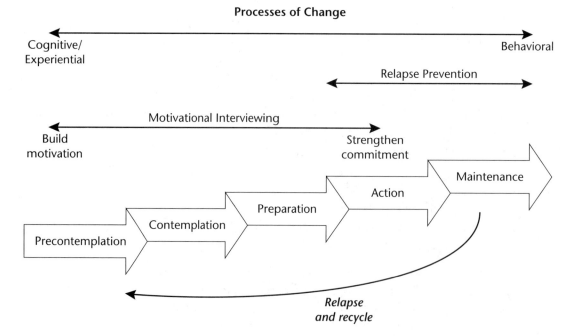

Figure 7.7 Integration of key concepts for understanding the processes of change.

Transtheoretical Model

In attempting to understand how people change health behavior, Prochaska, DiClemente and Norcross (1992) describe a progression through five stages: precontemplation, contemplation, preparation, action and maintenance (Table 7.5). Most people do not progress in a linear fashion through these stages. Instead, relapses are common, and one may recycle through the stages several times before achieving a long-term goal. A basic hypothesis is that change is most likely to occur if both the patient and the practitioner are focusing on the same stage of change and using the appropriate process for that stage.

Precontemplators may be largely unaware that a particular behavior (e.g., a fast-food, high-fat diet) may have long-term implications for their health (e.g., heart disease). Another subgroup within precontemplation (decided not to act) are those individuals who have made an explicit decision not to change a health behavior (i.e., they intend to continue cigarette smoking). In the **contemplation** stage, the individual recognizes or admits that a particular health behavior may be of concern, yet the individual is at the point of still thinking about change. Indeed, chronic "contemplators" may for many years think about changing a lifestyle behavior (e.g., losing weight, quitting smoking, starting an exercise program) but not take action to initiate this change. **Preparation** is the stage at which the individual is ready for change soon (e.g., in the next thirty days) and is beginning to seek advice (e.g., make an appointment with a family doctor). The **action** phase involves the initiation of the behavioral change strategy, and **maintenance** is operationally defined by the achievement of a goal for at least six months.

However, relapses are common, especially with addictive behaviors. At this point, the individual may recycle back to either contemplation or even precontemplation (denial). Prochaska and DiClemente (1986) found that, with respect to cigarette smoking, self-changers made at least three serious attempts to quit (revolutions through the stages of change) before they achieved long-term abstinence.

Olson (1992) provides an excellent discussion of psychological barriers faced by patients (Table 7.6) when they are not recognizing or thinking about a health risk (precontemplation), when they are ambivalent about change (contemplation), or when they are trying to maintain a behavioral goal (maintenance).

One of the most important features of the Stages of Change concept is that it encourages a far more realistic assessment of how individuals 'under-

Table 7.5   Key Concepts in the Transtheoretical Model

Stages of Change

Precontemplation: Has no intention to take action within the next six months

Contemplation: Intends to take action within the next six months

Preparation: Intends to take action within the next 30 days and has taken some behavioral steps in this direction

Action: Has changed overt behavior for less than six months

Maintenance: Has changed overt behavior for more than six months

Decisional Balance

Pros: The benefits of changing

Cons: The costs of changing

Self-Efficacy

Confidence: that one can engage in the healthy behavior across different situations

Temptation: to engage in the unhealthy behavior across different situations

Processes of Change

A) COGNITIVE/EXPERIENTIAL

Consciousness raising: Finding and learning new facts, ideas, and tips that support the healthy behavioral change

Dramatic relief: Experiencing the negative emotions (fear, anxiety, worry) that go along with unhealthy behavioral risks

Self-reevaluation: Realizing that the behavioral change is an important part of one's identity as a person

Environmental reevaluation: Realizing the negative impact of an unhealthy behavior or the positive impact of the healthy behavior on one's proximal social and physical environment

Self-liberation: Making a firm commitment to change

B) BEHAVIORAL

Helping relationships: Seeking and using social support for the healthy behavioral change

Counterconditioning: Substituting healthier alternative behaviors and cognitions for the unhealthy behaviors

Contingency management: Increasing the rewards for the positive behavioral change and decreasing the rewards of the unhealthy behavior

Stimulus control: Removing reminders or cues to engage in the unhealthy behavior and adding cues or reminders to engage in the healthy behavior

Social liberation: Realizing that the social norms are changing in the direction of supporting the healthy behavior

Adapted with permission from Prochaska, Redding and Evers (1997). In: Karen Glanz, Frances M. Lewis and Barbara K. Rimer (Eds.), *Health Behavior and Health Education: Theory, Research, and Practice,* 2nd ed. San Francisco: Jossey-Bass Publishers.

Table 7.6   Psychological Barriers to Behavior Change

RECOGNIZING A HEALTH RISK (PRECONTEMPLATION)

---

a) Denial or trivialization: no threat from overexposure to the sun

b) Perceived vulnerability: "I am different ... I won't get lung cancer from smoking"

c) Faulty conceptualizations: "I can tell when my blood pressure is elevated" (i.e., get headaches)

d) Debilitating emotions: fear of discovering I might have breast cancer as a reason for not having a mammogram

---

ATTEMPTS TO CHANGE (PREPARATION – ACTION)

---

a) Lack of knowledge: quitting an exercise program due to injury (no warm-ups, too intense workouts)

b) Low self-efficacy: lack of confidence about being able to refuse drinks at a social function

c) Dysfunctional attitudes: "I'd rather smoke and be thin than not smoke and get fat"

LONG-TERM CHANGE (MAINTENANCE)

---

a) Motivational drift: hard to keep focused on a low-fat diet over many years

b) Lack of perceived improvement: stop taking medications for asymptomatic conditions (e.g., hypertension)

c) Lapses: one or two cigarettes can trigger heavy smoking again

d) Lack of social supports: family members undermine the value of an exercise program

---

Adapted with permission from Olson (1992)

stand' their health risk behavior. This has extremely important implications for health care and health promotion initiatives. The vast majority of people with health risk behaviors are not in the action stage (Velicer et al., 1995):

- 10–20% prepared for action
- 40–50% contemplation stage
- 40–50% precontemplation stage

Yet, many prevention and behavior change initiatives, such as the Ask-Advise-Assist approach to smoking cessation (Glynn & Manley, 1989) are directed at the action stage. In a Health Maintenance Organization study, Orleans et al. (1988) surveyed cigarette smokers and found that 70% indicated that they would participate in a smoking cessation program. However, when a state-of-the-art smoking cessation program was offered, only 4% actually signed up! Similarly, in a study of home-based interventions for

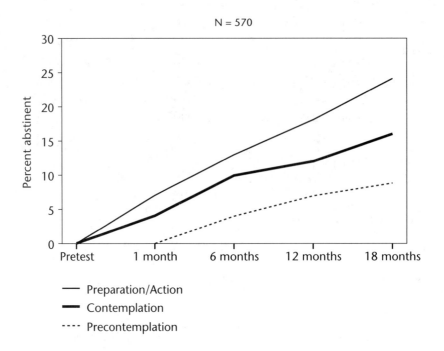

Figure 7.8 Smoking cessation rates over 18 months predicted by stage of change (N=570). Adapted from Prochaska et al. (1992).

individuals having problems with weight control, Schmid et al. (1989) successfully recruited only 3–12% of eligible participants. These studies support the need to 'match' intervention strategies with the individual's stage of change. When adherence to a recommendation is not followed, blame is often placed on the patient for being 'unmotivated' or 'resistant' rather than on the inappropriate focus of the intervention.

Prochaska et al. (1992) present evidence that stage of change predicts who will quit smoking cigarettes. In their 18-month follow-up study depicted in Figure 7.8, they found a dramatic difference in abstinence rates for individuals who were initially classified as being at either the precontemplation, contemplation or preparation/action stages. This study suggests that behavior change is not always the most appropriate outcome measure. Instead, a more sensitive criterion is whether the intervention shifts a significant proportion of individuals from one stage to the next. Too often, health professionals leap immediately into giving the patient advice on behavioral change strategies. They are less prepared in using effective strate-

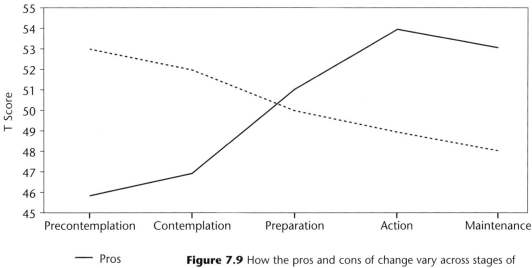

— Pros

---- Cons

Figure 7.9 How the pros and cons of change vary across stages of change for individuals looking at reducing dietary fat intake. T Score is a standardized metric having a mean of 50 and atandard deviation of 10. Data from Prochaska et al. (1994).

gies (e.g., decision balance) for building commitment to change for those individuals who are either in precontemplation or contemplation stages.

Prochaska et al. (1994) have found that there is a clear shift in an individual's assessment of the pros and cons as the individual advances along the readiness for change continuum. For instance, Figure 7.9 gives the pros and cons by stage of change for adopting a reduced-fat diet. As one moves through the stages, there is an increase in the reporting of the pros (good things) about changing the behavior and a decrease in the cons (not-so-good things). Prochaska et al., (1994) proposes that progression from precontemplation to action is a function of one standard deviation increase in pros of a healthy behavior and a 0.5 standard deviation decrease in the cons.

A basic tenet of the Transtheoretical Model is the sequencing of specific processes by stage of change (Figure 7.7). In a study of smoking cessation, Perz, DiClemente and Carbonari (1996) found evidence for matching processes of change with the individual's stage of change, i.e., engaging in experiential process activities during contemplation/preparation stages and shifting to behavioral process activities during action (Table 7.5). Rosen (2000) re-analyzed 47 studies of change processes across a range of health behaviors. Processes that varied **most** by stage were 1) self-liberation: committing to change, and 2) counterconditioning: substituting new behaviors.

However, Rosen (2000) found that the sequencing was not consistent across health problems:

- **Smoking:** cognitive processes were used more in earlier stages than were behavioral processes
- **Exercise Adoption and Diet:** use of cognitive and behavioral processes increased together

This reflects differences between ceasing an addictive behavior and initiating a health-enhancing behavior. The less one thinks about smoking after deciding to quit, the easier it is to abstain. However, active exercisers must continually think about their new behavior, including time and place for exercising, bringing necessary gear and clothes, involving a friend, taking care of aches or minor injuries.

Joseph, Breslin and Skinner (1999) provide a comprehensive review of the scientific literature over the past 15 years regarding the Transtheoretical Model. The model has proven to be of heuristic value for stimulating research on understanding the processes of change as well as for providing clinicians with an intuitively appealing model for guiding clinical practice based on the patient's readiness for change. However, questions are raised regarding the definition of concepts as well as the need for more evidence from longitudinal studies. The model, by itself, does not consider a patient's personal history, chronic course of a disorder and co-morbidities, socioeconomic status and the social environment—all of which can have a powerful impact on health behavior change. Similarly, Whitelaw et al. (2000) reviewed the status of evidence on stages of change and point out significant gaps in research. They caution that the popularity of the model may be skewing health promotion activities at the expense of considering other models and approaches.

Motivational Interviewing

This approach is particularly relevant for working with patients who are in the precontemplation or contemplation stages of change (Figure 7.7). Motivation has been traditionally viewed as a **trait** of the individual that is difficult to change. "It is the person's problem ... a reason why the patient did poorly in treatment." However, a contrasting view is that motivation is a **state** that is changeable (e.g., Miller, 1985). Both patient and practitioner play key roles in fostering a commitment directed toward changing a health behavior.

Miller and Rollnick (1991) describe five basic principles for enhancing motivation:

1. **Express empathy:** through listening rather than telling

2. **Develop discrepancy:** between where the patient is now (i.e., risk behavior) and where he or she wants to be

3. **Avoid argumentation:** do not try to convince patients by the force of your argument

4. **Roll with resistance:** rather than meet patient resistance head-on

5. **Support self-efficacy:** instill hope and support patients' belief that they can do it (change)

The use of these principles requires health practitioners to take a very different stance (e.g., nonconfrontational) with respect to the patient (Rollnick et al., 1999). The basic goals are to develop a 'shared' understanding of how the patient sees the health issue and to motivate the patient's commitment to change.

Miller and Rollnick (1991) divide motivational counselling into two major phases. The first phase, Building Motivation for Change, is directed at patients who are fairly early in their readiness for change (precontemplation). They may be reluctant about change or even show marked resistance at the outset. Using the eight related strategies summarized in Table 7.7, the aim is to work with the patient in ways that will tip the motivational balance in favor of change; that is, increase perceived positive benefits and decrease the perceived concerns of change. The second phase, Strengthening Commitment to Change, aims at consolidating the client's commitment to change and movement toward a decision to act. The seven strategies of this phase are described in Table 7.7.

Motivational interviewing has been studied with several populations, including community recruited subjects, patients at addictions treatment facilities and patients in medical care. The Motivational Interviewing website gives an updated list of research publications including outcome studies:

http://www.motivationalinterview.org/library/biblio.html

Overall, these initial studies support the effectiveness of motivational interventions: in some cases motivational interviewing is more effective than waiting list treatment controls, in other cases motivational interventions produce results that are equivalent to more intensive interventions.

Table 7.7   Strategies for Motivation Enhancement

BUILD MOTIVATION FOR CHANGE

- Elicit self-motivational statements
- Listen with empathy
- Question
- Present personal feedback
- Affirm the client's views
- Handle resistance
- Reframe the issues
- Summarize

STRENGTHEN COMMITMENT TO CHANGE

- Recognize readiness for change
- Discuss a plan
- Communicate free choice
- Consequences of action or inaction
- Information and advice
- Deal with resistance
- Make a plan

Source: Miller and Rollnick (1991)

Noonan and Moyer (1996) provide a review of 11 of these clinical trials. In the five studies where subjects were volunteers from the community, consistent evidence was found supporting the efficacy of motivational interviewing with respect to control groups (waiting list), and motivational interviewing produced results that were comparable with more intensive interventions (extended treatment including relapse prevention, six-week class and discussion group). Within the field of addictions treatment, consistent evidence supports the efficacy of motivational interviewing compared with a treatment control group. In the most comprehensive comparison of interventions in a multi-site randomized trial, project MATCH (1997) found that a brief motivational interviewing intervention (4 sessions) yielded excellent outcomes that were comparable with more intensive cognitive behavior therapy (12 sessions) or 12-step facilitation therapy (12 sessions).

Results to date in medical settings are mixed. Of three initial studies conducted in primary care, two found that motivation interviewing yielded results that were better than the control groups receiving no treatment, whereas one study found no such effect (Richmond et al., 1995). One possible explanation is that the study protocol had motivational interviewing occurring in the second session, whereas there was considerable drop-out of subjects (49%) before this session. Noonan and Moyer (1997) point out that poor compliance at initiation of treatment is one of the key target areas for motivational interviewing approaches and that previous studies have demonstrated the value of motivational interviewing for engaging clients in the treatment process (e.g., Brown & Miller, 1993; Saunders et al., 1995). This is supported by a recent study (Smith et al., 1997) in which motivational interviewing significantly enhanced adherence to program recommendations and glycemic control in a behavioral weight-control program with obese diabetic patients.

Monti et al. (1999) compare motivational and control interventions for addressing drinking problems in youth who attended hospital emergency departments. At six-month follow-up, they found that patients who receive the motivational intervention have significantly lower incidence of drinking and driving, traffic violations, and alcohol-related problems.

Further research is needed in health care settings to help us better understand the conditions under which motivational interviewing strategies are effective, either as a stand-alone intervention or as a component for enhancing adherence to a treatment protocol.

Relapse Prevention

When an individual takes action to change a health behavior, the most likely outcome is not long-term maintenance but rather relapse. Over 25 years ago in their review of the treatment outcome literature, Hunt, Barnett and Branch (1971) found that approximately 66% of all participants relapsed by the 90-day follow-up assessment in studies of habitual smokers, heroin addicts and alcoholics. Earlier approaches to treatment have tended to focus on making initial changes in behavior rather than on how to maintain these changes over time. What has resulted is a 'revolving door', where patients relapse and return again to treatment.

Marlatt and colleagues have taken the lead in advancing conceptual models and intervention strategies that address the maintenance of change through relapse prevention programs (Carroll, 1996; Marlatt, 1998; Marlatt & Gordon, 1985). Relapse prevention uses cognitive-behavioral strategies that focus on self-management skills for maintaining a desired behavioral change. Relapse prevention was initially developed for the treatment of addictive behavior, with abstinence as the primary goal. Subsequently, relapse prevention has been extended to a broader range of health behaviors and outcome goals consistent with a harm-reduction philosophy (Marlatt et al., 1993; Marlatt and Tapert, 1993).

According to Dimeff and Marlatt (1995), relapse prevention is based on four assumptions:

1. Different processes govern the action and maintenance stages of behavior change.

2. Relapse risks are complex and involve individual, situational, physiological and sociocultural factors.

3. Relapse and the process of recovery is ongoing and not an endpoint to be equated with treatment 'failure'.

4. Relapse prevention is most successful when the client (patient) confidentially acts as his or her own therapist following treatment (i.e., personal empowerment).

The relapse prevention model draws heavily on self-efficacy theory (Bandura 1997). For instance, when an individual enters a high-risk situation (e.g., a problem drinker at a cocktail party), the individual's sense of perceived control may be threatened. The cognitive, affective and interpersonal pressures culminate in the individual making a judgment (efficacy expectation) about his or her ability to cope with the risks of drinking at this event. If the person copes successfully, then this leads to an increase in self-confidence in dealing with other risk situations in the future. Conversely, if the individual does not cope adequately, then this leads to a decrease in the individual's confidence and fear about future risk situations (decreased self-efficacy). Marlatt et al. (1995) have proposed three types of self-efficacy (i.e., action, coping, recovery) that mark transition points in the stages of change (Table 7.4).

Relapse prevention strategies (Annis & Davis, 1991) begin with an analysis of the individual's high-risk situations. Then, the individual works through assignments that involve progressively more risky situations in their natural environment. In addition to the progressive development of skills and coping strategies, relapse prevention employs cognitive restructuring. An important distinction is drawn between a lapse, which can be defined as a slip that occurs in the process of changing an addictive behavior, and a relapse, which is a more complete return of the undesired behavior. The relapse prevention model encourages patients who experience a lapse to view this as a temporary setback, rather than as an indicator of total failure and return to the previous risk state.

Annis, Schober and Kelly (1996) developed a structured relapse prevention model for substance abusers that consist of five components: 1) assessment; 2) motivational interviewing; 3) preparation of an individualized treatment plan; 4) initiation of change counselling; 5) maintenance of change counselling. These components are matched to the stages of change continuum. Annis and colleagues evaluated this model and provide evidence on its effectiveness in substance abuse treatment (Annis, 1990; Annis et al., 1996; Graham et al., 1996; Moser & Annis, 1996).

In a review of 24 randomized controlled trials of relapse prevention, Carroll (1996) found that 9 of 12 studies of smoking and 3 of 6 studies of alcohol dependence report significant main effects for relapse prevention at both post-treatment and follow-up. Far fewer studies evaluate relapse prevention in marijuana cessation (one with no main effect), cocaine (three with no main effect, one with delayed effects), or other drug use (one of two found main effect). Carroll (1996) concludes that there is evidence for the effectiveness of relapse prevention over no-treatment control conditions. However, findings are mixed when compared with reference conditions. Although relapse prevention in these 24 trials did not appear superior to other forms of treatment, it did hold promise in reducing the severity of relapses when they occur, in extending the durability of acute treatment, and in patient-treatment matching.

Moving On

We have completed our examination of the need for health care reform and explored options for organizational change. Prevention and behavior change initiatives can significantly improve both clinical outcomes and health of the population served. But this requires fundamental integration of medical care and public health approaches. The next section provides a practical guide, the Five-Step Model, for transforming and continually improving the performance of health organizations.

Worksheet 7.1 Likelihood of Action Analysis

Name: _____   **Change Being Considered** _____

"This Person ..."	Rating	Rationale
1. Sees the health risk as serious and is personally concerned	1 = *yes* .5 = *somewhat* 0 = *no*	
2. Feels personally susceptible to the health risk	1 = *yes* .5 = *somewhat* 0 = *no*	
3. Believes the recommended change to be effective in reducing risk	1 = *yes* .5 = *somewhat* 0 = *no*	
4. Assesses the benefits (pros) to be greater than the costs (cons) of change	1 = *yes* .5 = *somewhat* 0 = *no*	
5. Believes that significant others (family, friends) think the behavior should be changed	1 = *yes* .5 = *somewhat* 0 = *no*	
6. Is motivated to comply with the other person's desire	1 = *yes* .5 = *somewhat* 0 = *no*	
7. Is in a context (environment) that is supportive of the action	1 = *yes* .5 = *somewhat* 0 = *no*	
8. Has the knowledge, skills and emotional coping responses to change	1 = *yes* .5 = *somewhat* 0 = *no*	
9. Feels capable of carrying out the action successfully	1 = *yes* .5 = *somewhat* 0 = *no*	
10. Wants to engage in the action because of personal choice	1 = *yes* .5 = *somewhat* 0 = *no*	
Index Score (total) = _____		

Part Two

Five Steps for Improving Organizations

Deming's 85:15 Rule: Approximately 85% of opportunities for improvement are in system changes, 15% are with people.

CHAPTER 8

The Five-Step Model

If you want to understand something, try to change it.

—Kurt Lewin

Overview

Most sailing races are won or lost at the starting gun. Misjudge a wind shift or get caught up in another boat's dirty air and you end up following everyone else around the course. The same is true of initiatives in organizational change—it is vital to have a clear start. This chapter presents a Five-Step Model for improving your organization. The model integrates macrolevel (top down) and microlevel (bottom up) approaches with practical tools for building a high performing organization:

Step 1. Generate motivation for organizational change (Chapter 9)

Step 2. Strengthen organizational capacity for improvement (Chapter 10)

Step 3. Identify strategic directions in prevention and behavioral health care (Chapter 11)

Step 4. Conduct a critical functions analysis of supports that help practitioners and patients change health behavior (Chapter 12)

Step 5. Improve performance using rapid cycle change and quality improvement tools (Chapter 13)

Sustain The Momentum. Apply the Five Steps in successive cycles to continue the improvement process, consolidate gains and prevent organizational drift (Chapter 14)

Getting the Right Start

What influences organizational improvement? Think back over the past year about changes that have occurred in your organization. Focus on a critical incident—one in which you felt a significant change occurred with positive or negative results. Perhaps a preventive care protocol was implemented for child immunizations, a risk factor screening tool was introduced during office visits, a new computer-based office system was set up, or on-site childcare services were established for patients and staff. These initiatives can improve patient outcomes and practitioner satisfaction.

Nevertheless, many organizations get stuck trying to make relatively simple changes. The following case study illustrates how the organizational climate (macrolevel) can stymie efforts to improve performance at the microlevel.

Case Study

Glenwood Family Practice Service is affiliated with an academic health sciences center located in a large city on the west coast of North America. The catchment area reflects an increasingly diverse population with respect to socioeconomic status and cultural background. Glenwood is trying to increase its emphasis on behavioral risk factors at both the individual and community level.

I met with the clinical manager, a nurse and several physicians to discuss their progress in improving behavioral health care. Six months previously, I had given a workshop on organizational and motivational approaches to behavior change. Today's meeting was to consider a quality improvement initiative for putting prevention into practice. Although the family physicians were interested, the clinical manager and staff were restrained about beginning anything new.

We discussed how using Hot Files could better support their practitioners. Hot Files are patient information guides stocked in folders on the walls of the examination rooms. As I began to describe the positive experience of another clinic (Dr. Paul Frame's Tri-County Family Medicine Services; see Chapter 4), the clinical manager stopped me. She had attempted to get this implemented six months ago without success. She believed that nursing and clinical support staff were already overstretched. Staff were quite concerned about taking on any additional responsibilities.

I mentioned that I saw brochures and self-care booklets in the Waiting Room. Would it be possible to have Hot Files stocked with appropriate brochures in each of the examination rooms? One of the physicians immediately spoke up that he would gladly do this himself since it would make his work easier to have appropriate material readily available. The clinical manager appreciated his good intentions but questioned whether he would follow through.

The issue had little to do with figuring out who could stock the Hot Files—this task was straightforward. A fundamental problem was evident with the organizational climate (macrolevel). Staff felt overextended and frustrated. In this time-pressured clinic, implementation of a microlevel improvement (Hot Files) took on immense proportions. The Glenwood case illustrates the need to approach organizational improvement from multiple levels.

The Five-Step Model

The ability to lead change requires energy, direction and practical tools. The Five-Step Model, by integrating the principles and tools of change, provides a dynamic means for leading change (see Chapter 1, Figure 1.1). Tom Nolan argues that three elements are vital for producing quality change: will, ideas and execution. To this we have added a fourth element: sustain through ongoing renewal (Table 8.1).

The Model is distinctive in several respects. First, it integrates key concepts with opportunities for change to achieve improvements that span macro- and microlevels in the organization (Figure 8.1). Second, each step provides practical tools for implementing and testing interventions. Third, the Model encourages team approaches using both 'top-down' and 'bottom-up' strategies for improvement. Fourth, the Model can be applied to a wide variety of behavior change and disease management programs. Fifth, the model can be applied to a range of health organizations and settings.

Step 1. Developing Motivation for Change (Chapter 9)

Too often, programs for organizational change are implemented without giving sufficient attention to building understanding and commitment to the improvement process throughout different levels of the organization. A model is described for differentiating organizations along a continuum ranging from a reactive to a high performing standard:

Reactive organizations lack direction and are caught up in the present, mainly 'fighting fires'.

Table 8.1   What It Takes to Improve Your Organization

The Basics	Guiding Framework	Tools	Key References
Will	**Step 1.** Build motivation for organizational change	*Your Organizational Prototype, Readiness for Change Analysis, Decision Balance*	Chapter 9 Kotter (1996) Stacey (1996)
	Step 2. Strengthen capacities for organizational improvement	***ACTSS:*** *Success Factors for Organizational Improvement*	Chapter 10 (1994,1999) Senge et al., (1990)
Ideas	**Step 3.** Identify strategic directions	*Stakeholder Needs Analyses, Environmental Scans SWOT, Analyses, Payoff Matrix*	Chapter 11 Bryson (1995) Bryson & Alston (1996)
	Step 4. Conduct a critical functions analysis	***CFA:*** *Critical Functions Analysis*	Chapter 12
Action	**Step 5.** Improve using rapid cycle change	*Aim Statement,* **PDSA** *cycles, Clinical Value Compass, Charts*	Chapter 13 Langley et al. (1996) Dever (1997)
Sustain	Maintain the momentum and consolidate gains	All of the above	Chapter 14 Kotter (1996) Senge et al. (1999)

Proactive organizations have a clearer sense of purpose, strategic goals and the required systems alignment to achieve results.

High performing organizations have a long-range vision linked with an emphasis on quality and continuous improvement that permeates all levels.

A fundamental principle of motivation underscores the discrepancy between where you are now and where you want to be. The self-study tool, *Your Organizational Prototype*, can be used to contrast individuals' and team's evaluations of how the organization is currently performing with how it should perform. The magnitude of this discrepancy when broadly communicated can be a powerful catalyst for generating momentum for change. This simple tool can be used in both bottom-up ways to 'mobilize the troops' for improvement initiatives and top-down approaches to solidify and demonstrate senior level buy-in to organization-wide improvement.

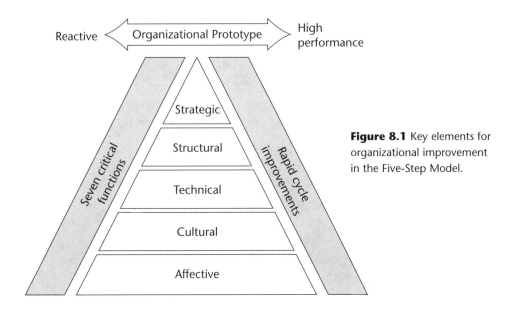

Figure 8.1 Key elements for organizational improvement in the Five-Step Model.

Step 2. Strengthen Organizational Capacity for Improvement (Chapter 10)

Organizations vary widely in their resiliency and capacity for change. High performing organizations incorporate new knowledge about the improvement process itself. Information systems and quality improvement methods are used on an ongoing basis. Five key dimensions (ACTSS) determine an organization's readiness for sustained efforts at improving performance:

- **Affective:** trust versus anxiety, ownership versus disengagement, pride versus demoralization
- **Cultural:** openness versus resistance to innovation, support versus obstruction of leadership
- **Technical:** knowledge about improvement models and tools, information technology systems to support initiatives
- **Structural**: resources and planning systems, performance appraisal and reward systems
- **Strategic:** initiatives linked to strategic directions, involvement of stakeholders

Underlying this model is an evaluation tool, *ACTSS: Success Factors for Organizational Improvement*, that can be used for organizational self-study and assessment. The *ACTSS* tool will help you assess an organization's capability to sustain efforts at improving its performance in behavior change and disease management programs. You can reapply this tool to monitor and set new priorities regarding an organization's capacity for improvement.

Step 3. Identify Strategic Directions in Prevention and Behavioral Health Care (Chapter 11)

High performing organizations achieve success by identifying and concentrating efforts on a small number of strategic directions. These directions shape what the organization is, where it is going and why. They provide a clear statement of the organization's intentions to develop behavior change aimed at prevention and disease management programs (Step 3), and they set the stage for effective decisions and actions to improve performance (Steps 4 and 5).

High performing organizations proactively scan their external environment for important trends and forces that affect their mission and performance. They understand who their primary stakeholders are, what these stakeholders need from the organization and how well these needs and expectations are being met. The organization concentrates efforts on achieving goals that capture opportunities in the external environment while balancing internal functions and structures. Specific objectives are addressed by continuous cycles for improving performance.

Strategic directions emanate from the organization's mission and mandate. They are identified by careful attention to both key stakeholders' interests and current and future forces in the organization's internal and external environment. Three interrelated activities, *Stakeholder Needs Analysis, Environmental Scans* and *SWOT* (Strengths, Weaknesses, Opportunities, Threats) *Analyses*, provide a sound basis for *Issue Identification*. These issues are framed positively as challenges that the organization can do something about. Finally, a *Payoff Matrix Analysis* is used to sort through various directions to identify those that are relatively easy to implement yet offer high impact for the organization. Without these functions the organization will inevitably be reactive in responding to forces and trends.

Step 4. Conduct a Critical Functions Analysis (Chapter 12)

Experience shows that even an expert practitioner working in a badly organized system will lose out to the system over time. This chapter describes seven critical functions that support practitioners and patients in achieving health behavior change. Each function encompasses a group of linked activities or processes that are directed at accomplishing a specific goal. For example, after a health status assessment is administered, information systems provide practitioners with the patient's risk factor profile before the consultation begins.

Critical functions can open a window of opportunity for practitioners; they make it possible to use motivational approaches effectively in behavior change and disease management programs. The critical functions include:

1. **Professional Development in Behavior Change:** individual (patient, practitioner) and organizational levels

2. **Priming/Prompting of Patients and Practitioners** to address prevention and behavioral risk factors

3. **Identification of Risk Behaviors:** screening tests and use of case-findings at the clinic and community/population level

4. **Continuing Care:** monitoring, re-assessment, provision of additional care

5. **Establishing Linkages/Networks Among Services and Resources** inside and outside the health setting

6. **Options for Help:** professional assistance, professionally led support groups, self-help groups and community resources

7. **Information Management:** system design and maintenance to support behavior change initiatives.

The *Critical Functions Analysis* (CFA) identifies opportunities for improvement as well as generates a database for assessing the impact of improvement initiatives.

Step 5. Improve Performance Using Rapid Cycle Change and Tools (Chapter 13)

Over the last few years, a variety of methods and tools have emerged that offer practical assistance to help individuals and organizations make 'rapid cycle improvements.' In rapid cycle improvement, one tests relatively minor changes. These changes are based on ideas from the *Critical Functions*

Analysis, from analogous practices in other clinics, or from the literature. Rapid cycle improvement helps practitioners make relatively minor but useful changes to their daily clinical routines, and this success lays a foundation for broader and continuing organizational changes.

A model and several tools and practices that assist teams in making rapid cycle improvements are discussed. We emphasize the importance of setting an aim for improvement. We describe a model for identifying a simple yet balanced set of outcome measures, the 'Clinical Value Compass', and we guide the reader through application of the *PDSA Cycle* (Langley et al., 1996), a method for making change. Several further tools are described: the process flowchart (used to identify work processes) and the run chart (useful for graphing outcome and process measures). The model and tools are illustrated by a team aiming to improve the care of diabetic patients in a family practice clinic.

Four elements that are common to successful initiatives include (Berwick & Nolan, 1998):

1. **Aim:** organizational improvement is not seen as an accident but as the result of a clearly intended aim

2. **Measurement:** data collection and feedback show that a system change has actually resulted in an improvement

3. **Good Ideas for Change:** multiple sources are drawn upon to identify opportunities and alternatives for change

4. **Testing:** ideas for change are promptly tested on a small scale, adjustments are made based on test results and redesigns are tested in an iterative fashion.

Sustain the Momentum (Chapter 14)

The Five-Step Model can be applied through successive iterations to keep the organization focused on sustaining improvement while addressing slippage and motivational drift. Most change initiatives emphasize what is needed for improving and transforming the organization. Far less attention is directed at preventing organizational drift and thus maintaining gains. Systems theory emphasizes the interconnections among forces that either drive or impede change. The very process of initiating change also activates counterforces and resistance to change. Senge et al. (1999) describe 10 such challenges:

- we don't have enough time for working on this change

- we need more help (coaching and support)

- this change isn't relevant to me

- leaders talk about change but don't demonstrate it by their behavior

- we feel exposed and anxious about this change

- what happens if it doesn't work (negative assessment)?

- we are already doing it right

- who is really in charge of this?

- how do we communicate success so others can build on it?

- where is this change leading us?

Sustaining momentum in organizational improvement hinges on addressing these challenges.

Renewal

To be successful over time, organizational improvement must emphasize 'renewal' over 'change'. The key is to get beyond 'change for change's sake'. Too often, change is driven by a perceived problem or threat or even the need to put one's stamp on the organization (e.g., re-engineering) as the 'change agent'. Scant attention is given to analyzing the pros and cons of change. What are the implications of a proposed change for the organization's stakeholders? How will we measure outcomes to see if desired improvements have actually been realized? How will we sustain improvements once they are achieved? Renewal is an adaptable and evolving process through which high performing organizations continually improve their ways of working. They move beyond reacting to challenges of the external environment and take charge of their own destiny.

Experience over many years in quality improvement underscores the following maxim: *"To improve you have to change, but not all change leads to improvement."* We concur and add that: *"not all improvement renews an organization."* To achieve organizational renewal one needs to sustain improvement cycles, infuse the organization with vitality and nurture regeneration and competitiveness. Organizational change of this special type is a building process. This vision is captured succinctly by R. H. Waterman (1987, p. 23):

> *Renewal, after all, is about builders. Many people can introduce change for change's sake and call it renewal. This is illusory. A builder, on the other hand,*

leads an organization to renewal that outlives the presence of any single individual, and revitalizes even as it changes.

Moving On

A critical step before initiating change programs is to assess and foster motivation for improvement throughout different levels of the organization. The next chapter describes a model for characterizing an organization's readiness for change and a tool for enhancing organizational motivation for improvement.

CHAPTER 9

Step 1: Developing Motivation for Change

Harvey Skinner and Richard Botelho

Even if you are on the right track you will get run over if you just sit there.

—Mark Twain

Overview

A fundamental technique for motivating change is to underscore the gap between where you are and where you want to be. In this chapter, three organizational prototypes are described. They vary with respect to their organizational character and ultimately their ability to provide preventive and behavioral health care:

- **Reactive organizations** lack direction, have poor morale and are caught up in the present 'fighting fires'.
- **Proactive organizations** are more supportive, have a clearer sense of purpose, and have systems aligned to achieve results.
- **High performing organizations** have excellent morale, a long range vision and emphasis on continuous improvement throughout the organization.

A self-study tool, *Your Organizational Prototype*, is described. It helps you assess your organization's current status (its position on the continuum), and it helps you define where you want your organization to be. This discrepancy can be used as a catalyst for organizational improvement. Two additional tools, *Readiness for Change Analysis* and *Decision Balance*, are described for building motivation for improvement at individual, team and program levels.

159

Building Motivation for Improvement

Many organizations find it difficult to create an imperative for change: to respond to the external and internal forces that influence an organization and that may even challenge it to reinvent itself. Organizational vitality is contingent on the ability to scan the external environment, set strategic directions, and align internal structures and processes to achieve performance goals. Although your organization may be doing 'OK' right now, resting satisfied with this achievement may be short-sighted. How do you stimulate motivation for organizational improvement? Berwick (1998, p. 60) emphasizes that "all improvement begins with the intention to change—with the whole-hearted admission that a gap exists between what is and what should be."

The following riddle illustrates the cumulative and exponential effect of change, and underscores the potentially dire consequences for an organization that ignores forces that challenge it to change (Conner, 1995):

Lily Pad Riddle

On day one, a large lake contains only a single small lily pad. Each day the number of lily pads doubles, until on the thirtieth day the lake is totally choked with vegetation. On what day was the lake half full?

Day 29 is the correct answer, since it takes 29 days for half of the lake to fill with lily pads. Only an additional day is needed for the lake to become completely filled with lily pads.

The diverse forces (positive and negative) described in Chapter 2 are the proliferating lily pads that health organizations face today. If these challenges are ignored, they accumulate as lily pads of lost opportunity that clog the organization's ability to navigate its future course. For instance, one part of the lake may be filling with lily pads driven by time pressures and constrained resources; in another part the lily pads arise from an increasingly diverse patient population (e.g., aging, ethnocultural, socioeconomic); emerging pathogens may spring up here or there as additional lily pads; another part of the lake raises lily-pads nurtured on the high costs of new medical and information technologies; and the risks of an organizational takeover or government-imposed restructuring may stimulate an alarming growth of lily pads throughout the lake. High performing organizations recognize and adapt to these changes long before alarm bells on Day 29 announce that the organization is in serious trouble.

What day is it for your organization? We have found this riddle useful in staff development workshops for uprooting complacency and stimulating an examination of forces (positive and negative) that are challenging the organization.

Organizational Prototypes

Health organizations are complex systems that can drift and become stuck in increasingly dysfunctional, chaotic states. Conversely, they can evolve toward creative and very productive forms able to apply broad-based actions to achieve their health care goals. How would you characterize your organization's current status and potential for improving performance in prevention and behavioral health care?

Following Nelson and Burns (1984), we distinguish three prototypes: reactive, proactive, high performing organizations (Figure 9.1). Key attributes of each are summarized in an analysis tool, *Your Organizational Prototype* (Appendix A), which can be used as a checklist for characterizing an organization. These prototypes help us understand the critical factors that lead to renewal and transformation of an organization (strike at the root) as compared with the protective factors that offer only minor adjustment and limited impact (trim the branches).

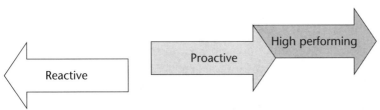

Figure 9.1 Three organizational prototypes. Adapted from Nelson and Burns (1984).

Reactive Organizations

Reactive organizations concentrate on the present, dealing largely with disease management and rehabilitation of patients. Everyone is consumed with pressing clinical concerns. Little time or resources are directed at prevention, let alone at the challenges of motivating risk behavior change. Leadership is either absent, laissez faire or highly controlling in form. Not much attention is given to professional development in new approaches to individual or organizational change. A sense of complacency pervades: *"this is the way it has always been done here ... things will never change"*. The organization focuses inward on satisfying the needs of its practitioners, who assume that they are providing quality care.

For instance, the organization described in Case 1 of the McVea et al. (1996) study (see Chapter 4) is a reactive organization that spends a lot of time just putting out fires. Considerable work is needed to shift this practice toward that of a proactive organization, an organization that can provide behavioral health care.

Proactive Organizations

Proactive organizations focus on prevention (e.g., health and disease screening, advice and education) in addition to disease management. Some outreach initiatives are taken for high risk patients. The leadership style is supportive of personal initiative and professional development. Attention is given to building and supporting a team that provides behavioral health care. Practitioners and staff feel a sense of commitment to both the clinical and disease prevention needs of patients and their families. Quality assurance programs are in place.

Case 2 of the McVea et al (1996) study describes a Proactive Organization that provides screening and early detection services guided by the implementation of general office systems.

High Performing Organizations

High performing organizations have a culture in which excellence permeates all activities of the organization. The leadership provides vision as well as practical strategies for implementing programs. The organization's core values and plans are clearly aligned with its long-range goals for prevention and behavioral health care. The focus is not only on individual patients and families but also on the population served by the organization (e.g., outreach initiatives targeted at high risk groups in the community). Emphasis is placed on preventive services and community health promotion that integrates individual and population health perspectives. Key to this approach is the ability to sustain the organization's efforts by using continuous improvement cycles.

Case 3 of the McVea et al. (1996) study exemplifies a high performing organization that not only has systems in place for preventive services, but also has practitioners who show enthusiastic leadership and skill in enhancing the motivation of patients. This practice strives to achieve a higher standard of excellence in preventive care than the practices of the other organizations. Similarly, the Group Health Cooperative of Puget Sound described in Chapter 5 provides a good example of a comprehensive health organization that emphasizes prevention on the population health level.

Note, it is important to distinguish between quality assurance and quality improvement perspectives. Proactive organizations emphasize quality assurance by identifying problems or deficits and taking necessary action to rectify them; that is, they cull the 'bad apples'. This may be thought of as a *raising the floor* approach to organizational improvement. In comparison, high performing organizations concentrate on quality improvement via ongoing efforts to enhance processes and promote excellence throughout all levels of the organization; that is, they cultivate 'good apples'. This positive emphasis may be described as a *raising the roof* approach.

Characterizing Your Organization

Your Organizational Prototype

Where is your health organization on the reactive-proactive-high performing continuum? Take a few moments to peruse the defining characteristics in the *Your Organizational Prototype* tool (Appendix A). Circle the descriptor in each row that best characterizes your organization's prevention and behavioral health care. For larger organizations, apply the checklist to distinct components (e.g., team, program, division, site). Then, use these data to produce a profile of the organization as a whole.

It is highly instructive to compare and discuss your assessment of the organization with colleagues at a team meeting, workshop or retreat. Have individuals plot their assessment on copies of the tool, which can be collated and displayed for feedback. Here are some questions to guide and stimulate discussion:

1. What are the organization's strengths and weaknesses?

2. How congruent are various components of the organization? Does one stand out?

3. How large is the discrepancy between where your organization is now and where you want it to be in 1–3 years?

Participants have found that this self-study exercise effectively raises their consciousness of the need for change; that is, it moves the possibility of change to the forefront. This is a vital step in motivating commitment to organizational renewal.

The aim of this exercise is to stimulate both individuals and teams to aspire to higher performing standards. Reapply this tool every six months or so in order to strengthen and monitor commitment to improvement. In large organizations apply this tool to different sectors and compare the findings. This comparison is often a stimulating warm-up to a multi-sector workshop or retreat on organizational change.

Case Study

As part of a continuing education program conducted by the local medical school, Dr. B., attended a workshop on organizational improvement. She was recently appointed physician-in-chief of the Lakeside Family Practice Center (profiled in Chapters 11–14). At the workshop, Dr. B. learned about ways to stimulate organizational change and decided to devote the next staff meeting to this topic. This weekly meeting included the Center's administrators and the full health care team (physicians, residents in family medicine, nurses, nutritionist, social worker).

Dr. B. began the meeting by giving a brief overview of the workshop she had attended and then asked staff to complete the *Your Organizational Prototype* tool. Being sensitive to differences in status and authority, she asked everyone to complete the *Your Organizational Prototype* tool anonymously. During a coffee break, the worksheets were collected and a quick overview prepared. Basically, the median score was computed for each rating, along with the lower 25th percentile and upper 75th percentile. These were plotted using different colors on a transparency copy of the worksheet.

The resulting profile was presented to the group using an overhead projector. A most interesting discussion ensued. Most staff rated the Center in the reactive to proactive range. This was not surprising given recent cutbacks in funding and increases in clinical demands due to their aging and ethnically diverse patient population. Although everyone wanted to increase prevention and community outreach, staff were under considerable pressure just fighting fires. Dr. B. was encouraged to see that the leadership style was characterized as coaching and inspiring. However, staff morale was low due to relentless time pressures and caseloads.

After some initial awkwardness, staff began to talk about various ways in which they could increase communication and improve the organization. Indeed, Dr. B. was intrigued by how the use of this opened up a lively discussion about the Center.

After the meeting, several staff approached Dr. B. Although initially apprehensive, they found the meeting helpful. It gave them an opportunity to talk about 'the system', offer suggestions, and discuss possible changes and improvements.

Readiness for Change Analysis (Worksheet 9.1)

Considerable advances have been made over the past decade in understanding the dynamics of how people change behavior (Chapter 7). Several concepts and associated tools can be readily adapted for use with organizations. In particular, it is important to identify variations among different sectors of the organization with respect to their readiness for change, including their members' agreement or disagreement over the pros and cons of change. In addition to identifying areas of readiness and resistance to change, members' analyses and discussions of their organization's challenges and potentials, if properly guided, can generate powerful momentum for improvement.

In attempting to understand how people change behavior, Prochaska et al. (1992) describe a progression through five stages: not thinking about change (**precontemplation**), being unsure or ambivalent about change (**contemplation**), ready to initiate change (**preparation**), taking steps toward the goal (**action**), trying to maintain change over the long term (**maintenance**). This popular model has been applied to a range of behaviors and contexts (Joseph et al., 1999).

Building on this model, Figure 9.2 depicts a readiness for change continuum. This can be used as a heuristic tool for guiding how you approach the organization about a proposed change (see case study below). Readiness for organizational change can be put into practice using Worksheet 9.1.

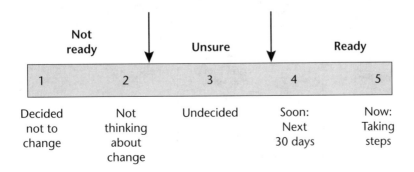

Figure 9.2 Readiness for organizational change.

Have the worksheet completed and then compare across key individuals and sectors of the organization. The Summary Table provides a convenient way to get an overall picture of the organization's readiness for change.

In addition to assessing readiness, consider individual differences in *confidence* and evaluation of the *importance* of a proposed change (Rollnick et al., 1999). It is not uncommon to find a discrepancy of opinion between senior management and staff regarding the importance of a particular change. For example, the chief information officer may see an integrated patient record and decision-support system as vital for improving accountability and outcomes, whereas clinical staff view this as a threat to their professional autonomy. Confidence denotes the sense that "we can do it" and builds on the concept of self-efficacy (Bandura, 1997). For instance, an organization may assess that it is very important to initiate a certain change (e.g., motivational counselling of patients) but doubt that it has the resources and skills to bring this about. Conversely, staff may feel very confident that they could accomplish a specific change (e.g., serve as a training site for health sciences students), yet view this proposed change as an inconvenience.

Decision Balance (Worksheet 9.2)

Decision Balance (Worksheet 9.2) is a versatile tool that can be used in both professional and personal contexts. The greatest value of completing a decision balance is that it facilitates getting all sides of the proposed change on the table. Often, individuals and groups tend to favor one or two aspects of a decision balance and fail to give sufficient attention to the others (Figure 9.3).

Consider the different perspectives of a practitioner and patient regarding cigarette smoking. The patient believes that smoking provides benefits such as helping him relax and control his body weight. Quitting would raise concerns about weight gain and the loss of a valued pleasure (sections 'a'

Figure 9.3 *Decision Balance* for comparing different perspectives on behavior change.

	Reasons not to change	Reasons to change
Stay the same	*Benefits*	*Concerns*
Change	*Concerns*	*Benefits*

and 'c' in Worksheet 9.2). On the other hand, the practitioner is more likely to focus on the reasons that the patient should quit smoking. These include the many health risks of cigarette smoking, such as increased incidence of lung cancer and heart disease, and the clear benefits that the patient would accrue from quitting (sections 'b' and 'd' in Worksheet 9.2). Completing a decision balance will reveal both sides of the issue. The process of completing the decision balance can be extremely valuable for achieving a shared understanding of the pros and cons of a particular proposed change. Depending on where the organization is regarding readiness for change, you will need to adapt your approach. Worksheet 9.3 provides a guide.

The following case study illustrates how a decision balance can both guide group discussion of a difficult issue and ensure that alternative perspectives on a proposed change are given due consideration.

Case Study: To Merge or Not?

Shortly after she assumed the position of physician-in-chief of the Lakeside Family Practice Center, Dr. B. was approached by the chief of the PMB Family Practice Center regarding a merger. The PMB Center was approximately twice the size of Lakeside in both staff and patient population. The PMB Center had an established and successful health services research program but was not as strong as Lakeside in collegiality and academic training. Both centers were under financial pressure and could benefit economically by merging administrative systems and clinical programs.

Dr. B. considered how ready the Lakeside Center was for a change of this magnitude. Indeed, she was unsure herself. Her initial analysis (using Worksheet 9.1) suggested that Lakeside was not ready for a change at this time. Although several physicians had talked about such a merger (they were colleagues of physicians at the PMB Center), most staff were not yet thinking about this type of change. Also, she wondered how Lakeside's patients would react to such a proposal. This would have to be managed carefully. On the other hand, she anticipated that their major funder (fee-for-service from a major insurance plan) would see economic benefits from such a merger.

Dr. B. raised this issue at the next staff meeting. Because most staff were not yet thinking about change, she needed to broach this issue carefully by focusing initially on consciousness-raising (see Worksheet 9.3).

The prospects of a merger generated a heated discussion. Several individuals voiced concerns about their Center losing its distinctiveness if they were to merge with the larger PMB Center. They liked the way things were at Lakeside, especially the friendly and supportive staff relationships and the excellent and much-appreciated care they provided their patients.

With the decision balance (Worksheet 9.2) in mind, Dr. B. directed the discussion to consideration of other aspects of the proposal: *"What would you see as some of the benefits if we were to merge with PMB?"* Staff began to acknowledge some possibilities, such as getting access to the computerized patient record and tracking system in place at PMB, as well as the benefits of academic rounds linking research and education. Then, Dr. B. posed another question: *"What concerns would you have if we decided to stay as we are?"* Initially, the discussion lapsed until one physician raised the point that Lakeside is having difficulty keeping up with advances in services. She noted that some of her patients had shifted over to the PMB Center because they liked the broader range of services offered at this Center (e.g., wellness and aging counselling).

By the end of the meeting, the mood among staff had shifted from initial scepticism about the proposed merger to a more positive, but cautious, consideration of possible benefits. Staff just did not want to be railroaded into a decision. They valued the opportunity to discuss all sides of the proposal. As a next step, Dr. B. suggested that a small task group be formed of key individuals from both Centers. This task group would complete an in-depth analysis of the possible benefits and disadvantages of merging, as well as discuss potential models for how a merger might be achieved. Their report would go to both Centers for review.

Postscript: Following the Task Group report and detailed negotiations, staff at both Centers voted decidedly in favour of the proposed merger.

About Choices

Success in sustaining motivation for improvement is contingent on having this aspiration permeate all levels of the organization. Change is best presented to individuals and teams as an option. Such an approach respects members' autonomy and supports their choice of a future organization that all can enthusiastically support (Ryan & Deci, 2000). In contrast, highly controlling ('top down') directives for change are likely to generate resistance and fizzle out once the pressure subsides (e.g., the CEO moves on to another organization). The following quotation from Peter Senge (1990, p. 225) captures the essence of this distinction:

Two fundamental sources of energy can motivate organizations: fear and aspiration. Fear, the energy source behind negative visions, can produce extraordinary changes in short periods, but aspiration endures as a continuing source of learning and growth.

Moving On

Given success at stimulating motivation for improvement, the next chapter describes five factors necessary for transforming your organization from its current prototype into its vision of a leading organization for the provision of prevention and behavioral health care.

Your Organizational Prototype

Instructions: Circle the number in each row that best describes your organizations's current functioning (focus on a particular level: unit, department, program or site).

	Reactive	Proactive	High performing
Focus	Primarily clinical 1 2 3	Prevention and clinical care 4 5 6	Clinical, prevention and health promotion 7 8 9
Level	Individual 1 2 3	Individual, some outreach 4 5 6	Individual, community and population 7 8 9
Time frame	Present "Fight fires" 1 2 3	Short/Medium term 4 5 6	Short/long, investing in future 7 8 9

	Reactive	Proactive	High performing
Leadership	Minimal or autocratic 1 2 3	Constructive 4 5 6	Visionary, inspiring 7 8 9
Influence mode	Controlling or laissez faire 1 2 3	Coaching 4 5 6	Empowering 7 8 9
Quality orientation	Informal Self-proclaimed 1 2 3	Quality assurance 4 5 6	Continuous improvement 7 8 9
Accountability mainly to	Professionals 1 2 3	Patients/ Clients 4 5 6	Patients, professionals and public 7 8 9

	Reactive	Proactive	High performing
Management style	Disorganized or rigid 1 2 3	Flexible 4 5 6	Synergistic, participatory 7 8 9
Communication	One-way, sporadic 1 2 3	Two-way 4 5 6	Multi-directional, continual 7 8 9
Professional development	Low priority 1 2 3	Optional, opportunistic 4 5 6	High priority, ongoing 7 8 9
Morale	Complacency, discouraged 1 2 3	Supportive, encouraging 4 5 6	High, self-sustaining 7 8 9

Worksheet 9.1 Readiness for Change Analysis

Change Being Considered: _____

Instructions: *Circle the number that best describes your organization's readiness for change. Have the analysis completed by distinct components (e.g. individuals, teams, programs, stakeholders) and then create a composite profile in the summary table below.*

Ready for Change

Not ready		Unsure		Ready
1	2	3	4	5
Decided not to change	Not thinking about change	Undecided	Soon: Next 30 days	Now: Taking steps

Summary Table

	Not Ready	Unsure	Ready
Key Individuals			
Teams/ Staff			
Programs/ Divisions			
Stakeholders (e.g., patients, payers)			
Other			

Worksheet 9.2 Decision Balance

Change Being Considered: _____

Instructions: List the most important reasons for the pros and cons of change. Start with a) Benefits of not changing.

Decision	Reasons Not to Change	Reasons to Change
Not Change	**a) Benefits** *What do you like about ...?*	**b) Concerns** *What are your concerns about ...?*
Change	**c) Concerns** *What concerns would you have if you were to change?*	**d) Benefits** *What are the benefits of changing?*

Worksheet 9.3 Tailoring Your Approach for Building Motivation

	Not Ready	**Unsure**	**Ready**
Aim	Consciousness raising	Acknowledge and clarify ambivalence	Strengthen commitment to change
Use the Decision Balance to ...	Look for a discrepancy between where the sector is now and could/wants to be	Explore the pros and cons of change	Make a plan based on shared under-standing of the pros and cons of change
Target:	*specify target:*	*specify target:*	*specify target:*
Key Individuals			
Teams			
Programs			
Stakeholders			
Other ...			

CHAPTER 10

Step 2: Strengthening Capacities for Improvement

Harvey Skinner and Richard Botelho

Change is often perceived as a perplexing jungle that many people, organizations, and even whole societies enter only to become entangled in the undergrowth of confusion and dysfunction.

—Daryl Conner (1995, p.xix)

Overview

Organizations, like the individuals within, vary widely in performance, resiliency and capacity for achieving their full potential. To achieve high performance, organizations must go beyond traditional approaches that rely mainly on professional knowledge and incorporate new types of knowledge about the improvement process itself. Five dimensions are essential for improving performance: Affective, Cultural, Technical, Structural and Strategic (ACTSS). A self-study tool, *ACTSS: Success Factors for Organizational Improvement*, is described that can help you assess your organization's capability to continually improve its efforts in prevention and behavioral health care. This model can be used repeatedly to monitor progress and to set organizational priorities.

Success Factors for Organizational Improvement

Many attempts at improvement get bogged down by 'the system', that is, held up through organizational inertia, team or departmental infighting, or lack of necessary skills and resources. Is your health organization able to make sustained efforts at improving its performance?

Often, a fairly straightforward modification can substantially improve an organization's performance. This may involve a change in patient scheduling or the reassignment of responsibilities and roles among health care team members. For example, extending the length of appointments by one minute on average resulted in a significant increase in general practitioners' discussions with patients about such health-related behaviors as cigarette smoking and alcohol consumption (Wilson et al., 1992).

To unlock their full potential and achieve a high performing standard, organizations must go beyond relying on professional knowledge and incorporate knowledge about the improvement process itself. Is your organization ready for making sustained efforts at improvement? Does it have the basics of this improvement knowledge in place? Five critical success factors (ACTSS) underlying this new approach, along with a self-study tool for assessing organizational readiness to engage in continuous improvement, are described in this chapter.

A New Knowledge Base for Improvement

Traditional approaches to improving health care apply professional knowledge developed by discipline-specific experts. Students are trained in the core knowledge of each specialty and apply this knowledge to improving health care. During the last 50 years a parallel knowledge base (e.g., CQI-TQM) that focuses on continual improvement has developed outside of the health care sector (Langley et al., 1996). Batalden and Nolan (1993) argue for the inclusion of the knowledge underlying continual improvement with traditional professional knowledge in health care. They describe four prerequisites for making continual improvement a top priority in a health organization: leadership, investment in improvement, professional subject matter knowledge, and knowledge for improvement (Figure 10.1).

Based on a review of the literature on CQI-TQM as applied in both health care and nonhealth care settings, Shortell and colleagues (Shortell, Levin et al., 1995) found that evidence regarding the overall effectiveness of quality improvement initiatives was inconclusive. Nonetheless, more successful implementations and potentially positive outcomes were associated with four dimensions: cultural, technical, strategic, structural. We have added a fifth dimension that addresses the affective climate, motivations and often powerful emotions that members have about the organization.

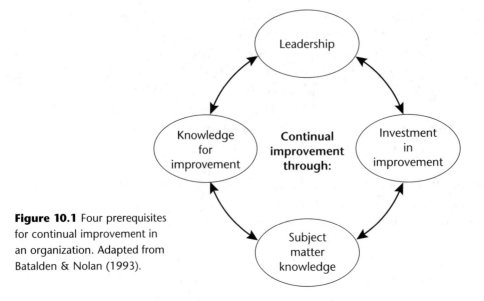

Figure 10.1 Four prerequisites for continual improvement in an organization. Adapted from Batalden & Nolan (1993).

The ACTSS framework (Figure 10.2) is useful for identifying organizational supports and barriers to improving performance. Specific examples of each dimension are given in the *ACTSS: Success Factors for Organizational Improvement* instrument (Appendix A).

Figure 10.2 Five critical factors for success in organizational improvement: the ACTSS framework.

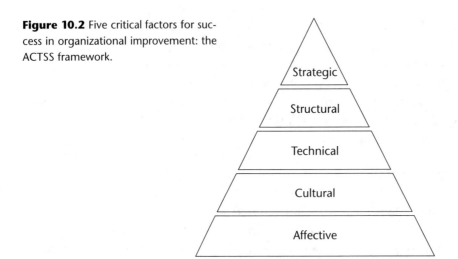

ACTSS Model

The following describes each of the elements of ACTSS:

Affective Dimension. Efforts at improving performance meet resistance in an organization that is undergoing rapid change such as restructuring, downsizing or re-engineering. Indeed, Michael Hammer (1993), who championed 're-engineering' as a blueprint for tearing down corporate structures and redesigning around key processes, now concedes that he underestimated the human costs. "When I first wrote about this I did not understand how hard it would be to do from a people point of view" (Hammer, 1999, interview in Toronto Globe and Mail).

A cornerstone of quality management is employee motivation. To achieve quality, organizations must drive out fear, so that everyone may work effectively (Edwards Deming, 1986). This climate of trust, belonging and commitment is difficult to achieve let alone maintain at a time when most health organizations are undergoing rapid and substantial change. Stacey (1996) argues that the denial of uncertainty and need to be 'in control' can protect us from anxiety for a while. But this defensive response, characteristic of reactive organizations where it is impossible to be in control over external forces, distant time frames and geographic spaces never works for long. The affective dimension is deeply rooted in individuals' sense of security, belonging and personal control over work. Members can have powerful emotions, positive and negative, about their organization, which fundamentally influence its capacity to sustain motivation for improvement.

Cultural Dimension. The culture of an organization encompasses important values, beliefs, norms and behaviors that either facilitate or act as barriers to improving performance. A key element for success is an organizational culture that facilitates empowerment of both professional and nonprofessional staff. For instance, Shortell, Levin et al. (1995) found that hospitals that emphasized teamwork, consensus building, adaptability and flexibility were significantly more advanced in improvement implementation activities, as compared with hospitals that had cultures emphasizing hierarchy and bureaucracy.

Technical Dimension. Information systems and data analyses can enhance knowledge about the concepts and tools for improving performance as well as aid in analyzing the organization's capability to support improvement initiatives. Success in improving performance involves employee training in the relevant principles and methods, adequate information systems, and senior management knowledge about quality improvement approaches. For example, Berwick et al. (1990) assessed that, of 21 projects in the National Demonstration Project for Health Care Quality Improvement, the 15 that had the necessary technical capacity were successful in applying basic tools of quality improvement.

Structural Dimension. Interconnecting an organization's quality improvement efforts multiplies the effect. For example, does the health organization have a designated unit that is primarily responsible for leadership and training in improvement initiatives? Berwick et al. (1990) highlight the importance of cross-functional teams that help the organization understand the interdependencies among people and processes across the continuum of care. Various structural challenges are summarized in the ACTSS tool (Appendix A).

Strategic Dimension. To what degree are quality-improvement efforts directed at the organization's core mandate and strategic directions? Several studies have found that this strategic dimension is most often lacking in quality improvement implementation (Ernst & Young & American Quality Foundation, 1992; O'Brian et al., 1994). Because of the critical need and the difficulty of involving physicians, Shortell, Levin et al. (1995) argue for the importance of focusing on strategically important clinical priorities such as improving diabetic management and self-care and ensuring compliance with new practice guidelines or regulations.

Specific challenges to improving performance tend to covary with an organization's experience in quality improvement (Shortell, Levin et al., 1995). In organizations that have not yet begun these initiatives, affective and cultural factors are most salient. For instance, staff anxiety and resistance to change may be high while the level of senior management commitment to continuous improvement is variable or conflicting.

At the early start-up stage, technical and structural barriers are most noticeable. Some illustrations include trying to define the scope of projects, establishing effective teams, and providing training in concepts and tools. In comparison, organizations at a middle stage of improvement tend to face more cultural and strategic challenges such as staff apathy and resistance or perceptions that improvement activities are not having an impact on the organization's core business (e.g., efficient medical services, financial success). At more advanced stages of improvement initiatives, challenges from all five dimensions tend to re-emerge but are more tightly interwoven. For example, the organization experiences difficulties in aligning performance appraisals with rewards as well as aligning budgeting and planning with the work of quality improvement.

Assessing an Organization's Capacity for Improvement

Continuous improvement initiatives are not always advisable for an organization. For instance, it is not an appropriate step for an organization when the 'roof has fallen' and all efforts are directed at dealing with a major crisis such as a takeover, merger or cash flow crunch. Continuous improvement initiatives are likely to fail if the organization lacks sufficient resources or the commitment of key decision-makers to make a sustained effort over the medium to long term. Thus, before embarking upon major initiatives aimed at improving performance, it is important to assess the organization's current capacity for making a sustained commitment to this process. Analogous to assessing a person's readiness or stage of change (Prochaska et al., 1992), one can evaluate an organization's readiness to undertake continual improvement.

The *ACTSS* instrument (Appendix A) is designed to help you assess the capacity and readiness of your organization for engaging in continuous improvement. The aim is to create a balance sheet of the organization's supports and barriers with respect to affective, cultural, technical, strategic and structural dimensions. For each dimension:

1. Generate (brainstorm) a list of strengths and barriers.

2. Discuss and prioritize the list.

3. Concentrate on the top three.

For larger organizations you can apply the *ACTSS* analysis to distinct organizational components, those for which an analysis makes the most sense in your situation (e.g., team, program, division, site). Use these data to produce a composite profile of the organization as a whole. Compare and discuss your assessment of the organization's readiness with colleagues at a team meeting or in a workshop format.

Building on work from Chapter 9 on characterizing your organizational prototype, the *ACTSS* assessment will enable you to get a good picture of the organization's strengths and readiness for continuous improvement. As well, it will point out specific aspects of the Affective, Cultural, Technical, Strategic and Structural dimensions that need to be addressed and bolstered. Moreover, the process of completing and then discussing results from *ACTSS* can be a powerful catalyst for building a team and strengthening commitments to continuous improvement.

The following case study illustrates the results of using this approach. It will help illuminate specific aspects of each dimension of *ACTSS*. We strongly encourage you to apply the framework to your organization so that you will have a firm grasp on the tools and uses of the ACTSS model.

Westbourne Case Study

Westbourne is a privately owned institution that offers services to clients with alcohol and drug problems. It is the major provider of these specialized treatment services for a local community of approximately 500,000 individuals, and it also plays a national role in addictions prevention, professional education and research. Westbourne has a total complement of 150 staff members from a range of health and social service disciplines. It holds contracts from both public and private sectors. However, Westbourne's level of public funding is shrinking, and it is under increasing pressure to be more entrepreneurial.

The board of directors of Westbourne has expressed interest in continuous quality improvement. Accordingly, an organizational change consultant was contracted to guide a one-day workshop with 20 staff members from various areas of the organization. Participants completed a self-study using the ACTSS model to evaluate Westbourne's readiness for sustained initiatives aimed at improving performance. Here are the results of their evaluation (a synopsis is presented in Figure 10.3).

Affective Dimension. One is immediately struck by staff friendliness and their pride in Westbourne's achievements locally, nationally and internationally: *"We are the best in preventing and treating substance abuse."* Staff have a fair degree of autonomy in making decisions regarding their work, and this contributes to a sense of personal control and lowers stress levels. Westbourne has experienced very little staff turnover. Although everyone senses that the pace of change has increased significantly, many have confidence that the organization can adapt successfully. However, further probing reveals that some staff are uneasy about the organization's future and their

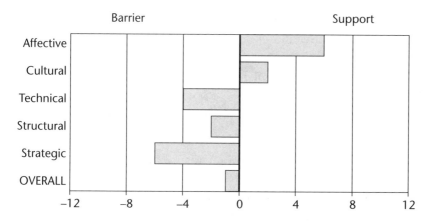

Figure 10.3 Profile of ACTSS success factors at the Westbourne Clinics.

own job security. One practitioner commented that *"Westbourne tries to remain aloof from the pressures and uncertainties driving health care reform rather than confronting them directly."*

Cultural Dimension. Westbourne has had a good reputation for meeting the needs of its patients and community clients. However, funding cutbacks from the public sector have resulted in the curtailment of services (especially inpatient services) often without providing a clear explanation to the community affected. Westbourne's leadership style would be characterized as closed and hierarchical. Most staff do not feel they have much understanding of, or input in, setting organizational priorities: *"New programs are started and existing ones cut back without much consultation ... The President just tells us."* For this reason, employees feel more and more disconnected: *"No one seems to know what is really going on around here."* At the workshop, discussions about improvement initiatives were not free-flowing, and this reflected a certain level of resistance. Many staff were unsure about the real purpose behind the workshop and worried that 'organizational improvement' could threaten their positions.

Technical Dimension. Staff at Westbourne are involved in ongoing professional development. Indeed, several provide training programs within Westbourne, in the local community and at a national level as part of the educational mandate of Westbourne. However, professional development is focused on individual level skills. Clinical staff are quite knowledgeable and have advanced skills in motivational approaches to behavior change. Several staff have taken the 'Trainers Program for Motivational Interviewing' given by William Miller and Steven Rollick (based on Miller & Rollnick,

1991; Rollnick et al., 1999). Yet, many did not appreciate how their highly developed skills for motivation enhancement with individual patients or clients could be applied at the organizational level. One participant underscored this in his take-home message from the workshop: *"I now see how my clinical skills in understanding resistance, effective communication and building commitment to change can be applied to the organization."*

Structural Dimension. It is not clear to staff that the organization has decided to undertake improvement initiatives nor is it clear whether improvements undertaken by staff will be considered in their performance appraisal and reward system as currently structured. The organization does not have a history of using project management concepts and mechanisms. Clinics within Westbourne tend to operate in isolation. Both the physical and psychological separation of these clinics hinders ongoing communication and sharing of quality improvement ideas and approaches. Thus, considerable work is needed to provide support for improvement initiatives.

Strategic Dimension. Most staff were unclear about the strategic directions of the organization: *"Do they really exist?"* one participant asked. Thus, it was difficult for staff to see how improvement initiatives could be directly related to any strategic directions. Certain key professionals (e.g., physicians) did not understand the need for organizational improvement: *"I am too busy providing quality care to my patients to think about organizational issues."*

This self-study reveals that Westbourne is at an early stage of readiness for making sustained efforts at continuous improvement. Clearer direction and commitment from senior management is a priority. However, Westbourne has a solid tradition of quality health care and is held in good regard by the community. Given a realignment in organizational supports and reward structures, staff could apply their considerable expertise in behavior change and professional development to the task of continuous improvement. Participants agreed that this self-study assessment played an important role in raising organizational consciousness.

Moving On

The next chapter describes a framework for achieving strategic goals in prevention and behavioral health care by keeping an organization's internal environment responsive to significant forces and trends in its external environment.

CHAPTER 11

Step 3: Identify Strategic Directions in Behavior Change

*Do you have a compelling vision of the future and
strategies for getting there?*

—John Kotter (1996)

Overview

High performing organizations achieve success by identifying and concentrating efforts on a small number of strategic directions. These directions shape what the organization is, where it is going and why. They provide a clear statement of the organization's intentions in prevention and behavioral health care (Step 3 of the Five-Step Model), and they provide a focus for effective decisions and actions in improving performance (Steps 4 and 5).

Strategic directions emanate from the organization's mission and mandate. They are identified by careful attention to key stakeholders' interests, as well as to current and future forces in the organization's internal and external environment. Three interrelated activities, *Stakeholder Needs Analysis, Environmental Scans* and *SWOT* (Strengths, Weaknesses, Opportunities, Threats) *Analyses,* provide a sound basis for *Issue Identification.* These issues are framed positively as challenges that the organization can do something about. Finally, a *Payoff Matrix Analysis* is used to sort through various directions to identify those that are relatively easy to implement yet offer high impact for the organization. Without these functions in place, the organization will inevitably be reactive in responding to forces and trends.

Why Focus on Strategic Directions?

Given the pace of change facing today's health organizations, successful performance is contingent on anticipating and adapting to the external environment. At the same time, many organizations are undergoing major changes to their internal environments due to factors such as: downsizing, mergers and restructuring, new technologies, professional stress and 'burnout', aging work force and early retirements, and initiatives in ethno-racial diversity. The capacity for resiliency distinguishes successful health organizations that assimilate these changes from those who become dysfunctional and suffer 'future shock' (Conner, 1995). Resilient organizations successfully absorb high levels of change by monitoring their external environment, eliciting feedback from key stakeholders and continually making internal adjustments to improve performance in an 'artful dance'.

This chapter presents some practical guides for aligning the organization's external and internal environments to achieve high performing standards. The aim of Step 3 is to help organizations specify clear intentions for achieving prevention and behavioral health care. Achieving this clarity of intention is based on a careful analysis of stakeholder interests and the forces in the organization's external and internal environments. These strategic directions provide a focus for decisions and actions in Steps 4 and 5 that will improve organizational performance.

Before describing activities and tools that lead to the specification of strategic directions, it is important to be clear about what makes an issue strategic. Bryson (1995, p.126) describes a litmus test for distinguishing strategic from operational issues. An issue is *strategic* when it has any of the following characteristics: commands attention of the organization's board and chief executives; is just coming onto or is about to come onto the organization's agenda for action; will have broad impact and must be dealt with throughout the organization; has large financial risk or opportunity; has significant consequences if not addressed; is highly sensitive or 'charged' for the organization and/or its community; and will require major action such as the development of new services/facilities, staff expansion or contraction, change in revenue structure or phasing out of existing services.

On the other hand, an issue is mainly *operational* when it has any of the following characteristics: requires action now, can be dealt with at a lower management level in the organization (e.g., line staff supervisor); will only have local impact in the organization; has minor financial risk or opportunity; does not require the development or closing of significant services or facilities.

In practice, these issues can be ordered along a continuum ranging from chiefly operational to primarily strategic. In this chapter we identify prevention and behavioral health care issues at the strategic end of the continuum.

Tools for Analyzing Your Environment

To operate effectively in today's fast-paced world, health organizations need to be alert to changes in the outside environment and to link their assessments of these external changes to internal strategic actions that can continually improve performance. Key external factors (Chapter 2) that can pose both opportunities and threats for health organizations include:

- Health care reform and restructuring

- New medical and information technologies

- Purchasers

- Regulators/Accountability

- Economic/Political climate

- Rise of patient consumerism

- Population changes

- Community needs

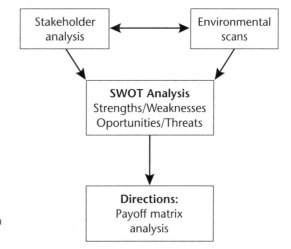

Figure 11.1 Analytic steps for identifying an organization's strategic directions.

Health organizations can use a five-part approach (Figure 11.1) to monitor and analyze their environments. Worksheets that have been adapted, in part, from Bryson (1995) and Bryson and Alston (1996) are appended to this chapter for each component. The five components:

1. **Stakeholder Needs Analysis:** understanding and satisfying stakeholders is fundamental to an organization's success

2. **Environmental Scans:** identify and monitor significant trends and forces that impact upon the organization

3. **SWOT Analyses:** assess the organization's internal strengths and weaknesses as well as the external opportunities and threats

4. **Issue Identification:** differentiate significant from less-significant options and directions in prevention and behavioral health care

5. **Payoff Matrix Analysis:** identify actions that will be relatively easy to implement and have high impact

Stakeholder Needs Analysis (Worksheet 11.1)

Maintaining the satisfaction of your primary stakeholders is fundamental to organizational success. Stakeholders (partners, associates, colleagues) are those persons, groups and organizations who have a 'stake' in the quality of the organization's functioning and services. It is useful to distinguish external from internal stakeholders. If this distinction is not made clearly or not made early enough in the process, then the stakeholder analysis can run into ambiguities, require time-consuming clarifications and risk losing momentum.

External stakeholders affect the organization but are not under the organization's direct control (e.g., patients, funders, regulators); indeed, some may actually control the organization via claims to accountability. Through their interest, investment in or benefit from an organization's services, outputs and resources, external stakeholders have a certain right to demand accountability. External stakeholders provide inputs as well as use outputs from the organization.

Internal stakeholders, on the other hand, are an integral part of the organization (e.g., practitioners, staff, administrators). They may be full-time employees or have a major portion of their time contracted with the organization (e.g., physician services).

It is essential to distinguish the relative importance of various stake-holders to the health organization. In practice, it can be a considerable challenge to achieve agreement about who the primary stakeholders are. Divergent perspectives often exist among different factions (e.g., practitioners versus administrators) and levels (e.g., line clinical staff versus senior administration) of the organization. You need to be fully aware of the potential magnitude of these differing perspectives and take steps to address them during the early stages of planning. The process of conducting a stake-holder analysis is a powerful means for building a shared understanding throughout the organization. As such, the process must be conducted in a way that is inclusive and supportive.

Bryson (1995) argues that if an organization is pressed for time in its strategic planning, then a stakeholder analysis is the single most important step to take. The aim is to understand who your stakeholders are, and to distinguish primary from secondary stakeholders. What criteria do they use for assessing your performance, how well are you satisfying them, and what do you need and expect from your stakeholders? In larger, multifaceted organizations, the various levels and sectors of the organization are analyzed before a general analysis is undertaken. A stakeholder analysis involves two basic elements.

Stakeholder Identification and Ranking. Identify your significant stakeholders and assess their relative importance to the organization for achieving its mission and mandate. First, have your planning team generate a list of stakeholders. Second, have members assess and discuss how important each stakeholder is to the organization for achieving its mission and mandate (e.g., use a five-point rating scale: 1 = slightly, 2 = moderately, 3 = fairly, 4 = highly, 5 = extremely important). Third, rank them by differentiating the primary stakeholders (e.g., top three) from less significant stakeholders.

We recommend that you compile a separate list for external and internal stakeholders and maintain this distinction in subsequent analyses. Any new direction (e.g., automated patient record system for preventive services) can be weighed in terms of its impact on and support of these primary external and internal stakeholders. This will provide valuable information for balancing the organization's internal and external environments and achieving a high performing standard.

Stakeholder Needs Analysis (Worksheet 11.1). It is necessary to understand stakeholder needs, that is, what they expect from you and how well your organization is meeting their needs. Have the planning team specify the criteria by which each primary stakeholder assesses the performance of your organization (use a separate Worksheet 11.1 for each stakeholder). Estimate how well your organization is performing in meeting these expectations. At this point, validate and revise this information by consulting with stakeholders. Do they agree with your analysis? This feedback is invaluable not only for identifying aspects that need improvement but also for strengthening the relationship with your stakeholders (i.e. you truly value their input and want to meet their needs). Finally, indicate on Worksheet 11.1 what your organization expects and needs from each key stakeholder.

Should your organization then alter its mission, your stakeholder analysis will help you anticipate and address any shifts in the relative importance of stakeholders. For example, you will be able to respond to questions and challenges from your stakeholders (e.g., patients, other practitioners, payers) should your organization shift resources from a clinical program in order to provide increased resources for preventive services and health promotion. It is important both to understand what changes in partnerships and collaborations will be needed and how to align these changed partnerships and collaborations effectively to accomplish this redirection of focus.

Environmental Scans (Worksheet 11.2)

High performing organizations have finely tuned sensors in place for monitoring and assessing trends in the external environment that can impact upon the organization. The purpose is to make sufficient lead time available for anticipating shifts and making necessary adjustments. This ability is exemplified by how Wayne Gretzky, arguably the greatest hockey player ever, approaches the game: *"I skate to where I think the puck will be."* Gretzky has an uncanny ability to avoid the congestion of players, sense how the play will unfold, and be out in the open to receive the puck and score.

Chapter 2 reviews major trends and forces affecting health organizations. Bryson (1995), among others, suggests using the acronym PESTE for categorizing these Political, Economic, Social (demographic) and Technical trends and forces. Additional categories may be useful for your particular organization, for example, Education and the natural Environment. Worksheet 11.2 provides a format for identifying and ranking external issues that are significant for your organization. An example of various PESTE forces experienced by the Lakeside Family Practice Center is given in Table 11.1.

SWOT Analysis (Worksheet 11.3)

SWOT analysis is a powerful and versatile tool for linking identification of external forces with actions necessary to the internal environment. The purpose is to provide information about the opportunities and threats facing an organization (generally external) relative to its strengths and weaknesses (generally internal). High performing organizations strive to take advantage of significant opportunities by building on their strengths, addressing threats and rectifying their weaknesses.

Using Worksheet 11.3, the planning team begins by listing strengths, weaknesses, opportunities and threats. Important sources of information include *Stakeholder Needs Analyses* and *Environmental Scans* (Worksheets 11.1 and 11.2). The planning team then performs an in-depth analysis as a basis for developing effective responses and action plans. Before they create an overall action plan the team conducts *SWOT analyses* of different levels or sectors of the organization.

Table 11.1 Environmental Scan for the Lakeside Family Practice Center

	CURRENT FORCES AND TRENDS
Political	Health care reform has shifted the focus from professional autonomy to public accountability. Practitioners are expected to move beyond an individual focus on the patient to include a population-based focus. Also, this shift will require the family practice center to provide data about the quality of care and services rendered to its patients and the local community.
Economic	Health care organizations are trying to reduce costs, improve quality and enhance access to patients in need. This economic pressure is creating unstable work conditions. Payers of health care expect the center to demonstrate value in the provision of care by improving their performance and range of services.
Social	Demographic changes in the community (aging population, ethnoracial diversity) are shifting the demand from acute care to chronic disease management and also necessitating that services be available in several languages. This is driving a fundamental change in how to address the health care needs of the center's patient population. A growing emphasis is being placed on prevention as a way of reducing the demand for unnecessary services.
Technical	The health care system is set up on an acute care model and is in the process of making a transition to a chronic care model such as disease management programs and using a population-based approach to risk behaviors. The Five Step Model described in this part of the book provides a framework for helping the organizations make this difficult transition.
Environment (physical)	Extensive development is underway in the center's catchment area that is resulting in increased air pollution, congestion on streets and highways, concerns over fresh water supply especially in peak summer periods, and strain on electrical energy supply. Thus, there are considerable threats on maintaining good standards in the local physical environment and quality of life.

Carrying out a *SWOT analysis* is a forceful catalyst for organizational improvement. It encourages team members to weigh external and internal factors, to consider present and future scenarios, and, in general, to think 'strategically'. Moreover, the SWOT process aligns two planning perspectives: 'outside-in' (accent on external factors) and 'inside-out' (accent on internal factors). Groups from different program areas can present and discuss their *SWOT analysis* at a workshop or retreat. This helps create a shared understanding of strategic issues and builds commitment to effective action.

A frequent observation when conducting *SWOT analyses* is that the same issue can be framed as both a positive and a negative factor. For instance, breadth of programs offered by an organization could be viewed as a strength (i.e., comprehensiveness) or as a weakness (i.e., resources stretched too thinly). Or, an external opportunity such as the possible merger with a highly complementary organization could, if not exercised, turn into a threat when this organization chooses to merge with your main competition. Explore and openly discuss this duality—it leads to a deeper understanding of the issue and stimulates the development of effective action plans.

The following example highlights results from a *SWOT analysis* conducted by a the Lakeside Family Practice Center. This organization is considering its current status and future directions in prevention and behavioral health care:

Internal Strengths. High commitment to providing continuous, comprehensive care to patients is an internal strength. Some notable successes in prevention have been achieved, such as a nurse-led immunization program that achieved very high immunization rates in children. Most staff appreciate the need to develop population-based approaches to health care and to incorporate continuous improvement methods that will enhance the overall performance of the organization.

Internal Weaknesses. Weaknesses are lack of experience, staff time, and technical capability for organizational change and continuous improvement. Everyone is feeling pressured to do more with less. Resources and professional development are needed regarding how to devise better programs for risk behavior reduction and behavioral aspects of disease management, how to employ teams for implementing such programs, and how to use methods (e.g., *PDSA cycles,* Chapter13) for continuously improving them. Also, information system upgrades are needed to assist clinical decision-making, support patient care and track performance over time.

External Opportunities. Professional development in continuous improvement methods is available at the affiliated hospital but not in the primary care setting. Lakeside has an opportunity to join with several primary care organizations to purchase a comprehensive information system for the clinical and behavioral management of diabetic patients. This system could also support community outreach and preventive programs for other chronic diseases.

External Threats. Payers are increasingly asking Lakeside for data demonstrating that they provide high quality care. Although the Center wants to expand its clinical and population-based programs aimed at reducing risk behaviors, it is concerned about the level of support it could expect from payers and its affiliated acute care hospital.

Strategic Issue Identification (Worksheet 11.4)

The stakeholder, environmental and SWOT analyses will generate a rich source of information about the issues that the organization faces. What makes an issue 'strategic'? According to Bryson (1995), an issue is strategic and compels action if:

1. The organization can realize a valuable opportunity to increase its performance and vitality and thereby prosper

2. There are significant consequences from failing to address it. In the extreme, the organization will perish if the issue is left unattended.

Worksheet 11.4 is designed to help you summarize these significant issues and evaluate the required level of organizational response. One approach is to form a broadly based team of members from different sectors of the organization who have been involved in the stakeholder, environmental or SWOT analyses. Have the team compile a 'short list' of issues gleaned from planning materials such as Worksheets 11.1, 11.2 and 11.3. For each issue, the team follows the process outlined in Worksheet 11.4. The issue is framed positively as a challenge that the organization is able and motivated to do something about. Team members list and discuss what makes each challenge important, and they discuss the consequences of failing to respond to each challenge. The team evaluates the priority of the challenges and urgency for action:

- **Immediate response**: cannot be handled in a routine way

- **Regular response**: issue is on the horizon but can be handled as part of usual planning cycles

- **No response**: monitor for future action.

This sequence is repeated for each issue on the short list. Finally, the issues are ranked according to their priority for action.

For example, Lakeside Family Practice Center may decide that immediate action is needed to improve their behavioral management of diabetic patients and their related community-based preventive services. This decision is driven by the following: 1) their academic mission to lead in the prevention and management of chronic diseases; 2) the threat of a managed care corporation expanding into their area; and 3) the opportunity of forming a partnership with a major health informatics company that wants to field test and refine a comprehensive system for diabetic patients.

Payoff Matrix Analysis (Worksheet 11.5)

This analysis provides an effective mechanism for sifting through strategic issues and deciding on those that have high impact (Senge et al., 1999). Have a team consider various ideas and directions for improving the organization in prevention and behavioral health care. These may be derived from issue identification analyses summarized in Worksheet 11.4. Review and then place each issue into one of four categories in the *Payoff Matrix Analysis* (Worksheet 11.5, Appendix B) according to its potential impact and ease of implementation:

a) High impact on the organization, Easy to accomplish

b) High impact on the organization, Difficult to accomplish

c) Low impact on the organization, Easy to accomplish

d) Low impact on the organization, Difficult to accomplish

Strategic directions that compel action are those in category 'a' followed by category 'b', taking into account their priority from the Strategic Issue Identification analysis (Worksheet 11.4). In our example, Lakeside, after a *Payoff Matrix Analysis*, may decide on the following directions:

1. Offer a series of professional development workshops on how to enhance motivation and lower resistance in the behavioral management of diabetic patients. The workshops would draw on Botelho (2001) and Rollnick et al. (1999). (High impact, easy to accomplish).

2. Undertake a partnership with the health informatics company for field testing and refining a comprehensive information system for the management of diabetic patients. (High impact, difficult to implement).

Moving On

Once strategic directions have been specified at a macrolevel (Step 3), we shift our attention in Steps 4 and 5 of the Five-Step Model to achieving microlevel objectives in prevention and behavioral health care. The next chapter describes seven functions that are vital for supporting practitioners and patients in health behavior change.

Worksheet 11.1 Stakeholder Needs Analysis

Stakeholder: _____

Importance: Primary or Secondary

Relation: External or Internal

What They Need From Us	What We Need From Them
How We Are Performing?	**Aspects Needing Improvement**

Worksheet 11.2 An Environmental Scan

What major forces and trends are having impact on your health organization in achieving its mission regarding prevention and behavioral health care?

	Currently	Near Future
Political	1. Identify issues 2. Rank them in importance and urgency	
Economic		
Social		
Technical		
Environment (physical)		

Worksheet 11.3 SWOT Analysis

Internal Strengths	Internal Weaknesses
External Opportunities	External Threats

Worksheet 11.4 Strategic Issue Synopsis

What Is the Issue?

Describe the issue concisely. Frame it as a challenge that the organization can and wants to something about.

Why Take Action?

List factors that make the issue important along with consequences of failing to address it. Draw upon findings from Stakeholder, Environmental and SWOT analyses.

What Is the Priority for Action?

Rate the issue/challenge according to its urgency and priority for action:

1. *Immediate response*: cannot be handled in a routine way

2. *Regular response*: issue is on the horizon and can be handled as part of usual planning cycles

3. *No response*: monitor for future action

Worksheet 11.5 Payoff Matrix Analysis

	Easier to Accomplish	Difficult to Accomplish
High Impact on the Organization	*a*	*b*
Low Impact on the Organization	*c*	*d*

CHAPTER 12

Step 4: Conducting a Critical Functions Analysis

HARVEY SKINNER, RICHARD BOTELHO, SHAWNA MERCER AND EILEEN deVILLA

Focus on Improving the Organization, Rather Than Blaming Individuals:

Opportunities for overall improvement most often lie in the design and implementation of organizational functions and processes, rather than in the scrutiny of an individual's performance.

—Joint Commission on Accreditation of Healthcare Organizations (1994, p.21)

Overview

Most practitioners recognize the value of being proactive in helping patients change health behavior. Yet, practitioners often work under relentless time pressure and in inefficient or poorly organized systems. How can we renew health care settings to assist practitioners and patients in behavior change?

This chapter describes seven critical functions and a corresponding tool, *Critical Functions Analysis (CFA)*, for supporting practitioners and patients in behavior change (see Appendix A also). Each function encompasses a group of linked activities or processes that are directed at accomplishing a specific goal in health behavior change. For example, a computerized health status assessment provides practitioners with the patient's risk factor profile in a timely fashion before the consultation begins. Integration of the critical functions in a dynamic system will 'open the window' of opportunity for practitioners to be more effective agents of change. The seven critical functions are:

1. **Professional Development in Behavior Change:** individual (practitioner, staff) and organizational levels

2. **Priming/Prompting of Patients and Practitioners:** to address prevention and behavioral risk factors

3. **Identification of Risk Behaviors and Related Complications:** using screening and case-findings in clinical encounters and at the community/population level

4. **Continuing Care:** monitoring, re-assessment, additional care and follow up

5. **Linkages/Networks Among Services and Resource Options:** within and outside the health setting

6. **Options for Help:** professional assistance, support groups that are professionally led, self-help groups and community resources

7. **Information Management:** feedback to patients and practitioners and systems to support behavior change initiatives.

Working in Disorganized Systems

What would a health care organization look like that optimally supports practitioners and patients in behavior change? Let's take a mental walk through your setting.

As you open the door and enter the reception area, are posters and pamphlets in sight that signal the importance of promoting health and preventing disease? Have patients been sent individualized letters reminding them about specific health issues, and is this linked with a clinical flow sheet outlining recommended activities? Consider ways in which patients receive risk factor screening and assessment. Is this routine built into the intake process, perhaps using computer technology? Do you find that you are doing a good job in some areas (e.g., cigarette smoking), while other areas could be improved (e.g., identifying excessive drinkers)?

As you walk through the clinical setting, consider occasions when assessment feedback is given in a timely fashion to clinical staff and patients. During clinical encounters, do practitioners have time to listen to patients' concerns and engage in motivational counseling? Are risk factors outlined and a menu of options available to aid in discussing risk modification with patients? The menu of options might include: professional assistance, support groups, self-help and community resources. Are effective linkages established among members within the health setting as well as between the health setting and the local community? Are you organized to monitor patients' progress in risk behavior change, and to provide additional care when needed? Who is responsible for maintaining contact and updating records in patients' charts?

Ongoing professional development is critical in today's fast changing environment. Are you given sufficient opportunities to keep abreast of clinical guidelines and the latest approaches to health behavior change? Although there may be great pressure on the health organization to change, are you given sufficient training and professional development in understanding what initiatives are most likely to produce effective outcomes in prevention and health promotion?

How does your organization measure up?

I have not failed 10,000 times.
I have successfully found 10,000 ways that don't work.

—Thomas Edison

As described earlier in Chapters 2–5, there is considerable evidence that prevention and behavioral health can lead to significant gains in improving health, while controlling health care costs. Yet, something is amiss. Despite the proliferation of protocols and clinical guidelines for behavioral health care, these initiatives are not being implemented broadly: note the 'one size doesn't fit all' reaction to the Put Prevention Into Practice Program (McIlvain et al., 1997; McVea et al., 1996).

Blaming the practitioner is counterproductive. Most causes of trouble and most possibilities for improvement come from the system. If you put practitioners into a system with limited supports, then the system will win most of the time. Rather then blaming practitioners as 'bad apples' for failing to put prevention and behavioral health care into practice, our efforts will be far better rewarded by focusing on producing good systems (Berwick, 1998).

In this chapter, we describe seven critical functions (Figure 12.1) practitioners and patients need in order to effect health behavior change. Success at implementing prevention and behavioral health care programs is strongly influenced by the degree to which the seven critical functions are in place and renewed through continuous improvement cycles. We describe the *Critical Functions Analysis (CFA)* tool and illustrate it with a case study of a family practice center.

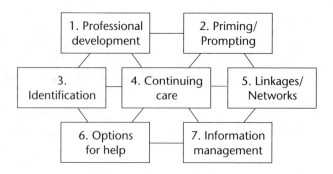

Figure 12.1 Seven critical functions for supporting practitioners and patients in health behavior change.

Seven Critical Functions

Each function encompasses a group of linked activities or processes that are directed at accomplishing a specific goal in behavioral health care (see specific items in the *CFA* tool, Appendix A). Their integration in a program of continuous improvement provides a fundamental approach to organizational renewal and a substantial support to practitioners and patients in achieving prevention and health behavior change. Items for the *CFA* tool were developed for use in a wide range of settings. The *CFA* allows for even greater modification, and you are encouraged to modify, add or delete processes/activities in the *CFA* to make it most suitable to your organization.

Table 12.1 Internet Links and Evidence-based Reviews for the Seven Critical Functions

Cochrane Collaboration: *http://hiru.mcmaster.ca/cochrane*

NHS Centre for Reviews and Dissemination: *http://nhscrd.york.ac.uk*

SoL International: *http://www.sol-ne.org/ne.html*

American Medical Association: *http://www.ama-assn.org*

HealthWeb Evidence-based Health Care Page: *http://www.uic.edu/depts/lib/health/hw/ebhc*

Canadian Medical Association: *http://www.cma.ca/*

Health Canada's Clinical Guidelines for Preventive Health:
http://www.hc-sc.ca/hppb/healthcare/pubs/clinical_preventive/index.html

Canadian Task Force on Preventive Health Care: *http://www.ctfphc.org*

HealthLinks (clinical practice guidelines):
http://www.hslib.washington.edu/clinical/guidelines.html

American Medical Informatics Association: *http://www.amia.org*

MD Computing: *http://www.mdcomputing.com*

Institute for Health Information: *http://www.ihi.org*

Table 12.2   Resources for Preventive Services

Put Prevention into Practice Education and Action Kit

Contains research-tested material and tools for:

    Patient reminder postcards

    Patient chart flow sheets

    Colored chart stickers and self-sticking removable reminder notes

    Prevention prescription pads

    Mini records for patients:

        Personal Health Guide (adults)

        Child Health Guide

Source: U.S. Government Printing Office (202-783-3238)

American Academy of Family Physicians Materials

Put Prevention into Family Practice Kit (# 1999)

Vital Signs Series

    Patient Satisfaction Surveys (# 754)

    Implementing and Measuring Clinical Prevention Services (# 755)

    Patient Tracking Reminder Systems (# 756)

    Medical Records Documentation (# 757)

    Assessing and Improving Your Cost-Effectiveness (# 758)

Source: AAFP order Dept. (1-800-944-000.)

    Website (*http://www.aafp.org*)

Make Every Visit Count

This guide for delivering preventive care 'on the run' focuses on opportunities to immunize children and gives advice on addressing reasons why children aren't immunized.

Source: U.S. Centers for Disease Control (FAX: 404-639-8828) or write to

    The Healthy Policy Group

    8905 Fairview Road

    Silver Springs, MD 20910 USA

    or National Immunization Program, CDC

    1600 Clifton Road NE, Mailstop E34,

    Atlanta, GA 30333 USA

Table 12.1 gives a synopsis of website links, including evidence reviews (e.g., Cochrane Collaboration) for the seven critical functions, and Table 12.2 lists sources for resource material (e.g., patient reminder postcards, self-assessment questionnaires, colored stickers and flowcharts).

Professional Development in Behavior Change

Goal: Provide all individuals in the health care organization (practitioners, staff, administrators) with continuing education and specific training in health behavior change at both individual and organizational levels.

An ongoing, comprehensive and interactive program of professional development is the most pivotal function for achieving a high performing organization in preventive services and behavioral health care. We can't maintain a high level of quality and effectiveness in the 2000s using approaches of the 1960s. Professional development targeted at individual, team and organizational learning can renew and transform health organizations.

A high performing organization has a carefully designed program of training and continuing education opportunities in place. Practitioners are offered knowledge development and skill-based learning exercises for lowering patient resistance and strengthening their motivation to change (Botelho et al., 1999; Rollnick et al., 1999). Emphasis is placed on adapting to patients' readiness for change as well as on the use of powerful tools such as the *Decision Balance* for enhancing motivation (See Chapter 9, Worksheets 9.1 to 9.3). Also, clinical staff are offered training in using motivational approaches in patient contacts (e.g., answering telephone inquiries, scheduling appointments) and in fostering teamwork. Administrators and managers receive continuing education to increase their knowledge regarding the need for and effectiveness of motivational interventions. They are informed of the supports and potential barriers that practitioners and patients face, and they are taught how to strengthen organizational commitment to behavioral health care initiatives. Finally, ongoing training involving all members of the organization focuses on increasing and supporting teamwork.

In addition to structured educational programs, a variety of self-directed learning materials are available. This ranges from a resource library of books and audio/video tapes on motivational approaches to distance learning courses and conferences. Regular meetings are held (formal and informal) among practitioners and staff to review progress in applying behavior change strategies. The organization arranges for advisors or facilitators when expertise is needed to address special issues of motivation, resistance and teamwork. Finally, the organization reinforces this positive learning and encourages individuals to continue using motivational approaches (e.g., 'Motivator of the Month' citation) and to maintain excellence in performance (e.g., annual recognition award).

A parallel set of processes is directed at professional development in understanding organizational change. Here we focus on the use of specific tools for improving performance and on the role of teams to achieve continuous quality improvement (Langley et al., 1996).

Although most attention tends to be given to physicians and nurses, receptionists and other clerical staff play vital roles. The clinic receptionist is typically the first point of contact for patients. With proper training and support, receptionists can be effective in helping to motivate patients by fostering a warm and caring environment. Essex and Bate (1991) found that a receptionist using only four hours a week and requiring minimal supervision was able to audit and provide feedback on practice goals for immunizations, pap smears, hypertension and smoking, diabetic follow-up, mental illness, screening the elderly, and availability of appointments. Moreover, this new responsibility resulted in an increase in job satisfaction.

Priming and Prompting

Goal: Stimulate both patients and practitioners to initiate relevant activities regarding health promotion and motivational interventions for behavioral health care.

Priming: Start by ensuring that a prominently displayed mission statement gives a clear message regarding your organization's commitment to preventive health services and health promotion. Posters, pamphlets and even videotapes in the reception area signal the priority you give to health promotion. One study of patients in a general practice setting found that most patients (82%) reported that they had noticed posters in the waiting room (Ward & Hawthorne, 1994). Presenting patients with a simple card that lists health maintenance concerns was found to stimulate patients to seek health information and advice (Saunder et al., 1996).

Another suggestion is the use of buttons. For example, a 'Key Into Health' button was worn by staff and was given to each patient upon completing the *Computerized Lifestyle Assessment* in a family practice center (Skinner et al., 1985a). The fanciful nature of the computer man on the button helped to diffuse some patient anxieties about computerized assessment. Moreover, individualized feedback from the assessment resulted in a two- to threefold increase in patients' intentions of raising a health concern (e.g., alcohol use) with their doctor (Skinner et al., 1985b). Dr. David White, a family physician, provides another example. He is renowned in his area for the use of buttons addressing potentially sensitive topics such as wife assault:

There's NO excuse
WIFE ASSAULT
It is a Crime

Dr. White (1991, p.1108) writes, "wearing this small piece of plastic provided me with more concrete results than anything I had read or heard about wife assault, probably because it made communication easier."

Prompting: Routine reminders to patients and practitioners are a simple, yet powerful, way of increasing the provision of preventive care. For example, a health-maintenance reminder letter is sent routinely to patients in the Tri-County Family Medicine sites (Frame, 1995). Szilagyi et al. (2000) reviewed 41 studies of patient reminders for improving immunization rates and found that 80% (33 studies) were effective. These studies spanned a range of baseline immunization rates, patient ages, settings and vaccination types. Increasingly, computer programs are available that link medical records with patient tracking and monitoring components (Frame, 1995). Several such systems have been tested in primary care settings and have resulted in a significant increase in the provision of preventive health services (Frame et al., 1991, 1994; McPhee et al., 1991).

Rosser and colleagues (1991) compared the effectiveness of three computerized reminder systems:

1. Physician reminder printed on the encounter form before an office visit

2. Telephone reminders to patients from the practice nurse

3. Letter reminder to patients signed by their physician and nurse describing procedures that are overdue.

In comparison with a control group, all three reminder systems significantly improved the delivery of preventive services; the telephone and letter reminders proved more effective than the physician reminder. In addition to computer-based reminders, many office systems such as Put Prevention into Practice include chart stickers and flow diagrams.

Identification of Risk Behaviors or Related Complications

Goal: Health risk behaviors and/or related complications are identified accurately, systematically and promptly. This includes case findings within clinical encounters as well as behavioral health and risk factor assessments conducted on a community/population basis.

Comprehensive guidelines have been prepared for both adults and child-adolescent preventive screening, and a host of practical tools are available (Table 12.2). Yet, in many health care organizations these tools are not used on a routine basis. This prompted Blum and colleagues (1996), in their study of the quality of adolescent health screening, to conclude: "Don't Ask, They Won't Tell." Indeed, the percentage of recommended screening questions asked varied from 20% in a private practice to approximately 60% in a community teen clinic.

In comparison, Skinner et al. (1985b) underscored the value of including a comprehensive lifestyle assessment in clinical practice. For instance, seven out of ten family practice patients indicated a health concern regarding nutrition; one out of two indicated a concern regarding physical activity; and one out of three indicated concern regarding body weight (Skinner, 1994). This prompted Skinner et al. (1985b) to conclude: "Just Asking Makes a Difference." Hence, a high performing health organization integrates health and risk factor assessments at various stages in the clinical encounter.

Specific areas to be covered by a protocol to identify risk behaviors and related complications would be tailored to issues that are most relevant to the community served by your particular health care setting. On the basis of a health profile of the patient population, compiled perhaps with data from the local public health authorities, the health organization can identify protocols that best suit its practice. Risk factor assessment is integrated into the intake process and repeated at regular intervals to monitor the patient's status. Acute care visits are used as opportunities to discuss health behaviors and their effects on the patient's well-being. This is particularly important with younger patients who tend to seek health care for acute conditions, rather than for preventive services. Including it with the more traditional medical history and clinical examination, facilitates health behavior assessment. For example, Robinson et al. (1995) found that including smoking status as a vital sign on patient charts significantly increased the likelihood that physicians would discuss smoking cessation with patients.

Following this goal, health organizations ensure that they use validated instruments whose diagnostic accuracy has been assessed in clinical settings. Also, mechanisms are in place to contact nonresponders and no-shows, so that their assessment status can be ascertained. The health setting would also maintain a register of specific diseases and risk behaviors (e.g., diabetes and weight control) for the patient population. These data form the basis for special outreach initiatives, based upon health and risk factor assessments conducted using mailed out questionnaires. Thus, the health organization is able to monitor and adapt to shifts in the health and risk profile of its patient population.

4. Continuing Care

Goal: Maintain continuity in the provision of care based on clinical guidelines and extending throughout the organization's involvement with the patient.

With this goal in mind, the organization establishes standards of practice for behavioral health issues based on published clinical guidelines (e.g., U.S. Agency for Healthcare Research and Quality website: *www.ahcpr.gov*) or recommended protocols. A patient record of specific risk behaviors is kept and regularly updated. In providing continuing care, motivational enhancement approaches are used during successive clinical encounters. Moreover, staff are aware of and use motivational approaches in their interactions with patients (e.g., telephone contacts). Since many individuals are not at a point where they are prepared to take action with a specific risk behavior, the patient's readiness for change is monitored over time and appropriate interventions used to help the patient build a stronger commitment to change. A follow-up process is well organized for specific risk behaviors, and systems are in place for providing additional information and care when needed.

Significant use is made of telephone contacts. Studies have shown that telephone-based care can help improve the patient's health status and reduce utilization of medical services (Brown and Armstrong, 1995; Wasson et al., 1992). Information technologies, such as the Internet and interactive voice systems, offer significant opportunities. For example, Friedman et al. (1996) found that a computer-controlled telephone system improved medication adherence and blood pressure control in hypertensive patients.

Finally, a tracking system is in place to monitor patient attendance at referred sites. Block (1996, p.49) identifies 11 capabilities of a patient tracking system:

1. Creates a data base of all patients in the practice, using demographic data from existing computer billing files

2. Tracks any patient risk factor, condition or test

3. Permits physicians to design their own rules for screening patients based on age, sex and other characteristics

4. Produces appointment forms or other prompts to remind physicians about needed interventions during office encounters

5. Maintains immunization records for children

6. Generates lists of patients who are overdue for care, including patients who have abnormal tests

7. Prints customized letters and mailing labels for patient reminder notices

8. Documents physician efforts to remind the patient

9. Exports data to files that can be read by other data base and spreadsheet programs

10. Produces statistical reports by doctor, service, and test result, and insures that report card requirements are met

11. Uses inexpensive and readily available computer hardware, with a convenient user interface.

Linkages/Networks Among Service and Resource Options

Goal: Well developed linkages/networks that cover a range of risk behavior and preventive service needs are maintained among service providers and resources both within and outside the health setting.

With this goal in mind, the organization provides a broad range of services and resources for practitioners and patients to deal with risk behaviors and behavioral health care. In a high performing organization, the necessary linkages are in place that enable ready access to such services. Specific referral criteria for these services and resources are maintained and updated, and advice is available for patients regarding which services to undertake. Specific individuals are assigned responsibility for developing and maintaining linkages both within and outside the health setting. The organization takes particular care in maintaining links with community health organizations, public health departments, social services and specific community groups.

Options for Help

Goal: There is ready access to a variety of interventions and options for different health issues.

A key element of motivation enhancement is to have various options available to accommodate the patient's needs and preferences. The patient's chosen behavior change is respected whenever possible. Practitioners are able to schedule additional needed time with a patient to address a behavioral issue. Additional professional assistance (e.g., nutritionist, health educator) is also available. It is particularly important to offer as wide a range of options as possible, including professionally led support groups, self-help/peer education groups, and community-based resources (e.g., diabetic association).

Facilitating self-care is an important goal, since studies have found that people can evaluate and treat up to 80% of symptoms themselves, without ever seeking professional care. For example, the Kaiser-Permanente HMO gives all their members a *Health Wise Handbook*, which provides information on prevention, when and how to self-treat, as well as when to seek professional care.

Borkman (1999) describes the various components of self-help and mutual aid, and ways these link with professional care. A resource book on how physicians and nurses can stimulate and support self-care is available from Health Canada, Health Promotion and Programs Branch (1997). This study reviews research literature and professional practice issues, as well as describes exemplary programs and tools for practitioners (contact Health Canada Publications, Brooke Claxton Building, Tunney's Pasture, Postal Locator 0913A, Ottawa, Ontario, Canada K1A 0K9. FAX 613-941-5366).

Patients will have access to a range of helpful approaches and philosophies. This might include women-focused groups or mutual support groups that take a harm reduction or an abstinence approach to substance abuse. Kyrouz and Humphreys (2000) review research on the effectiveness of self-help and mutual support groups covering a range of topics including: mental health, weight loss, addictions, bereavement, diabetes, caregivers, elderly, cancer and chronic illness (available at *http://www.mentalhelp.net/articles/selfres.htm*). They conclude that most studies have found important benefits when comparing participants with non-participants (controls), and when data are collected on multiple occasions (longitudinal studies).

Information Management

Goal: Timely access to comprehensive information supports prevention and behavior change initiatives. Such information should include risk factor data and feedback on the provision of care. The database must be regularly upgraded.

Practitioners need ready access to the risk factor profiles and health status of their patients. Increasingly, this information is made available using integrated computer systems, whereby practitioners can quickly check data using a computer terminal in the clinical examination room. Research has shown that giving patients timely and individualized feedback from lifestyle and risk factor assessments increases their intention of discussing concerns with their practitioner; it also leads to behavior change. Therefore, risk factor profiles should be easily accessible and must be regularly maintained and updated.

In a high performing organization, the information system gives practitioners feedback on their adherence to practice standards (clinical guidelines). In particular, practitioners and staff are given routine feedback regarding their performance in prompting patients regarding risk factors, identification rates of risk behaviors and complications, use of interventions, and provision of a variety of options for help. The individualized feedback given to practitioners is a powerful way to shape their behavior.

A high performing organization analyzes its information system needs and assesses the supports necessary for behavior change. Such an organization has the appropriate technology and the personnel with expertise in system design, development and implementation. A comprehensive study by the U.S. National Research Council (2000) called *Networking Health* provides an in-depth and forward-looking analysis of the Internet's capabilities for a wide range of health applications.

Recent research supports the value of computer-based preventive care systems as aids to providing preventive services and improving health status (see Chapters 15–18). For instance, Shea et al. (1996) conducted a meta-analysis of 16 randomized controlled trials of computer-based clinical reminder systems in ambulatory settings and found that computer reminders improved preventive practices for vaccinations, breast cancer screening, colorectal cancer screening, and cardiovascular risk reduction. Krishna et al. (1997) reviewed clinical trials of interactive patient education systems. Positive results were found, especially for diabetes education studies.

Using the Critical Functions Analysis Tools

How can you get an hour's worth of value out of a 10-minute patient encounter? The *Critical Functions Analysis (CFA)* is designed to help you determine how your health care setting can best achieve such a goal. Your interest may be a specific health issue, such as tobacco prevention and cessation, or a broad range of health issues, such as a healthy heart program with multiple components: nutrition, activity, tobacco, alcohol, stress.

A copy of the *CFA* booklet and instructions for its administration and scoring are given in the Appendix. The *CFA* generates a database useful for determining how well the organization is performing, as well as for identifying opportunities for improvement. The cycle for improving performance, depicted in Figure 12.2, provides a framework for using the *CFA* in a systematic program that merges design, measurement and improvement tools (Joint Commission on Accreditation of Healthcare Organizations, 1994). A critical functions analysis consists of two components:

1. Quantitative ratings of processes/activities that are essential for each critical function (Step 2 in Figure 12.2)

2. Qualitative analysis regarding organizational strengths, weaknesses and suggestions for improvement (Step 3 in Figure 12.2)

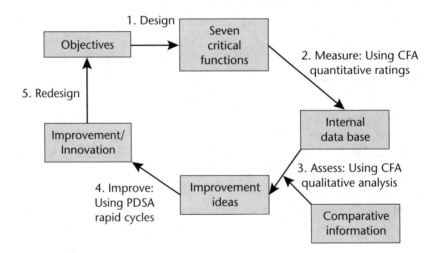

Figure 12.2 Using the *Critical Functions Analysis* in a cycle for organizational improvement. Framework adapted from the Joint Commission on Accreditation of Healthcare Organizations (1994).

The *CFA* is used to generate a data base on current performance and to help identify areas for improvement. Moreover, the process of completing a *CFA* can play a key role in stimulating interest and commitment to organizational renewal. The quantitative ratings yield measures of organizational performance that can serve as benchmarks:

1. Comparing the success of intervention for a given activity over time (e.g., smoking cessation)

2. Comparing two activities within a setting (e.g., smoking cessation with physical activity programs)

3. Comparing two (or more) settings providing the same given activity (e.g., child immunization rates at two sites of a health maintenance organization).

The qualitative analysis identifies areas of strength within each critical function as well as specific deficits that can be targeted for improvement. Both components of the *CFA* taken together provide a powerful tool for organizational self-study and quality improvement initiatives.

Case Study: Smoking Cessation and Physical Activity

The Lakeside Family Practice Center serves a diverse, multicultural patient population, and is linked to five community health centers in a large metropolitan city. Lakeside is located within an academic teaching hospital. The clinic staff includes physicians, residents in family medicine, nurses, a nurse manager, a social worker, a nutritionist and receptionists. Practitioners have expertise not only in family medicine but also in a wide variety of heath-related fields, such as physician behavior, motivational interventions, addictions, nursing management, health administration and medical education.

The *CFA* was used to evaluate Lakeside's activities regarding two health issues that are routinely encountered and managed in primary care: smoking and physical activity. Since many of the medical staff have extensive training and research interests in substance abuse and smoking cessation, counselling is a key activity at Lakeside. One half-day per week is reserved for the Smoking Clinic during which patients are provided with professional assistance and counselling on smoking cessation. In addition, the smoking clinic provides opportunities for medical residents to receive train-

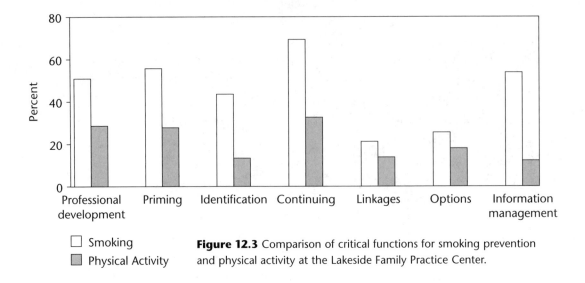

□ Smoking
▨ Physical Activity

Figure 12.3 Comparison of critical functions for smoking prevention and physical activity at the Lakeside Family Practice Center.

ing and develop skills in smoking cessation counselling. Physical activity counselling, although considered important by staff, is not a high profile activity. Such counselling is generally provided on a case-by-case basis (i.e., when the physician feels that it is of significance or when the patient specifically requests it). This difference in priority between smoking cessation and physical activity counselling is reflected in the overall *CFA* profile for the seven critical functions (Figure 12.3).

The following section highlights various strengths and needed improvements for each function. Table 12.3 summarizes suggestions for improvement resulting from the *CFA*. These suggestions are then brought forward to Step 5 (Chapter 13) for priority setting and rapid cycle improvement initiatives.

Professional Development in Behavior Change

Individual Level. Training and continuing education with respect to smoking cessation is made readily available to clinical and administrative staff at Lakeside. This includes resources for self-directed learning (especially books and other written materials), formal teaching sessions, and clinical rounds on, and regular discussions of, patient motivation and resistance. The use of motivational approaches for smoking cessation is encouraged through regular

Table 12.3   Suggestions for Improvement
at Lakeside Family Practice Center

Professional Development

- Continuing education activities applied to broader range of health issues, not just those of special interest to staff physicians.
- Teaching rounds specifically dedicated to organizational change and continuous improvement.
- Learning resources on the use of information technology and its applications for clinical care, prevention and health promotion.

Priming and Prompting

- Procedures similar to those used for the smoking clinic need to be introduced for other health issues
- Consider investing in a computer system that may be used for priming and prompting activities
- Discuss importance of role modeling by staff of healthy behavior and ways this can be integrated into the Center.

Identification of Risk Behaviors or Related Complications

- Develop standardized assessment forms/protocols for new patients, routine health visits and acute care or illness visits. Responsibility for conducting health behavior assessments need not fall to the physicians but may include other clinic staff.
- Population-based assessments (e.g., surveys) and outreach initiatives to ensure that the Center remains sensitive and responsive to needs of the community it serves.

Continuing Care

- Emphasize how motivational counselling skills generalize to areas other than smoking, and ensure that these skills are more widely applied.
- Implement routine follow-up and other modalities for the provision of care: e.g., by telephone, mail, interactive voice technology or e-mail.

Linkages and Networks

- Comprehensive list of services and resource options made available to both clinic staff and patients.
- Actively seek out what is available in the community and maintain an updated list of these linkages.
- Explorer linkages to other community groups (i.e., not just Community Health Centers). Look for collaborations that provide new options for programs on health behavior change.

Options for Help

- Referral options for a variety of health issues (including smoking cessation and physical activity counselling) should be investigated.
- Options should reflect a broad range of approaches or philosophies that are compatible with different needs/beliefs of the population served.

Information Management

- Access and feedback processes should be consistently applied to all health behavior change activities, not just to substance abuse programs.
- Regular feedback to all practitioners to ensure continuous improvement in facilitating health behavior change.
- Evaluate which aspects of the clinic structure and programs support health behavior change and which do not.

---

observation and evaluation of staff interactions with patients. Unfortunately, significantly less education and training is provided for counselling patients with respect to physical activity. Although the teaching sessions on smoking cessation may include principles that are applicable to any type of behavior change, there are few resources—and less encouragement—for staff to engage in physical activity counselling.

Organizational Level. Although Lakeside is a teaching center for family medicine residents, there is little in the way of training or education on organizational change, teamwork and continuous improvement. Although these concepts may be touched on in teaching rounds, the use of continuous improvement protocols is not actively encouraged.

Points of Pride. Lakeside is a training site for residents in family medicine, and staff physicians are involved in addiction research. As a result, behavior change—especially smoking cessation—is a major focus of the training and educational activities. Weekly teaching rounds present opportunity for professional development for all clinical staff. Clinical staff receive considerable training on motivational counselling and its applications to smoking cessation.

Areas Needing Improvement. As evidenced by staff education on smoking cessation, Lakeside is capable of providing professional development at the individual level. Lacking is the application of such training to other health issues such as physical activity. Virtually all professional development activities are conducted at the individual level. Very little training is provided on organizational change and continuous improvement. There is no formal training regarding use of information technology. Staff who are interested must find resources themselves and on their own time.

Priming and Prompting

Materials-Related, Location-Related. Posters and pamphlets on a variety of health issues are in abundance in the waiting areas. Although most were available only in English, some were available in other languages. However, there is significantly more material available on smoking and smoking cessation than on exercise or physical activity. This imbalance is evident in other priming and prompting activities.

Practitioner and Staff-Related. Specific practice protocols and record keeping methods provide staff with prompts for smoking cessation activities. In addition, during the weekly Smoking Clinic, staff routinely provide pamphlets and other written materials on smoking cessation to their patients. Similar activities are not routinely conducted with respect to physical activity counselling.

Points of Pride. The information sheet completed on a patient's initial presentation at the Smoking Clinic and standardized forms used during subsequent visits serve as excellent reminders for staff to inquire about a variety of smoking-related issues. Staff feel they are very sensitive to substance use/abuse issues and are more capable than are many other practitioners in recognizing and managing these issues. Given the ethnic diversity of the population served by the Center, special efforts are made to obtain brochures, pamphlets and other patient information in a number of languages.

Areas Needing Improvement. With respect to smoking cessation, Lakeside is conducting priming and prompting reasonably well. However, these activities are not conducted for other health issues, specifically physical activity counselling. Lakeside has not taken sufficient advantage of information technology systems for priming/prompting. There is little evidence of role modeling of healthy behavior by clinic staff.

Identification of Risk Behaviors or Related Complications

Clinical Encounter-Based. Although all patient charts include a sheet on which past medical history and health behaviors can be recorded, there is no standardized procedure by which health behavior assessment is incorporated into the intake process. There is an informal practice of asking about various health behaviors that is left to the discretion of individual physicians. However, the staff interviewed at Lakeside indicated that due to their interest in substance use/abuse, smoking is one health behavior that is generally assessed at both the initial patient visit and at subsequent visits. Both the social work and medical staff felt that their sensitivity to issues such as smoking, alcohol use and illicit drug use was one of their strengths in dealing with risky health behaviors. In addition, the medical residents at Lakeside receive a considerable amount of training on detection and management of substance use/abuse and addiction.

Community/Population Based. Lakeside does not routinely engage community-based activities for the identification of risk behaviors.

Points of Pride. Screening for substance abuse (especially tobacco use) during the clinical encounter is routinely done.

Areas Needing Improvement. Standardized screening processes for new patient intake, routine health care visits and acute care/illness visits should be implemented. Creation of standardized screens that are appropriate to the population served will require a risk factor assessment of the community.

Continuing Care

Lakeside staff feels that they are well-versed in motivational counselling techniques and that these techniques are regularly applied during the Smoking Clinic. Follow-up activities and the provision of additional care and information for Smoking Clinic patients is provided solely in person. There is little evidence of regular continuing care activities for exercise counselling.

Points of Pride. Staff physicians believe that motivational counselling is the "key to smoking cessation counseling." As a result, they emphasize motivational approaches in their Smoking Clinic sessions.

Areas Needing Improvement. Ensure that motivational counselling and appropriate follow-up activities are conducted for all health behavior change issues, including physical activity counselling. Follow-up activities and additional care for patients is only provided in person.

Linkages and Networks

In general, Lakeside has good links to other health care professionals in the teaching hospital and to five Community Health Centers (CHCs) in the area (i.e., primarily through medical referrals). However, little effort is made to form and maintain active links specific to smoking cessation activities or to counselling on physical activity. Although all clinic staff are well-informed about the Smoking Clinic, there is little, if any, training regarding other internal and/or external resources available for patients; the same is true for physical activity counselling. Thus, referrals to the Smoking Clinic either from CHCs or from within the teaching hospital occur fairly regularly, while referrals from the Family Medicine Center to other smoking cessation programs happen rarely, if ever.

Points of Pride. Lakeside has formal linkages to other health care practitioners in the teaching hospital and to five CHCs in the vicinity.

Areas Needing Improvement. Links with other health care practitioners and resources in the community are not used as effectively as they might be. While referrals are occasionally made to the smoking clinic from nearby CHCs, Lakeside generally does not refer patients to outside agencies for smoking cessation counselling. Similarly, there are a limited number of referrals made by clinic staff to outside agencies for exercise and physical activity programs. Lakeside needs a system that would regularly update the community resources and services available. Little use is made of information technology for linkages to other practitioners and health agencies.

Options for Help

Despite Lakeside's associations with local CHCs, the Center's staff tries to provide individual professional assistance rather than refer patients to support groups or other outside agencies. This is especially true for smoking cessation because the staff feels that their Smoking Clinic is one of the best smoking cessation options available in the community. In fact, during our interviews, staff indicated that the Smoking Clinic is the only option initially offered to patients who indicate interest in smoking cessation.

Although there is no formal 'Physical Activity Clinic', staff indicated that they would be happy to provide individual professional assistance on exercise to their patients and, if necessary, to investigate other options in the community.

Points of Pride: Lakeside is well known in the area, and its Smoking Clinic is well known to other medical practitioners in the hospital. Various members—staff physicians, family medicine residents, nurses, a nutritionist and a social worker—lend their professional expertise to the smoking clinic on a regular basis.

Areas Needing Improvement. The Smoking Clinic is the only option that is routinely provided to patients who are interested in smoking cessation. Explore other options. Expand options for exercise counselling beyond the individual counselling provided by health practitioners within Lakeside.

Information Management

Access and Feedback. Due to the high level of staff awareness and interest in addictive behaviors, access to patient information on smoking status and feedback to practitioners on their performance in the smoking cessation program are readily available. In contrast, access to up-to-date information on patients' level of physical activity and feedback to practitioners on their exercise counselling activities is rather limited.

System Design and Maintenance. Although needs analyses regarding systems and supports for behavior change activities have not been conducted, plans to introduce a computerized system for patient tracking and record maintenance are currently underway.

Points of Pride. Smoking status and motivation to quit are routinely assessed and recorded. Family medicine residents, in particular, get extensive feedback on their clinical performance, especially within the smoking clinic.

Areas Needing Improvement. With the exception of substance abuse, the access and feedback processes are not well-conducted. Lakeside has no system for analyzing its structure and how that structure supports behavior change.

Moving On

The *CFA* gives us a list of specific areas and opportunities for improvement (Table 12.3). Our next step is to decide which specific area(s) will be targeted and to follow that with an improvement initiative (Steps 4 and 5 in Figure 12.2). Chapter 13 describes a practical framework and provides the tools needed to make rapid cycle improvements.

Step 5: Improvement Using Rapid Cycle Change

G. ROSS BAKER

If you always do what you've always done,
you'll always get what you always got.

Paul Batalden, M.D.

Overview

This chapter describes practical tools that assist teams in making the rapid cycle improvements. The team begins by setting an aim for the improvement cycle. Then, a simple, yet balanced, set of outcome measures is identified to guide improvement. The process of making change is guided by the PDSA (Plan-Do-Study-Act) model. Several important tools are often used, including the process flowchart to identify work processes and the run chart for graphing outcome and process measures. These models and tools are illustrated using the example of a team aiming to improve the care of diabetic patients in a family practice clinic. We discuss how the model and tools can be incorporated into daily work, making improvement part of everyday activity. Finally, we address the integration of these improvement methods with the seven critical functions outlined in Chapter 12.

Practitioner's Guide to Rapid Cycle Change

Pressures on health care practitioners to provide more services or produce better outcomes with existing, or declining, resources has become commonplace. Creating a more effective practice and using resources more wisely is not an easy task. Motivation to change and knowledge of effective alternatives are necessary, but not sufficient, to those seeking better performance. As many practitioners have discovered, good intentions wilt in the face of ceaseless caseloads and limited resources.

Many practitioners have good ideas for improving their practices, yet find it difficult to bring these ideas into action. Over the last few years, a variety of methods have emerged that offer help to individuals and organizations to make rapid cycle improvements. This chapter describes a strategy, **rapid cycle change,** and practical tools for helping practitioners improve their work.

Rapid cycle improvement emphasizes making a series of small changes that are tested to see if they work. While each change is small in scale or focus, collectively these small changes create large improvement. Specific ideas for change may come from the *critical functions analysis* (CFA, Chapter 12), observations on practices in other clinics, and/or gleaned from the literature.

Establishing an Aim for Improvement

The first activity of any team is to establish a clear aim for its work. When others, such as clinic managers, give team goals, the team's early clarification of these goals ensures that its efforts are not wasted on unnecessary work. Especially when a team defines its own project, it is important to spend time crafting an aim statement. As team members involve themselves in the issues and begin to test small-scale changes, the aim statement provides a reference point for checking reasons for each new activity. In this way, members prevent misunderstandings about the purpose and scope of their work. New members and leaders reviewing the team's activity can quickly orient themselves by referring to the aim statement.

Good aim statements begin by identifying the population of interest, for example, patients with diabetes treated in the Lakeside Family Practice Center. The aim statement should be relatively brief, performance-related, and restricted in scope. Aim statements should not offer solutions or point at causes of problems, nor should they include aims that are beyond the team's responsibilities. The diabetes team might develop this aim statement: "To improve the outcomes and reduce the costs of caring for the diabetic patients who are enrolled in our clinic." This statement neatly clarifies the goals and orients the activities of the team.

Even with a clear aim, many teams discover that their activities drift from their original targets. After working for a period on a project, they lose sight of the purpose that brought the team together. One common drift is that from a focus on change to an interest in measurement. For example, a team that begins work on improving care for diabetic patients might get sidetracked by its data collection and lose sight of opportunities to make changes that improve care. Good data suggest what changes are useful. But some teams get so involved in studying patterns in their data and devising additional analyses that they neglect to test changes that may improve outcomes. Team leaders can refer to the aim statement as a way to shift the team's emphasis back to improving care.

Thomas Nolan and his colleagues (Langley et al., 1996) have suggested that one way to develop an aim statement is by asking the question, "What are we trying to accomplish?" This question helps the team create a general aim statement that guides the specific activities carried out by the team. Teams may also specify more detailed aims to target particular subpopulations or specific outcomes. For example, the Lakeside team may discover that a high percentage of patients with Type II diabetes have high hemoglobin A1C (HbA1C) levels and need yearly eye examinations. As a result, the team develops a specific aim for this issue. This narrowing of focus results from the teams' review of data and from trying out specific changes aimed at improving care. Until these systems are well-understood and data point toward more specific needs, the team should begin with a general aim statement, before moving to identify specific areas where changes are needed.

The Clinical Value Compass Worksheet

In many health care organizations there is an ongoing debate concerning critical outcomes: should emphasis be on reducing costs or improving quality of care? This discussion often leaves practitioners arguing that suggested changes will undermine quality of care and administrators contending that the failure to control costs will undermine the long term health of the organization—hence the ability of practitioners to deliver care. Both sides are right: the key to ensuring value requires consideration of both quality and cost. Consequently, measures of health care must include an array of different outcomes.

One way to accomplish this goal is to create a balanced array of outcomes on the *Clinical Value Compass* created by Nelson and his colleagues (Nelson and Mohr, 1996). The *Clinical Value Compass* incorporates four types of health care measures: 1) clinical outcomes; 2) functional health status; 3) satisfaction with care; and 4) costs, including direct costs to the providers and organizations and indirect costs incurred by the patient, family,

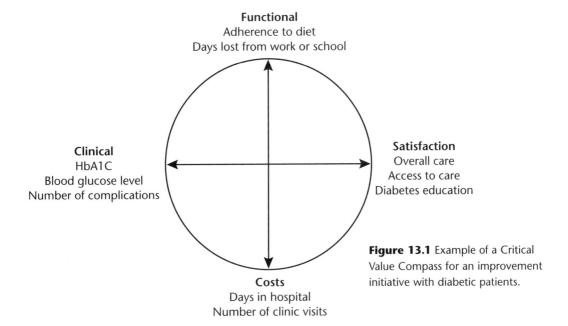

Functional
Adherence to diet
Days lost from work or school

Clinical
HbA1C
Blood glucose level
Number of complications

Satisfaction
Overall care
Access to care
Diabetes education

Costs
Days in hospital
Number of clinic visits

Figure 13.1 Example of a Critical Value Compass for an improvement initiative with diabetic patients.

employer and community. An example of a *Clinical Value Compass* for diabetic patients is given in Figure 13.1. Monitoring shifts in the array of values in the *Clinical Value Compass* provides a way to understand the impact of changes made to improve care. Teams can use the measures from the *Clinical Value Compass* to decide whether to extend successful changes, abandon changes that have little or no effect, or modify changes that are only partly successful. *Clinical Value Compass* measures and the changes developed from them are useful for improving the outcomes of individuals or groups of patients.

The *Clinical Value Compass* is not intended to offer an exhaustive set of measures. Rather, the goal is to select a small number which are readily available, or which can be collected at an affordable cost. This measurement strategy provides a balanced set of measures; it is not meant to define all possible outcomes. Nelson suggests that 4 to 12 measures are sufficient to get started. Since measurement often requires additional effort, it is important not to overwhelm staff with new measurement responsibilities. Guidelines on how to use the *Clinical Value Compass* to identify and evaluate changes are summarized in Table 13.1.

Table 13.1   Tips on Using the *Clinical Value Compass*

- Begin by specifying the specific population or group for which you wish to identify outcomes (e.g., teenage males who smoke who were seen in this clinic during the last year).
- Craft a general aim statement which outlines the purpose of your work (e.g., to improve the outcomes and reduce the costs of diabetes care for patients in our clinic).
- Identify the specific measures on the *Clinical Value Compass* starting with clinical outcomes that are more familiar to clinicians.
- Brainstorm a list of measures for each type of outcome.
- Select a small number of measures in each compass point taking into account the kinds of information now available and the costs and opportunities associated with collecting new measures.
- Where possible select commonly used measures to make it possible to compare results with other groups attempting similar changes.
- Focus on getting *useful* measures. Often there will be questions about the reliability and validity of measures—but these measures will not become reliable and valid unless they are used.

Understanding the Processes of Care

To improve outcomes, it is necessary to change the ways care is delivered. Short-term improvements can be gained by exhorting staff to work harder and avoid errors—but such demands rarely make a long-term difference because they have limited impact on the ways in which work is done. Few problems are the result of individual errors or inattention to instructions; most stem from poorly planned or ineffective work patterns. All work involves a series of steps or processes. A work process may produce less than optimal outcomes because of erroneous or insufficient process knowledge or process skills. What are the various work processes that lead to a particular outcome? What are their problems or potentials? What changes could be made? How do you achieve these changes and teach staff the new processes?

Since most work processes are the responsibility of more than one person, it is important to create a way for individuals who have responsibilities for tasks at different stages of the work process to share their knowledge. To understand the process of care, it is useful to create a process flow diagram (Figure 13.2), which graphically depicts the sequence of steps in the process. Teams can create a flow diagram in an hour or less that provides an overview of the steps in the process. This diagram provides a means to understand how care is currently provided and offers a way for

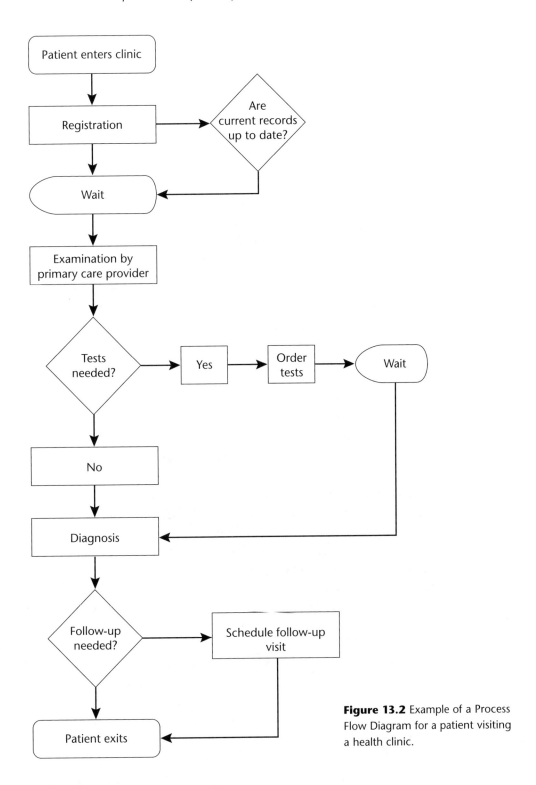

Figure 13.2 Example of a Process Flow Diagram for a patient visiting a health clinic.

Table 13.2   Tips on Flowcharting

- Diagram the process as it currently works, not as it is *supposed* to work
- Use the common flowchart symbols
- Agree on the use of the flowchart before starting
- Choose start and endpoints which represent areas that are under control of team members
- Draw a high level (or medium level) diagram representing the process in 8 to 12 steps
- Add more detail in areas where there are delays, errors or other events that suggest need for change
- Working with Post-It notes makes it easy to add steps or alter the process without redrawing.

team members to identify problems, including waste. Waste results from any activity that does not add value to the final result of the process. For example, patients are often asked for the same information repeatedly, or staff complete reports or forms which are never used. When work processes are documented on a flowchart it is easier to identify which activities are crucial for patient care and clinic administration and which are redundant or not needed.

Flowcharts can also identify bottlenecks or other process problems that limit staff effectiveness. A bottleneck is a step in a process that limits the capacity of the system as a whole. For example, if patients are waiting to register with a receptionist while physicians are idle, then patient registration is a bottleneck restricting the flow of patients into examination rooms. Flowcharts of clinic activity point to changes that could improve the effectiveness and efficiency of everyone's work.

Flowcharts are one of the most frequently used improvement tools. But the construction of highly detailed flow charts can be time-consuming and distract teams from accomplishing their goals. Therefore, it is important to agree on when and how to construct a flowchart and what level of detail is needed to achieve the team's goal. Tips on using flowcharts are given in Table 13.2.

Once the team has diagrammed the process of care as it currently exists, it is often easy to see where changes might be made. For example, a team analyzing how to improve diabetes care may realize that only some patients receive educational materials and motivational counselling. In charting the process, the team realizes that different practitioners hand out materials at varying points during the office visit, while some practitioners fail to distrib-ute these materials at all. Making the process visible helps to identify where process changes should be made. By diagramming the care process, team members can discuss the advantages of providing education materials in practitioners' offices or at the reception area after the visit. The flowchart also helps to identify opportunities for motivation enhancement counseling. Process flow diagrams also help teams decide where to collect data and to determine whether these changes have led to improvements in outcomes.

Testing Changes: *The PDSA Cycle*

Work cannot improve unless changes are made in processes. Yet, not all changes yield improvements. How can we safely test new changes to learn which ones actually improve outcomes? The *PDSA (Plan-Do-Study-Act) cycle* provides a simple but powerful method for testing change (Figure 13.3.) This method is useful both for individual changes that improve personal habits and for large-scale changes that improve care for patient groups. The four steps in the PDSA cycle are as follows:

1. **Plan:** Planning the change

2. **Do:** Carrying out the change

3. **Study:** Analyzing the results of the change and comparing them to pre-dictions

4. **Act:** Making changes permanent or identifying new changes to test.

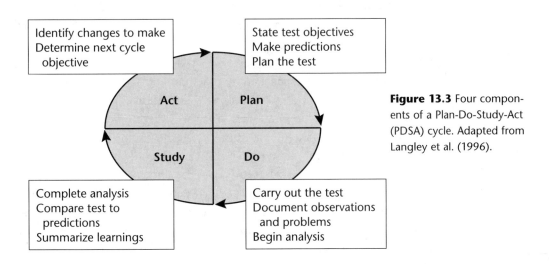

Figure 13.3 Four compon-ents of a Plan-Do-Study-Act (PDSA) cycle. Adapted from Langley et al. (1996).

The simplicity of the *PDSA cycle* makes it easy to learn but also tempts some to reject the process as obvious and not valuable. The *PDSA cycle* is a powerful tool in planning and carrying out change. It provides a way to translate ideas into action by testing improvements and studying the results of these tests. *PDSA cycles* can be used to decide which of several proposed changes will lead to a desired improvement, to evaluate the degree of improvement that results from a specific change, to test whether a change that works in one environment will work in a different setting, and to discover which combination of changes will work best.

In our diabetes example, the Lakeside team may decide to improve patient care by increasing the number of adult diabetes patients who receive foot examinations. Team members agree that practitioners often fail to include foot examinations when examining patients. The team identified a number of different ways to change this behavior: a reminder to practitioners about the need for foot exams, information to practitioners on the number of diabetic patients who had their feet examined, and the creation of an examination checklist attached to the patient's chart. One team member suggested that an easier way to remind practitioners to check feet in the course of the examination would be to have the clinic receptionist request that all diabetic patients remove their shoes and socks, prior to seeing their practitioner. This suggestion created debate among team members about the feasibility of such a change, the difficulty of ensuring that patients were reminded, and whether patients would object to walking around barefoot. While innovative, the idea of creating a visual cue for the practitioner might not work in practice. To test this idea, the team agreed to try it for two weeks. During this time, all diabetic patients would be asked to remove their socks and shoes in the examination room prior to meeting with their practitioner. Receptionists would tally the number of diabetic patients so instructed, and charts would be reviewed to determine the number of these patients whose feet were checked by practitioners. The team would examine the results of this study to determine if this change improved practice.

The four steps of the *PDSA cycle* must be linked. Ignoring one or more steps undermines the usefulness of the tool. One common failure is lack of attention to the 'study' phase of PDSA. In our urgency to move on to new ideas, it is easy to overlook what can be learned from earlier tests of change, including those that did not succeed. This knowledge can be helpful in identifying other changes to test. The study phase is key to rapid learning because individuals and teams that devote time to understanding why ideas work, or don't work, build knowledge about the systems in which they are

Table 13.3   Tips on Using PDSA Cycles to Test Changes

- Try tests on a small scale: identify how small a test can be and still be meaningful.
- Make predictions about the results of each test to identify why the test will be successful.
- Identify the measures you will use to assess whether change is an improvement.
- Take time for reflection on the results of each test of change to identify why the change did not work or how it could work better.
- Plan who will be involved in carrying out the change. Make sure that those responsible can coordinate their activities.

testing changes. Even when changes work, their effects may prove limited or diminish over time. In such cases, we need to identify how to amplify and sustain their results. How could the change be made stronger? Thus, even when a change is only partly successful or unsuccessful, we gain knowledge that can assist in our ongoing efforts.

In the case of foot examinations for diabetic patients, the team may discover that the clinic receptionist is too busy to remember to check if the patient who registers is a diabetic. Is there someone else who might be more effective in carrying out this task? Could the patients be recruited to remind the receptionist? Good ideas often require further reflection and refinement before they work effectively in practice. The *PDSA cycle* provides a quick method for teams to test these ideas in practice. Table 13.3 provides tips on using *PDSA cycles*.

The *PDSA cycle* allows us to improve a system of care step by step. Many individuals and teams who want to change face the obstacle created by their desire to make the 'perfect change'. Rather than trying out a change that may be partially successful, change efforts are often delayed until we are certain that the change will solve the total problem. Unfortunately, this time may never come! The PDSA method encourages us to try changes on a small scale in order to test whether they work, and then to modify these changes and add other changes to improve the results we gain from small scale testing. By 'small-scale', we mean focusing on a limited number of individuals, a small number of patients or a few practitioners, rather than testing across the whole clinic and aiming for results in days or weeks rather than months or years. A lot of knowledge can be gleaned from very small samples.

Teams that use *PDSA cycles* learn how to make changes by engaging in ongoing cycles of testing, studying the results of these tests, and then trying new ideas. The more tests of change, the greater the likelihood that we will learn what works. Beginning on a small scale and then expanding as we learn ensures that the resources needed to test change are minimized, while the learning from these tests of change is rapid. This method of 'learning by doing' is similar to the pattern of clinical learning that practitioners use in their daily practices as they test new approaches for managing problems.

By focusing on small-scale changes and building a reflective study step into the test of each change, the PDSA model offers the opportunity to build knowledge through multiple cycles. For example, the diabetes team at Lakeside is aiming to reduce HbA1C levels among Type II diabetic patients. Some practitioners do not know how many such patients have elevated hemoglobin A1Cs. Thus, the team may focus their first cycle on collecting data on the current HbA1C levels for Type II diabetic patients. Based on this information, the team then decides to learn from a small number of these patients why they have such high hemoglobin A1C levels. The results of this study show a range of reasons including drug non-adherence, lack of exercise, poor diets, and failure to show up for appointments. Instead of trying to solve all these problems, the team decides to try out two different interventions on a small scale to see if they can improve the HbA1C levels for these patients. For the first intervention, the team focuses on the Type II diabetic patients of two practitioners in the clinic. The charts of these patients are reviewed and a list is generated of all patients who have not seen their primary care provider in the last six months. Clinic nurses call 20 of these patients to ask them about their health and to remind them that they need to have regular visits to assess their diabetes. In the second test, carried out concurrently with the first, a group of Type II patients are given glucometers and provided with group instruction on their use. Baseline HbA1C tests are taken, and patients adjust their diets according to the results of their glucometer self-assessments. Each test is tried for three months, and then the team reviews the results of these pilot studies to see if they have an impact on the HbA1C levels of these groups of patients.

Based on the information obtained in each cycle, the team makes a decision about the next test of change. At each cycle, the team must decide whether to abandon this effort (and select a new idea for change), modify the change based on its current performance, increase the scope of the change, or propose its implementation. Table 13.4 provides a worksheet for PDSA cycles that includes a set of questions that teams can use to guide their activities.

Table 13.4   Sample PDSA Worksheet for Documenting a Cycle

Team members: Smith, Wayne, Chang, Morrison & Andrews.

Date begun: February 1, 2001

PLAN

What are the specific aims of the cycle?

To test a new diabetes education booklet that provides information on diet, exercise and smoking behaviors.

What measures do we need to collect to know a change is an improvement?

Measures of patient knowledge, HbA1C levels, blood glucose levels.

What are the predictions about this change?

Patients who receive the booklet will be more knowledgeable about diet, exercise and smoking and will demonstrate better control of their diabetes.

What specific change will be tested?

The booklet will be distributed to patients of Dr. Morrison and Dr. Wayne for the next 3 months. Nurse educators will call the patients a week later to see if there are any questions about the booklet.

Who will do what to carry out the change?

Dr. Morrison and Dr. Wayne will hand out booklet to patients. Booklet will be placed in patient charts by receptionist to be handy to the physicians when they examine diabetic patients.

What tools and training are needed?

None

DO

How will we know that each step of the change is completed?

The receptionist will track the number of booklets distributed to patients each day in a log.

Who will monitor and check the progress of the change?

The diabetes nurse educator will post the data on number of patients given the booklet and current clinical outcomes for the patients.

What are we learning as we change?

We missed several patients who were not identified as diabetes patients.

STUDY/CHECK

What were the results of the test? What did our measures of the test tell us? How do they compare to our predictions?

There was a small improvement in the HbA1C levels of the patients who received the booklets and a change in their knowledge levels. These are in line with our predictions. However, not all patients found the information useful.

If the results were different from our predictions, why do we think they were different?

Some patients did not think that the information applied to them.

What did we learn about the work process we were making changes on?

It is difficult to ensure that patients receive education materials and that they read them.

ACT

Should we abandon this test because it did not work?
No. Some improvement is seen in patients receiving the booklet.

How can we refine the test to improve results?
Some patients may require more information about the risks to them of not changing their behaviors.

What new tests could we try?
Provide information to patients on their HbA1C and blood glucose levels at the same time they receive the pamphlet and at regular times thereafter.

(For successful tests) what do we need to do to ensure that this change can be successfully implemented on a wider scale?
We should continue to test this change before wider implementation.

Adapted from Scholtes (1988, pp.5,46,47); Langley et al (1996, p.62); Nelson et al. (1998).

Collecting and Displaying Data

Groups working on improvement generally need two types of data. First, they need data from the *Clinical Value Compass*, that is, the outcome measures they have selected. These measures provide a concrete set of indicators of progress. Because the *Clinical Value Compass* measures are balanced they also indicate when gains in one type of measure (such as costs per encounter) are achieved at the expense of other types of outcomes (such as lower patient satisfaction or higher blood glucose levels.) Second, teams need data to measure the improvements achieved by the changes they are testing. For example, in tracking and phoning Type II patients who have not had a clinic visit in six months, the measure of change would include the percentage of such patients subsequently seen in the Lakeside clinic. This information is useful in assessing the impact of change and in designing new tests of change.

Once a team has selected its *Clinical Value Compass* measures, the team defines its variables and determines the sources of its data. Operational definitions require clearly specified methods for reliably identifying, classifying and measuring a variable. Specific and clear instructions must be given to data collectors to insure consistency. Plsek (1994) has outlined key questions a team should answer in designing data collection (Table 13.5). Working through these questions ensures that data collection will provide information useful for assessing the results of tests of change.

Table 13.5   Planning for Data Collection

1. What question do we need to answer?
1. What data tools do we envision using?
2. What types of data do we need in order to construct these tools and answer the question?
3. Where in the process can we get the data?
4. Who in the process can give us the data?
5. How can we collect the data from these people with minimum effort and minimum chance of error?
6. What else do we need to capture for future analysis, reference and traceability?

Source: Plsek (1994)

Data are usually recorded on data sheets or check-sheets. A data sheet is any form for recording data that is subsequently analyzed and then interpreted, while a check-sheet is a form that is directly interpreted. Clear directions are necessary to ensure consistent and reliable transfer of information onto these forms.

Once we have decided what question to answer, how to define the measures, and what processes are needed to collect data, it is useful to test

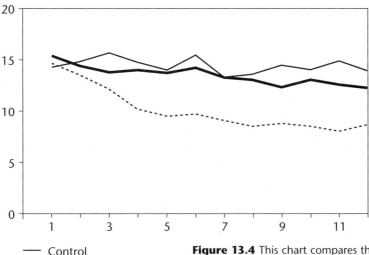

— Control
■ Nurse follow-up
---- Patient self-assessment

Figure 13.4 This chart compares the blood hemoglobin results over 12 months from a control group of diabetic patients with two groups: one where nurses call to remind patients to make clinic appointments, and a second where patients are given glucometers to test their blood sugar levels and monitor their diets where needed..

Table 13. 6 How to Construct and Interpret a Run Chart

A run chart (or line graph, as it also called) is used to examine the pattern of variation in a sequence of measures that vary over time. The run chart makes the variation visual such that a quick examination of the chart will reveal the presence of trends. The run chart can be used with any data that vary over time, such as patient clinical outcomes (blood sugar measures or weight) or utilization measures (numbers of patients seen in a clinic or waiting times for an appointment).

Constructing a Run Chart

Run charts require sets of data that include measures of the variable of interest (e.g., weight) for a specified sequence of time (e.g., weeks.) The data are plotted onto a graph with two perpendicular lines that intersect. The vertical axis show the changes in the variable of interest while the horizontal axis shows the time. Often, it is useful to set the bottom of the vertical axis at 0 to avoid misinterpreting small changes in the vertical axis that are magnified if the overall scale is limited. Data are plotted in time sequence. Both the vertical axis and the horizontal axis should be labeled and the values (units of measures) clearly specified. Provide a title that communicates the data provided in the graph.

Interpreting a Run Chart

The chart should be examined for trends and shifts in measures. However, it is important not to interpret each fluctuation as the result of a single cause (e.g., the training given to receptionists may explain only part of the change in the waiting time for appointments). Variation (fluctuation in the data) usually results from a combination of causes that are difficult to untangle. Moreover, collecting data often draws peoples attention to the variable of interest, creating change.

Runs of eight or more consecutive points on one side of the median indicate an unusual event (a statistically significant change.) Similarly, a sequence of seven or more points continuously increasing or continuously decreasing indicates a trend in the process. (When reviewing graphs for these trends omit entirely any points that repeat the preceding value. Such points do not add to the length of the run, nor do they break it.)

Many practitioners have found that keeping run charts (paper and pencil run charts are often sufficient) on key variables of interest to them helps them identify trends immediately. Similarly, patients can keep run charts of key clinical measures that offer them an easy way to monitor their health.

A more sophisticated graph, the control chart, provides additional information to interpret continuous data.

the process of data collection. For instance, if patient charts are the data source, pull a few charts to see if the information can be easily found.

When you have determined your data source and the means of collecting that data; you must also plan how you will report the data. To make the information as easy to interpret as possible, it is useful to display the data graphically. Run charts (also called line graphs) are particularly useful in displaying data since they show changes in performance over time. An example of a run chart is given in Figure 13.4. This chart shows the results of the two changes tested by the team over 12 months. Run charts can be computer-generated or hand-drawn; they are easy to construct; simple to interpret; and easy to update. Table 13.6 provides important tips on how to construct and interpret run charts. Carey and Lloyd (2001) provide a comprehensive guide to data collection techniques and statistical methods for testing variation using run and control charts.

Linking Improvement Cycles with the Critical Functions Analysis

The *Critical Functions Analysis* CFA (Chapter 12) evaluates an organization's essential supports to practitioners and patients for making health behavior changes. The *Critical Functions Analysis* provides an organization with information about where it is performing well and where additional attention is needed to optimize performance. The *CFA* also provides the organization with ideas that might be used to improve performance. For example, results of the *CFA* in the Lakeside case study, described in Chapter 12, provide suggestions for improving care at that clinic.

Which ideas for change should you address first? Organizations need to prioritize what they want to improve and which potential improvements should be tested. One method for doing this is through multi-voting. Multi-voting is a technique for selecting improvement needs; it takes all members' interests into account. Because they reflect this consensus, selected projects will have the support of the entire team. Instructions for multi-voting are provided in Table 13.7. A second approach for prioritizing the project is to use the Payoff Matrix Analysis (Worksheet 11.5 described in Chapter 11.).

Activities selected through multi-voting need to be assigned to improvement teams. Since staff time is limited, each team should work on

Table 13.7   Multi-Voting

How to conduct a multi-vote on suggestions for improvement from conducting a Critical Functions Analysis CFA (Table 12.3, Chapter 12)

1. First, generate a list of the items (suggestions for improvement) and number each item.

2. If two or more items seem very similar, combine them, but only if the group agrees that they are the same.

3. Each member of the group is given a number of votes equal to one-third of the total number on the list. Members silently select the items they wish to vote for.

4. Carrying out the voting by having each member place a mark next to the items selected (adhesive dots also work well).

5. Tally the number of votes for each item, placing those with the largest number of votes on a new list.

6. Keep the final list as a source of ideas for future projects.

Table 13.8   Getting Started: Tasks for the Team's First Meeting

In getting started, teams need to accomplish the following in their first meeting:

1. Team members need to introduce themselves and learn about the background and experiences of others on the team. These introductions help create a 'team' which can work effectively together. The information gathered should be recorded since it will assist in identifying which members have the skills or knowledge needed for specific tasks. These introductions may also demonstrate that representatives are needed from other areas of the organization.

2. Teams need to review the results of the *Critical Functions Analysis* (Chapter 12) to see the specific comments in the areas they have been asked to work. They also need to identify (and, if possible, review) other information and data on these issues. Team leaders should collect and summarize such materials, circulating them prior to the first meeting.

3. Teams need to develop an aim statement and measures on the *Clinical Value Compass*. The clinical value compass measures will be adapted to the population under study. In selecting these measures, the team needs to identify ways to assess whether the changes it selects and implements lead to improvement in the activities and supports identified by the *Critical Functions Analysis*.

4. Finally, teams need to brainstorm the next steps in their work and create a rough work plan for the team. These next steps, which will be accomplished in the weeks to follow, might include developing a flowchart that provides a view of the process which the team hopes to improve. Additional data may need to be collected. One or more team members may need to assess what data currently exists and what information may be available from sources outside of the organizations. One or more individuals should be assigned responsibility for the task and a date established when the task should be completed.

These four tasks can be accomplished if team members are prepared for this work by circulating an agenda and asking them to prepare for the meeting. The team leader needs to ensure that team members have been given some background information about the diabetes patients. How many are there? What do we know about their current health? Do we see any current opportunities for improvement? What are other organizations doing to improve diabetes care? The goal of this information is to help team members understand why there is a need to focus on diabetes and the extent to which there are unrealized opportunities to improve care.

one or two of these priorities areas. Choose team members with knowledge and responsibilities applicable to the team's area of focus. Each team will need a leader and a facilitator. The team leader manages the team: calls meetings, handles administrative details, oversees preparation of reports and presentations, and acts as the main contact person for the rest of the organization. The team leader should be someone who is very familiar with the organization's work processes, and who is interested in improving the organization's support for health behavior change.

In some organizations team leaders also act as facilitators, helping groups work more effectively with the methods and tools described above. Frequently, organizations select distinct individuals as facilitators. These individuals are experienced in helping groups work effectively and in teaching flowcharting and other tools to team members on a 'just-in-time' basis. Since facilitators focus on helping teams carry out work rather than on contributing knowledge of the work processes, some organizations select facilitators from other departments or divisions.

At the first meeting the team should establish its agenda and its pace of work. Team leaders must demonstrate that the time will be well-spent; that the team's efforts will lead to improved outcomes. First on the agenda is the formation of a clear aim. Following this, the team begins to outline its work; the specific activities it wants to undertake. An initial successful meeting creates momentum for change and an eagerness to identify and test changes that will transform the organization. The team's key tasks for this first meeting are outlined in Table 13.8.

Three Guiding Questions

Rapid cycle improvement provides a method and tools for moving from the evaluations offered by the *Critical Functions Analysis* and other good ideas to improved outcomes. Langley and colleagues (1996) suggest that such improvement be guided by three critical questions:

1. What are we trying to accomplish?

2. How will we know that a change is an improvement?

3. What changes can we make that will result in improvement?

Teams test the changes they select using the Plan-Do-Study-Act method. The methods and tools outlined in this chapter help to answer these questions and to work through *PDSA cycles* (Table 13.9.) Based on their test results, teams may choose to test other changes, to implement the successful change, or to focus on a new area. Worksheet 13.1 (Appendix) can be used as a template for guiding and documenting a change cycle.

While each of these steps seems simple in theory, our experience shows that obtaining results may not be easy. Keeping the aims clear, selecting relatively limited changes, keeping the test times short, reflecting on results, and trying multiple changes concurrently are some of the lessons we've learned by working with teams using these methods. Change initiatives benefit from local champions (practitioners who lend assistance and moral suasion) and senior leaders to clinic managers when, for example, can pro-

Table. 13.9 A Model for Improvement
and Rapid Cycle Improvement Tools

Three Guiding Questions[*]	Methods and Tools
1. What are we trying to accomplish?	Aim Statement Tips for the Team's First Meeting Multi-Voting
2. How will we know a change is an improvement?	*Clinical Value Compass* Flowchart Run charts
3. What changes can we make that will result in improvement?	*Critical Functions Analysis* Experience Research Literature Guidelines
Testing Change	*PDSA Cycles* *PDSA Worksheet* Data sheet Run charts

[*]For discussion of the three questions see Langley, Nolan, & Nolan (1994) .

vide resources, remove barriers and stimulate opportunities for change. A list of additional resources that can help teams carry out this improvement work follows.

Additional Resources on QI Tools

Batalden and Stoltz (1993), Bemowski and Stratton (1998), Berwick (1998), Brassard and Joiner (1995), Brassard and Ritter (1994), Institute for Healthcare Improvement (1996), Joiner (1994), Juran Institute (1989), Langley, Nolan, and Nolan (1994), Leebov and Ersoz (1991), Nelson, Splaine, Batalden, and Plume (1998), Tague (1995), Wheeler (1993).

Moving On

So far our presentation of the Five-Step Model has emphasized what is needed for changing and transforming the organization. Yet, the process of initiating change also activates counterforces of resistance to this change. The next chapter addresses how you can sustain the momentum and anchor change by applying the Five Steps in successive cycles.

WORKSHEET 13.1 Guiding Questions for Documenting a Change Cycle

Team members: _____

Date begun: _____

_____

Plan
_____

What are the specific aims of the cycle?

What measures do we need to collect to know a change is an improvement?

What predictions do we make about this change?

What is the specific change that will be tested?

Who will do what to carry out the change?

What tools and training are needed?

_____

Do
_____

How will we know that each step of the change is completed?

Who will monitor and check the progress of the change?

What are we learning as we do the change?

Study/Check

What were the results of the test? What did our measures of the test tell us? How do they compare to our predictions?

If the results were different from our predictions, why do we think they were different?

What did we learn about the work process we were making changes on?

Act

Should we abandon this test because it did not work?

How can we refine the test to improve results?

What new tests could we try?

(For successful tests) what do we need to do to ensure that this change can be successfully implemented on a wider scale?

CHAPTER *14*

Sustaining the Momentum for Positive Change

Every movement is being inhibited as it occurs.

—Humberto Maturana

Overview

Your organization has embarked on an ambitious journey of improvement in behavior change, using the Five-Step Model as a guide. But, after some initial successes ('picking the low hanging fruit'), enthusiasm wanes and your progress falters. You need to attend to an oft-neglected area, slippage or motivational drift. How do you stay the course?

This chapter outlines the dynamics of complex adaptive systems and the inherent challenges of sustaining change. It describes how to apply the Five-Step Model through successive iterations to keep the organization focused on improvement and maintenance.

Managing the Downside of Change

Kurt Lewin (1951) provides a lucid metaphor for understanding the organizational change cycle. The challenge is to thaw the current mode of operations, transform the organizational processes and structures, and then freeze the organization in this new form (Table 14.1). Usually, organizational thawing and transformation of this sort requires much personal energy but also generates a lot of emotional heat! Early results may be impressive, but will they last? There is a tendency for many organizations to stop at this juncture. Others get sidetracked and move on to another initiative.

High performing organizations, on the other hand, ensure that the gains from improvement initiatives are sustained. This is essential to completing the cycle of change facilitated by the Five-Step Model (see Figure 1.2).

243

Table 14.1   Leading and Sustaining Change

1. Unfreezing

Establish a sense of urgency

Create a guiding coalition

Develop a vision and strategy

Communicate the vision for change

2. Transformation

Empower broad-based action

Generate short term wins

Consolidate gains

Stimulate more change

3. Freezing

Identify positive (supports) and negative (barriers) forces

Develop strategies for sustaining change

Adapt the organizational structure (rewards)

Anchor new approach in the culture

Adapted from Kotter (1996) and Lewin (1951)

We often underestimate how difficult it is to make change last. Indeed, under normal circumstances most individuals and organizations have only limited capacity or energy to focus on, let alone achieve, substantial change. This capacity, our 'change space', is depicted in Figure 14.1. The key to making change last is to unstick the old behavior in our 'habit space', move into our change space where our old behavior is transformed, and then embed (freeze) that new behavior once again in our habit space. To learn the new behavior, we need to make the most efficient use of the limited energy available in our change space.

For example, consider the typical experience of dieting as a way of achieving healthy weight control. Many people try the latest fad diet, often lose weight initially, but have real difficulty maintaining their goal. Few succeed for any length of time despite the claims and missionary zeal of proponents of the latest diet. Why does the maintenance of a healthy weight ellude most dieters? Most regimens overemphasize weight *loss*, when they need to pay far more attention to healthy weight *maintenance*. Maintaining a healthy weight requires learning new behaviors that are

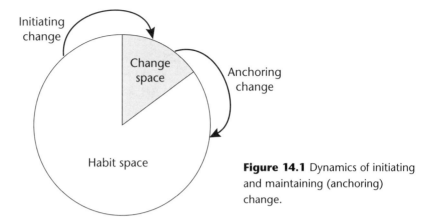

Figure 14.1 Dynamics of initiating and maintaining (anchoring) change.

embedded in one's habit space (e.g., balanced diet, smaller portions, regular exercise).

Similar dynamics are at work in health organizations. For instance, a common approach to stimulating change is to undertake a strategic planning exercise. Initially, staff enter the exercise with enthusiasm stimulated by the passion of the team leader. A new aim is articulated, goals are set, analyses of stakeholder interests and environmental scans result in a number of strategic directions (see Chapter 11), and an action plan is mapped out. This planning exercise often culminates in a retreat in a pleasant surrounding some distance from the day-to-day pressures of the organization. Staff feel energized and return to the organization with intentions to carry out the plan.

They make some initial progress. But gradually the change effort loses momentum as staff get caught up in their day-to-day responsibilities and pressures. Things drift back to the way they 'always were' with few signs of improvement. Younger staff feel frustrated, while veterans shrug their shoulders—"We've seen this before!"

The lesson: In any improvement initiative, give early and ongoing attention to both the barriers and supports (e.g., reinforcements) needed to maintain change. Use Worksheet 14.1 at the end of this chapter to guide this analysis and identify solutions.

Understanding Complexity

Heath care organizations are complex adaptive systems. This is quite evident when you walk into a busy clinic, attend a staff meeting on a heated issue, or develop a process flowchart of patient encounters. Complexity is especially striking whenever you try to change the system. Insights from complexity science (or chaos theory) help explain why many change programs fail to produce change that sticks. Some key references on complexity science in health care include: Goldberger (1996), Waldrop (1992), Dooley and Johnson (1995), Stacey (1996) and Zimmerman et al. (1998). Also, visit the Santa Fe Institute website (*www.santafe.edu*), which is a center of complexity science. An up-to-date listing of complexity websites is compiled by VHA (*www.vha.com*).

Lifecycles. Zimmerman et al. (1998) describe four lifecycles of organizations: birth (exploration), maturity (conservation) creative destruction, and renewal (mobilization). This model is useful for appreciating and understanding the natural cycles that organizations go through. Considerable attention has been given to the S-curve, which describes the birth, growth and maturity phases of an organization's history. This analysis, however, is incomplete. Organizations are complex systems that can also adapt through phases of partial destruction and renewal.

The history of IBM is a classic example of organizational transformation through five major eras (*www.ibm.com/ibm/history*). Incorporated in 1911 as the Computing-Tabulating-Recording company, IBM began with the manufacture of tabulating machines for census data. During the Great Depression of the 1930s, IBM prospered while others floundered by using innovative business tactics and stressing the importance of the customer. During and after World War II, IBM reinvented itself, taking first steps toward electronic computers: the IBM 701 in 1952 was the first large computer based on vacuum tubes, and the IBM 7090 in 1959 was the first fully transistorized mainframe. Then, in 1964, the System/360 was introduced as the first large computer to use interchangeable software and peripherals (e.g., magnetic tape and disk drives). However, in the 1970s IBM lost ground with the advent of minicomputers (e.g., VAX by Digital).

IBM rebounded in 1981 with its personal computer (64k RAM and $5\frac{1}{4}$ inch floppy disk), but IBM struggled. It was slow to appreciate the fundamental shift underway in the PC era as computers were being placed in the hands of millions of people. IBM lost ground to upstart companies such as COMPAQ and Apple. Then, in 1993, IBM for the first time in its history found a new leader, Louis Gerstner, from outside its ranks. He was able to transform IBM's focus from a producer of hardware to providing integrated services and networked computing. This has positioned the company well for the Internet revolution—or at least it seems so at present.

IBM illustrates how a high performing organization goes through cycles of birth, maturity, creative destruction through loss of market share, and then a renewal process focusing on new aspects of the industry. The rise, re-invention and current dilemmas of Apple or Intel provide other examples of complex adaptive organizations undergoing lifecycle transformations.

Health care organizations are undergoing similar dynamics, challenged by rapid developments in technology, changes in population diversity and needs, rising costs, and globalization (cf., Chapter 2). The lifecycle model provides a useful heuristic for understanding the dynamics of health organizations over time.

Two Organizations in One. Stacey (1996) argues that organizations actually consist of two organizations: the **legitimate system** which includes the formal hierarchy, rules and roles, and the **shadow system** denoted by the informal, behind the scenes, power networks and communication grapevines. The legitimate system is the public face as depicted on the organizational chart and described in the mission statement, the *words*. In contrast, the shadow system reflects *deeds*—how the organization gets things done through the informal power structures, brokers and hallway communication systems. This distinction is very important for gaining a deeper understanding of how the organization truly works. The shadow system is often where much of the organization's creativity and resistance reside. Just listen to the conversational buzz in the cafeteria, where staff discuss good ideas on how to turn the organization upside down!

How the legitimate and shadow aspects interact influences the organization's capacity for the type of change discussed in Chapter 2. When the legitimate and shadow systems are aligned, the organization is most capable of incremental improvement (level one) change (Argyris et al., 1985; Watzlawick et al., 1974). When they are operating against each other, the organization is on the verge of chaos and is capable of transformative (level two) change and creativity (Plsek, 1997).

Motivational Drift. In complex systems, the forces (Figure 14.2) that drive positive change (individual motivation and organizational supports) are counterbalanced by negative forces (individual resistance and organizational barriers). When the positive forces for change succeed, the negative forces must still be kept at bay; the organization must resist slippage or motivational drift by keeping the organization focused on sustaining improvement.

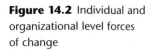
Figure 14.2 Individual and organizational level forces of change

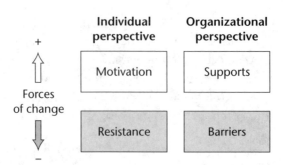

Senge et al. (1999) highlight the need in systems dynamics to deal not only with the growth processes but also with the limiting processes. Most change initiatives emphasize what is needed for improving and transforming the organization. Far less attention is directed at preventing drift and maintaining gains. Systems theory emphasizes the interconnections among forces that either drive or impede change: the positive and negative forces in Figure 14.2. The very process of initiating change also activates counterforces and resistance to change.

Senge et al. (1999) describe 10 such challenges and provide a wealth of strategies for addressing them (Table 14.2).

Sustaining and anchoring change in organizational improvement depends on fully addressing these challenges up front, in the planning of an improvement initiative. High performing organizations use multistep processes that create sufficient direction and energy to overcome inertia and resistance; they deal with the limiting or negative forces (Figure 14.2).

Leading Change

Kotter (1996) describes an eight-stage process for leading change that is summarized and expanded in Table 14.1. He draws a fundamental distinction between leadership (inspirational vision) and management (controls and attention to details). Success requires attention to both—the left and right hands of an organization working in harmony.

The initial challenge is to generate motivation and energy for change. One strategy for generating a sense of urgency is to use the Lily Pad exercise described in Chapter 9; this is a way of getting the organization unstuck. The change initiative itself needs to be led by a core group (guiding coalition) that can work together effectively and has the mandate and tools to accomplish the task. A key element for creating motivation and momentum for change is to create a vision that is broadly communicated

Table 14.2   Ten Challenges for Producing Change
and Strategies to Overcome Them

Challenges of Initiating

- We don't have enough time for working on this change.
- We need more help (coaching and support).
- This change isn't relevant to me.
- Leaders talk about change but don't demonstrate it by their behavior.

Challenges of Sustaining Transformation

- We feel exposed and anxious about this change.
- What happens if it doesn't work (negative assessment)?
- We are already doing it right.

Challenges of Redesigning and Rethinking

- Who is really in charge of this?
- How do we communicate success so others can build on it?
- Where is this change leading us?

Source: Senge et al., (1999)

and then shared by the group. A compelling vision involves a 'stretch' between where the organization is now and where you want it to be (use *Your Organizational Prototype* tool, Chapter 9). These first four elements are part of unfreezing the organization.

The next four elements address the transformation phase. Obstacles are addressed and support systems and structures are put in place to guide the changed vision. Emphasis is placed on generating short-term gains by selecting improvement opportunities that will be relatively easy to implement yet offer high impact (use Worksheet 11.5 in Chapter 11). Initial gains are consolidated, important lessons are learned, and the guiding coalition continues its focus on producing more change, especially change entailing improvement initiatives that may be more difficult to implement yet offer great benefits to the organization.

Following successful transformation, the organization now focuses on sustaining or freezing the gains made from improvement initiatives. Careful attention needs to be given to individual and organizational barriers and the reinforcements needed for maintaining change (e.g., timely and individualized feedback to practitioners and managers, communication of improved services to stakeholders including patients and funders).

Case Study

Approximately two years after the merger of the Lakeside and PMB Family Practice Centers to form the new Pacific Health Services (described in Chapter 9), a colleague visited Dr. B. Over dinner the colleague asked, *"How are things going in the new organization?"* Dr. B. spoke about some early successes, enhancing preventive and clinical services as well as providing a broader academic training site for the local university.

Then, she shared her frustrations. Implementing a much-heralded computerized patient booking, medical record and tracking system was way behind schedule. She couldn't keep a good information technology manager, and even the consultants kept changing. Staff where complaining that this new 'sophisticated' system was actually inferior to the old one.

Also, Dr. B. recounted events from a stalled effort to recruit a physician for a new role in expanding their community outreach activities. Although there was apparent agreement on the position description prior to the search, a review of potential candidates created an uneasy split among members of the search committee. Members aligned with their previous organizations (Lakeside versus PMB). This test of a broader vision for the new center revealed that considerable ground had been lost. The enthusiasm expressed by staff at their planning retreat 12 months ago had waned, and their efforts at improvement had faltered.

Although, when viewed from a high level after the merger, Pacific Health Services appeared to be functioning well, significant problems were still evident in the swamp of day-to-day activities. Dr. B. was encountering major challenges in sustaining momentum.

Anchor Change with the Five-Step Model

The Five-Step Model provides resources, a guide, and a toolbox for achieving success on the demanding journey into continuous improvement. Yet, these steps by themselves are not enough—to achieve organizational renewal the complete model must be applied through successive iterations.

Step 1 underscores the need to build motivation throughout all levels of the organization. Thereby the organization fosters support and reduces barriers for maintaining renewal efforts over the long term. Step 2 considers whether the organization has the requisite capacities (ACTSS dimensions) in place and is ready for the journey. These capacities for organizational improvement are also fundamental for sustaining gains and dealing with organizational drift. Versatile tools such as the *Stakeholder Needs, SWOT* and *Payoff Matrix Analyses* described in Step 3 keep the organization's external and internal environments aligned for achieving strategic directions in prevention and behavioral health care. Repeated applications of the *Critical Functions Analysis,* Step 4, will generate 'high leverage' ideas for improvement, whereupon the rapid cycle change model, Step 5, gives a practical and powerful way to achieve them.

Thus, the real power of the Five-Step Model derives from the mutual reinforcement of macro- and microlevel systems in the organization. For instance, efforts to ensure that organization-wide capacities are in place for supporting improvement increases the likelihood that a specific *PDSA Rapid Cycle* initiative at a microlevel will be successful. This *PDSA Cycle* success, when widely publicized, feeds back to enhance overall commitment to continuous improvement in the organization.

An organization is successful at sustaining performance over the long haul when change gets rooted in its norms and values (habit space of Figure 14.1). This entails a fundamental shift in organizational culture. Three activities for fostering an organizational culture that are conducive to ongoing, long-term improvement include:

1. **Leadership:** Openly talk about the renewed purpose of the organization (division, department or unit), and take steps to reinforce values underlying the new approach.

2. **Teamwork:** Build trust, cohesion and cooperation through a climate that reinforces mutual respect, open communication and group results.

3. **Feedback and Rewards:** Provide group and individualized feedback on results showing that new approaches work better than old practices, and reward sustained accomplishments, not just short-term results.

Visit Our WebSite.

As described in Chapter 19, we have developed an Internet website that you can access at: *http://www.HealthBehaviorChange.org*. This website is designed to be your 'virtual' partner in organizational renewal. Try it out!

The website provides self-directed learning resources and workshops where you can advance your knowledge and skills in using the concepts and tools from the Five-Step Model. Of particular note is the *Discussion*

Board where you can interact with the author and others engaged in organizational improvement. This forum serves as a timely way to work and learn together using the book's tools. For example, you can join a study group that is conducting a *Critical Functions Analysis* of its organization. This will enable you to share questions and experiences in a group with others who are tackling similar problems.

Keep a Long Term Perspective

Amid the initial enthusiasm for improving organizations, one can easily lose track of how difficult it is to produce the fundamental change that is needed in health care today (Chapter 2). Substantially increasing prevention and behavioral health care from both a clinical and public health perspective will be a 'stretch' for most organizations. This transformation of health organizations to *'Promoting Health'* will take a long-term commitment spanning 5 to 10 years. The commitment will need to outlast initial leaders and be carried forward in the vision and core values of the organization. Otherwise, gains from specific improvement initiatives (e.g., PDSA cycles) will evaporate and staff will become disillusioned.

Wisdom gained from the World Health Organization's European Healthy Cities Project (1992) is germane. In reviewing this experience, Hancock (1993, p.12) underscores the need to take a long-term perspective in producing fundamental change:

> It is important to realize that change takes time: perhaps two to four years to change structures and processes, three to six years to develop healthy policies, four to eight years to create healthy settings, and five to ten years to see this reflected in health gains. This is because it takes time to overcome political concern, bureaucratic tradition, community scepticism, professional resistance, and the scarcity of resources.

Moving On

We are in the midst of rapid developments in information technology, including the Internet and beyond. This is having profound influences on how the public and health care providers access health information and how patients interact with practitioners and health organizations. As well, information technology offers new channels or sites for the delivery of services (e-Health). The next section provides an overview of these developments with particular attention to opportunities for increasing prevention and behavioral health care.

Worksheet 14.1 Sustaining Organizational Improvement

Positive Forces	Strategies
a) Individual motivations: *list three*	*Describe options for building on each*
b) Organizational supports: *list three*	

Negative Forces	Strategies
a) Individual resistance: *list three*	*Describe options for addressing each*
b) Organizational barriers: *list three*	

Part Three

e-Health: The New Role of Information Technology

80% of the Technologies that we will still be using 20 years from now have yet to be invented.

—Prediction by many futurists

CHAPTER 15

Information Technology to Support Practitioners and Patients

Technology Must Be More Useful Than Dazzling

Don't get too caught up in technology, while ignoring the people who use it. You get so enamoured in the technology and its capabilities, you forget to sit back and ask why someone else would care.

—Peter Eddison, Fulcrum Technologies

Overview

We are in the early stages of e-Health: a fundamental transformation of how health information and health care are delivered using information technology. Comprehensive systems are available for key processes such as prompting patients and practitioners, automated records, patient tracking, and timely feedback to patients and practitioners. These systems are typically 'in house'. However, the explosive development of Internet technology has ushered in a new era of linkages and networks locally, nationally and internationally. Both patients and practitioners can access comprehensive health information on the Web, and innovative models are being tested for the delivery of health services online. In this chapter, we provide an overview of advances in information technology that are relevant to the seven critical functions (Chapter 12) and health behavior change. In particular, we focus on using the Internet for organizational change, telemedicine and telehealth applications.

Subsequently, Chapter 16 takes an in-depth look at the use of expert systems, such as *Pathways To Change*, for tailoring behavior change interventions to the person's readiness for change. Chapter 17 illustrates the use of the Internet for health applications with youth, through a description of websites developed by the TeenNet project. Finally, Chapter 18 examines the immense potential and current applications of the Internet for self-help and mutual aid. Also, guidelines are given for helping consumers navigate and assess quality of health information on the Internet.

e-Health: The Future of Health Care

We have crossed the threshold into a whole new 'site' for health care and health promotion termed electronic based e-Health or cybermedicine. Eysenbach et al. (1999) describe cybermedicine as "the science of applying Internet and global networking technologies to medicine and public health". It is estimated that by 2010 more than 30% of physicians' time will be spent using information technology (IT) tools and more than 20% of in-office visits will be eliminated as patients communicate and are monitored using the Internet (PriceWaterhouseCoopers, 1999a).

More and more, the Internet is being used as a key source of health information by both public and practitioners. Reviews of this fast breaking field are given in the *Networking Health* report by the U.S. National Research Council (2000) and the *Future of the Internet* by Mittman and Cain (1999). *The British Medical Journal* (*http://bmj.com*) and *Journal of the American Medical Association* (*http://jama.ama-assn.org*) are also good sources of reviews and empirical studies on information technology and health care.

Rapid Growth

The Internet has grown rapidly since the development and spread of e-mail and the World Wide Web. Indeed, the Internet has grown much faster than any other media format in history. For example, it took 30 years for radio and 15 for television to reach an audience of 60 million people. It has taken the Internet a mere five years to do the same. In fact, during the past three years (1997–2000) alone a total of 100 million new users went online. New cross platform access points, such as Web-ready cellular phones, are expected to grow even faster with one billion users predicted by 2003, surpassing for the first time the total usage of personal computers (Carroll & Broadhead, 1999).

Despite this technological growth, the oldest and perhaps simplest application, e-mail, remains the most popular Internet tool. Estimates for the year 2000 suggest that on a typical day 10 billion e-mail are sent across the globe. This is expected to explode to upwards of 35 billion per day by the year 2005 (IDC, 2000).

The Internet is and will be increasingly international as it grows. In the year 2000, for the first time ever the number of international users outpaced North American users. It is predicted that by 2003 Chinese will surpass English as the most commonly used language on the Net (Carroll and Broadhead, 1999). As of September 2000, there were an estimated 377.65 million users worldwide. Here is how they break down by region (NUA, 2000):

Africa	3.11 million
Asia/Pacific	89.68 million
Europe	105.89 million
Middle East	2.40 million
Canada & U.S.	161.31 million
Latin America	15.26 million
TOTAL	**377.65 million**

To keep on top of the latest Internet usage statistics worldwide, the best current source of information is NUA, an Irish nonprofit organization that is the world leader in Internet-usage surveys (*http://www.nua.ie/surveys/how many online/index.htm*).

Health Applications

The success of health organizations is fundamentally influenced by the way they manage communication. Successful organizations value contributions and sharing of ideas from all members (practitioners, administration, support staff) and clients (patients, communities, funders, regulators). Information technology, especially the Internet, offers significant benefits for improving communication and developing innovations that produce behavior change. Several Health Maintenance Organizations (HMOs) have explored providing 'infoscriptions' (approved health information sources online) to ensure that their insured patients are receiving good quality and reliable information (Goedert, 1997; Morrissey, 1997).

The U.S. National Research Council (2000) report draws seven major conclusions regarding health applications of the Internet (Table 15.1). Although the Internet can support a diverse range of applications, the study concluded that security, quality and access are critical needs that are not being met by today's Internet. Also, the study found that many health organizations are not well-prepared to adopt Internet-based applications.

An Internet site connecting units within and outside the health organization can provide 'one-stop information shopping' for practitioners and patients alike. However, accessing computerized information is only a first step. The real power of information technology lies in its ability to connect individuals and programs in ways that stimulate sharing and mixing of ideas (Milio, 1996). This fosters creativity and excellence in achieving quality performance. The Internet takes this process to new heights by enabling information sharing and idea mixing on a scale previously not possible. It provides an environment that is graphically appealing, anonymous, nonjudgmental, mutually supportive, accessible 24 hours a day, and paced at the user's speed (Paperny, 1997; Thomas et al., 1997; Turner et al., 1997).

The Future Today

Internet-based services such as interactive voice and video-phone technology will link practitioner and patients in an ongoing, dynamic relationship. Patients and practitioners will have access to high-quality health information and computerized records across multiple sites: hospitals, primary care, and home. Patients' health status will be closely monitored using assessment systems, which incorporate evidence-based guidelines for managing risk behavior and chronic disease. Patients will have access to their records at any time and can leave questions for their practitioners. Practitioners will receive updates on the changing characteristics of individual patients and patient groups based on risk behavior (e.g., cigarette smoking) or disease state (e.g., diabetes). As well as providing relevant health information, these technologies can provide motivational interventions to assist patients and practitioners in behavior change (see Chapters 16, 17 and 18).

These technologies will provide ongoing, individualized feedback to both practitioners and patients in ways that continuously improve quality of care and system performance. Practitioners will have feedback about their performance and their patients' outcomes, and they can compare this to others within their own setting, locally, regionally, or nationally. Patients will also have access to performance indicators so they can then make informed decisions about selecting a health care practitioner and organization. The following example illustrates how information technology can influenced the behavior of both the patient and practitioner.

Case Study

For several years Dr. S. at the Lakeside Family Practice Center has been treating Mr. D., a 35-year-old self-employed electrician, for recurrent gout. Mr. D. misses a few days of work with each episode of gout. Just before his doctor's appointment, Mr. D. is asked to complete a *Computerized Lifestyle Assessment,* or CLA (Skinner, 1994). This self-administered assessment takes 20–30 minutes and provides both graphic feedback and a printed report of strengths and areas of concern, risk, or both.

When Mr. D. sees Dr. S., the first thing he says is, *"You know, this thing tells me that I'm overweight, and I'm not sure about that."* He was puzzled by the assessment. Dr. S. reviews the CLA feedback and explains what the Body Mass Index (BMI) means. He then asks Mr. D. *"What do you think?"*

Mr. D.'s view changes. He starts talking about how he might lose weight: *"I probably could lose at least 10 or 15 pounds ..."* and he continues, *"Well, you know, I could ask my wife not to put dessert in with my lunch."* Mr. D. starts off puzzled by the CLA assessment that describes him as overweight. By the end, he understands that his weight is a health concern.

Dr. S. appreciates the CLA assessment of Mr. D.'s risk behaviors and its objective feedback about his health. The CLA saved Dr. S. time by identifying Mr. D.'s health issues, and it helped Mr. D., rather than his doctor, set the agenda for discussion.

This example shows how CLA facilitated the identification and discussion of body weight as a health concern for this patient. The provision of immediate and personalized feedback, using both computer graphics and printed reports, primed the patient to talk about this sensitive issue with his doctor. Also, the CLA prompted the doctor to address body weight as a risk behavior. This sets the stage for motivational counselling and follow-up at subsequent appointments.

Matching Technology to Your Needs

Information technology can fundamentally support health promotion and delivery of health care at individual, organizational and population levels. However, the scope and pace of technological development presents a challenge for deciding which technology to use, for which purpose, with which population, and in which setting. A study by the U.S. National Research Council (2000) has found that many health organizations are not well prepared to adopt Internet-based applications. And although the Internet can

Table 15.1   Main Conclusions from U.S. National Research Council (2000) Study on the Internet and Health Applications

CONCLUSIONS

Conclusion 1. The Internet can support a wide range of applications in consumer health, clinical care, health care financial and administrative transactions, public health, professional education, and biomedical research. The networking capabilities needed to support these applications are not unique, but they do reflect distinctive characteristics of the health environment.

Conclusion 2. Security and availability are critical technical needs for health applications of the Internet and are not adequately met by today's Internet.

Conclusion 3. The quality of service needed by a number of high-end health applications will not necessarily be deployed soon across the Internet in a form that meets the needs of the health industry.

Conclusion 4. Ensuring widespread access to the Internet is essential to achieving its promise in health applications.

Conclusion 5. Technical advances are needed across many areas of information technology (not just networking) if the potential of the Internet is to be achieved in support of health applications.

Conclusion 6. Health care organizations are ill-prepared to adopt Internet-based technologies and applications effectively.

Conclusion 7. A number of difficult public policy and regulatory issues constrain the adoption of Internet-based health applications by health organizations and consumers. Some of these issues are specific to the health sector; many others extend beyond the health sector but require the health community's active participation in their resolution.

support a diverse range of applications, the study concluded that security, quality and access are critical needs not being met by today's Internet. The seven major conclusions by the U.S. National Research Council regarding health applications of the Internet are outlined in Table 15.1.

The Seven Critical Functions Model described in Chapter 12 can help you match technology to your prevention and behavioral health care needs. The following section highlights various applications of information technology according to each critical function (Table 15.2).

Professional Development in Behavior Change and Disease Management

In general, technologies that support professional development focus on the individual level rather than the organizational level. There are numerous examples of Internet-based programs used for continuing education and training. Computer technology can be used to facilitate access to sources of medical knowledge and information, providing details on relevant courses, events and conferences and access to current journal articles (e.g., MEDLINE, Cochrane Collaboration Systematic reviews).

Table 15.2   Technology Options for the Seven Critical Functions

---

1. PROFESSIONAL DEVELOPMENT

Internet Web-based modules for training and/or instruction purposes

Computer conferencing for open discussions among health care providers

E-mail for one-to-one and one-to-many communication and information dissemination

Facsimile messages for information dissemination

Distance learning using satellite-based delivery of training courses or cable television 'narrowcasting'

Computerized medical records may be linked to MEDLINE and other sources of medical information

---

2. PRIMING AND PROMPTING

Computer-based health tracking or medical record systems that generate regular provider and/or patient reminders for preventive care procedures. For example:

   HTRAK – Tri-County Family Medicine, N.Y.

   Check-Up – American Cancer Society

   Practice Partner – Physician Microsystems Inc., Seattle, WA

   Cancer Prevention Reminder System – University of California, San Francisco

---

3. IDENTIFICATION

Internet- and computer-based interactive interviews; can be administered in the clinical setting or by telephone (using interactive voice response technology) and can be used for assessment of various risk factors/conditions

   Computerized Lifestyle Assessment (Skinner, 1994)

   PRIME-MD computer administered version of Primary Care Evaluation of Mental Disorders (Kobak et al., 1997)

Computerized medical records for identification of health issues that require attention

   Care4th Medical Record System (Med4th Systems Limited, Milwaukee, WI)

   Practice Partner Patient Record System (Physician Microsystems, Inc., Seattle, WA)

---

4. CONTINUING CARE

Telephone care as a substitute for routine clinic consultation and/or follow-up.

Interactive voice technology, such as the Telephone-Linked-Care (TLC) system that monitors patients with chronic diseases, health behavior counselling and care-giver support (Friedman et al., 1997)

Telephone follow-up for elderly, ambulatory patients in a general internal medicine clinic (Wasson et al., 1992)

'Phone-in Clinic' replacing in-person consults and home visits in a general practice setting (Brown & Armstrong, 1995)

---

5. LINKAGES

Computer networks for distance linkages, such as long-distance consults using interactive video technology (Crump & Pfeil, 1995).

   Kansas University Medical Center – distance consults for rural areas using interactive video technology

   Texas Tech MedNet – connects 37 counties in west Texas to Texas Tech Health Sciences Center (for information provision and dissemination, consultation and diagnostic services and continuing education)

6. OPTIONS

Behavior change programs tailored to readiness for change, such as the *Pathways To Change* system (Chapter 14) and CyberIsle website (Skinner, 2000)

Patient education software on health issues such as asthma, diabetes, and hypertension (Krishna et al., 1997)

Computer-based networks that provide health information and communication services (provider-patient and patient-to-patient communication)

ComputerLink – a public computer network that provides users with an electronic encyclopedia of illness-specific information, communication services (electronic bulletin board and e-mail) and a decision-support system

Canadian Health Network – like ComputerLink, this Canadian network, provides users with access to information on a variety of health issues and with communication services (online forums, electronic bulletin board)

CHESS – an information, communication and decision-support network for patients with HIV

Stanford Health-Net – a computer-based health promotion network including e-mail, electronic bulletin board, information and referral listings and a self-help information library

7. INFORMATION MANAGEMENT

Computer-based health tracking systems or computerized medical records can allow ready access to patients' risk factor profiles and health status.

Data from the computerized medical record can be used to generate a Health Maintenance Report for specific patients (Nilasena et al., 1994)

Computerized medical records can be used for monitoring at the organizational and individual provider levels, thereby facilitating the feedback process. Information may be made available to both health care providers and to clients.

Computerized medical record systems such as **Practice Partner** (Physician Microsystems, Inc.) or **Care4th** (Med4th Systems Ltd.) can provide data on practice patterns of health care providers which, in turn, can be used for providing feedback.

Health Plan Employer Data Information Set (HEDIS 2.0) – a project of the National Committee for Quality Assurance (a nonprofit accrediting body for managed care organizations) aimed at producing organizational 'report cards' for customers.

The Cochrane Library is an electronic data base and publication (available on CD-ROM and via the Internet) set up to provide access to evidence-based research reports and guidelines for persons providing and receiving care; those involved in research, teaching, and funding; and administrators at all levels. The Cochrane Collaboration has developed in response to a call by Archie Cochrane, a British epidemiologist, for systematic up-to-date reviews of evidence-based research. The Cochrane Centre was initially opened in 1993 at Oxford University. Since then, it has rapidly evolved into a comprehensive international organization. Primary contacts for the Cochrane Library websites are:

■ United Kingdom: *http://www.cochrane.co.uk*

- United States: *http://www.updateusa.com/clibhome/clib.htm*
- Canada: *http://hiru.mcmaster.ca/cochrane*

The Cochrane Centre now includes centers in 15 countries with 6000 members working in over 50 topic-based review groups; these include cancer, child health, primary health care, complementary medicine, health care of older people, physical therapies and rehabilitation, vaccines, and quantitative and qualitative research methods.

While the Internet continues to grow as a source of information for professional development, the Internet's multimedia and communication technologies are changing the structure of professional development. For example, electronic mail has increased and accelerated communications between caregivers, while computer conferencing and satellite technology have made distance learning a feasible alternative to the traditional method of classroom or lecture-based teaching. Table 15.3 provides a list of websites for continuing education and clinical guidelines.

Priming and Prompting of Patients and Practitioners

Computer-based health tracking and medical systems initially introduced to assist with billing, may be used to record data on preventive services provided to patients and for generating reminders for practitioners to provide follow-up and/or preventive care services. At present, information technology is used primarily for practitioner and staff prompting. Only a few applications described in the literature allow patients to use information technology to prime and prompt health-related activities.

Computer technology can tailor information to specific patient needs, preferences, and even cognitive style of learning (Bental et al., 1999; Bull et al., 1999; Dijkstra & De Vries, 1999; Jimison, 1997; Strecher, 1999; Street & Rimal, 1997). Strecher (1999) reviewed 10 randomized trials of tailored smoking cessation materials and found that 6 of the 9 interventions that promoted smoking cessation across stages of change had positive effects.

Identification of Risk Behaviors and Illness-Related Complications

A computer-based interactive interview can identify health risk behaviors and illness-related complications. This is the major technology currently supporting screening activities. The *Computerized Lifestyle Assessment* (Skin-

Table 15.3   Selected Websites for Professional Development

ELECTRONIC PUBLICATIONS

Directory of Scholarly and Professional E-Conferences

http://www.n2h2.com/KOVACS/index.html

Emory MEDWEB: Electronic Publications

http://WWW.MedWeb.Emory.Edu/MedWeb/

Browse under the keyword *Electronic Publications* for an extensive list of links to electronic publications sorted by subject

WebMedLit

http://www.webmedlit.com/

Monitors a number of medical journal websites, providing links to the updates sorted by topic

British Medical Journal

http://www.bmj.com

Provides up-to-date access to the weekly medical journal in an online format; includes options for choosing topics that you can be e-mail updated each week as new resources appear

INFORMATION ON CME EVENTS AND COURSES

AMA's CME Locator

http://www.ama-assn.org/iwcf/iwcfmgr206/cme

Provides access to a data base of continuing medical education activities.

Continuing Medical Education Directory

http://www.crha-health.ab.ca/clin/cme/cmedir.htm

A directory of organizations and individuals involved in Continuing Medical Education in Canada.

ONLINE COURSES AND INTERACTIVE LEARNING RESOURCES

Continuing Medical Education

http://www.oma.org/cmeprog/cmeded.htm

A collection of Web resources including interactive software and electronic forums from the Ontario Medical Association's Continuing Medical Education Program for Rural and Isolated Physicians

Virtual Lecture Hall

http://www.vlh.com/

Online continuing education courses for physicians.

The Interactive Patient

http://medicus.marshall.edu/medicus.htm

This interactive WWW teaching tool from the Marshall University School of Medicine simulates a patient encounter

PractitionerNet.org

http://www.practitionernet.org

Online resources for adolescent health practitioners, including online courses and autosearching features

HealthBehaviorChange.org

http://www.healthbehaviorchange.org

Online courses and resources for preventive health practitioners.

PRACTICE/CLINICAL GUIDELINES

National Guideline Clearinghouse (NGC)

http://www.guideline.gov

NGC provides access to evidence-based clinical practice guidelines

Cochrane Collaboration

http://www.cochrane.co.uk (UK)

http://hiru.mcmaster.ca/cochrane/ (Canada)

http://www.updateusa.com/clibhome/clib.htm (U.S.)

Provides access to the Cochrane Reviews of evidence-based research for all areas of health care

CMA: CPG Infobase

http://www.cma.ca/cpgs/

Database of clinical practice guidelines from the Canadian Medical Association

CMA: Clinical Practice Guidelines

http://www.cma.ca/webmed/cpg.htm

A collection of Clinical Practice Guidelines on the Web from the Canadian Medical Association

Agency for Health Care Policy and Research (AHCPR): Clinical Information

http://www.ahcpr.gov/clinic/

Provides access to a selection of Agency for Health Care Policy and Research (AHCPR) supported clinical practice guidelines, quick reference guides for clinicians and consumer guides

PATIENT INFORMATION

Canadian Health Network

http://www.canadian-health-network.ca/

Healthfinder

http://www.healthfinder.org/

NOAH: New York Online Access to Health

http://www.noah.cuny.edu/

Sympatico Healthy Way

http://healthcentralsympatico.com/home/home.cfm

Virtual Hospital

http://www.vh.org/

Table 15.3   Selected Websites for Professional Development, *continued*

SELF-HELP/MUTUAL SUPPORT

American Self-Help Clearinghouse

http://www.selfhelpgroups.org

The national clearinghouse for self-help groups, organizations and centers in the United States

Self-Care Central

http://www.healthy.net/home/index.html

A collection of online self-care and self-help resources including groups, mailing lists, directories and articles

The Self-Help Resource Centre (SHRC) of Greater Toronto

http://www.selfhelp.on.ca

Includes links to self-help resources on the Internet

DocTom's Online Self-Care Journal

http://www.healthy.net/home/tomonline/

This online journal includes an overview of online consumer health information, including self-help communities, by Dr. Tom Ferguson, Senior Associate at the Center for Clinical Computing, Harvard Medical School.

EVALUATING WEBSITES: RELIABLE HEALTH INFORMATION

JAMA – Journal of the American Medical Association

http://jama.ama-assn.org/

A number of articles related to the quality of Web health information are available on the site, including *Rating Health Information on the Internet Navigating to Knowledge or to Babel?* (Jadad & Gagliardi, 1998)

BMJ – British Medical Journal

http://bmj.com/

Including *Published Criteria for Evaluating Health Related Web Sites: Review.* (Kim et al., 1999)

OMNI Guidelines for Resource Evaluation

http://omni.library.nottingham.ac.uk/agec/evalguid.html

Guidelines used by OMNI (Organising Medical Networked Information) to select and evaluate biomedical Internet resources

Health on the Net Foundation (HON)

http://www.hon.ch/

Includes information on HON's Code of Conduct. The HONcode was established to help unify and standardize health information on the Web

ner, 1994) is one such computer-based tool that can be used in the clinical setting to identify risky health behavior and elicit patient concerns. Furthermore, with interactive voice technology, screening need not be confined to the clinical setting. For example, Kobak et al. (1997) demonstrate that a computer-administered telephone interview is an effective method for identifying psychopathology in primary care patients. The computerized medical record, which can facilitate identification of health issues that require medical attention, represents another technological advance to support screening activities.

Continuing Care

Although an older information technology, the telephone remains one of the most powerful communication tools. Studies indicate that the provision of health care through telephone communications, in many cases, is a viable alternative to routine clinic consultation or follow-up (Brown & Armstrong, 1995; Wasson et al., 1992). Indeed, studies show that increased use of telephone-based care in the management of selected patients may increase continuity and efficiency of care and improve patient satisfaction (e.g., by reducing time spent travelling to the clinic and time spent waiting). Efficiency is improved because telephone consults may be provided more frequently than office visits and can save time for both the patient and provider. We profile a comprehensive Telephone-Linked-Care (TLC) system later in this chapter.

Computer-assisted communication provides patients with another avenue for communication and another means to access health care services delivery. Balas et al. (1997) reviewed 80 trials assessing the impact of electronic communication between clinical health providers and patients. They found that computerized communication, telephone reminders, and interactive telephone information systems provide improved continuity of care by improving access to health care and supporting the coordination of clinician activities. Distance-medicine activities, facilitated through computer interventions, enable greater continuity of care and facilitate clinician coordinated care activities (Balas et al., 1997).

Linkages and Networks Among Services and Resources

In the past, access to specialized care was limited to major cities. With the advent of computer networks, however, the provision of long-distance health care using interactive video technology has become a reality. Indeed, telemedicine, the provision of health care services in an interactive fashion to one or more patients by one or more providers at locations remote from the patient, has been used to facilitate long-distance cardiology, radiology, and psychiatric consults (Crump & Pfeil, 1995). E-mail and other electronic communications provide opportunities for enhanced physician-patient communication by providing detailed feedback in text form, thus reducing the possibility of verbal misunderstanding. The American Medical Informatics Association recently published guidelines for physicians who use e-mail in clinical practice (Kane & Sands, 1998); they believe that e-mail can provide a useful means of enhancing patient-practitioner communication. Reviews of the related literature find a demonstrable correlation between effective physician-patient communication and improved patient health outcomes (Balas et al., 1997; Stewart et al., 1995). Provider prompting/reminder systems, computer-assisted treatment planning, patient education, and patient treatment reminders are interventions found successful in addressing primary care needs (Dijkstra & De Vries, 1999).

Westberg and Miller (1999) state that current information technology applications for primary care can provide valuable and timely information to assist in primary care. Although some current technologies are still not ideal for providing certain forms of information, Westberg and Miller find that such technologies are being developed. Currently there exists a variety of Internet-based decision support systems to aid physicians, and the affordability and usability of such systems are rapidly improving. Such applications of information technology into primary care practice can enhance physician awareness and complement health promotion education.

Options for Help

Computer software packages designed to provide patient information and education are among the many options currently available to patients. Information support networks, which can also facilitate access to health information, have the added benefit of communications services. Through the use of electronic bulletin boards and electronic mail, users can communicate with both providers and other patients throughout the world. By facilitating patient access to health information in a format that is both interesting and convenient for patients, computerized educational methods can go a long way towards promoting patient autonomy and feelings of control.

Patients can use the Internet to answer health-related questions, access current research, connect to community resources and communicate with others (some website links are given in Table 15.3). Many patients create their own web pages, outlining their experiences and providing links to resources they find valuable. The following websites were developed by patients:

- Irritable Bowel Syndrome (IBS) Self Help Group: *http://www.ibsgroup.org/*

- Lymphovenous Canada: *http://www.lymphovenous-canada.com*

- North American Chronic Pain Association:
  http://www.chronicpaincanada.org

In addition to accessing health information via the Internet, patients are using the technology to connect to other individuals to share common experiences, and provide each other with advice and support. The online self-help community includes conferencing systems, bulletin boards, list servers and chat groups (see Table 15.3).

To date, over 60% of national and international self-help groups and organizations are accessible over the Internet (Madara & White, 1997, p.93). There are several advantages to online self-help: ease and convenience, anonymity, increased access to support groups for rare conditions, and few physical barriers or restrictions. Online self-help's most significant contribution is shifting consumers from passive information recipients to actual producers of knowledge and information. Online self-help provides its users with a means of support, a source of practical and technical information, a way to share experiences and ideas, and a potential means of empowerment. Similar to the Community Networking movement, exemplified by FreeNets and the Tele-Communities, online self-help may lead to wider efforts of advocacy.

Also, many websites are devoted to specific health conditions and rare disorders, for example:

- Canadian Organization for Rare Disorders *http://www.cord.ca*

- National Organization for Rare Disorders *http://www.rarediseases.org*

- American Cancer Online Resources *http://www.acor.org*

- Dystrophic Epidermolysis Bullosa Research Association of America - a rare skin disorder *http://www.debra.org*

The Internet has significantly helped patients and practitioners concerned about rare disorders and orphan diseases. Patients scattered throughout the world, patients with rare diseases, have been brought together with the advent of online communities and discussion forums. In several instances such online communities have helped patients and practitioners to improve research and treatment.

There are also a number of health 'megasites', both public and private, that provide access to a comprehensive range of information and communities:

- Canadian Health Network *www.canadian-health-network.ca*
- Adam *www.adam.com*
- Diagnosis Health *www.diagnosishealth.com*
- Health Central *www.healthcentral.com*
- Health Finder *www.healthfinder.com*
- Mayo Clinic Health Oasis *www.mayohealth.org*
- Sympatico's HealthyWay *www.healthcentralsympatico.com/home/home.cfm*

The information on these sites ranges from very general to clinically specific and allows patients to access information at their level of need.

In addition to accessing health information via the Internet, patients are using the technology to connect to other individuals to share common experiences and provide each other with advice and support. The online self-help community includes conferencing systems, bulletin boards, list servers and chat groups (see Table 15.3).

There are a variety of technology-based intervention options for guided self-change, such as the *Pathways To Change* program described in Chapter 16 and the Smoking Zine website for youth smoking prevention and cessation described in Chapter 17. Computer-tailored interventions have been developed for behavioral self-control of drinking problems (Hester & Delaney, 1997), physical activity promotion (Bull et al., 1999), smoking cessation counselling (Ramelson et al., 1999), as well as for promoting patient self-help (Bental et al., 1999; Dijkstra & De Vries, 1999).

Information Management

Technology to support information management includes health tracking systems and computerized medical records. Such systems allow ready access to patient risk factor profiles and health status. Furthermore, many of the computerized medical record systems are designed for recording the practice patterns of health care providers. This type of monitoring—which can be done at both the organizational and individual provider levels—can be extremely useful for providing feedback to individuals and organizations.

Shiffman et al. (1999), in a review of computer-based clinical practice guideline implementation systems, found that guideline adherence improved in 14 of the 18 systems reviewed, and documentation of clinical activities improved in all four of the related studies reviewed. Computer-assisted reminder systems for implementing clinical practice guidelines have shown higher improvement rates than those that rely on physician recall for implementation (Worrall et al., 1997). Both of these review articles have been assessed by the Cochrane Collaboration.

Palm-held, miniaturized computers offer considerable potential for continuing care, in particular for providing accurate feedback to both patients and practitioners. For example, Shiffman and colleagues (Stone & Shiffman, 1994) have conducted a program of research in behavioral medicine that they call 'Ecological Momentary Assessment' (EMA). The EMA methods are used to monitor key behavior and moods in a patient's natural environment. The investigators assess the covariation between two behaviors, such as smoking and drinking (Shiffman et al., 1994), and evaluate the prevention of relapses by having participants monitoring their environmental and personal cues to smoking (Shiffman et al., 1995, 1996). Although still at a research stage, the practical applications are many. For example, Collins et al. (1998) uses this EMA technology to assess drinking and related behaviors for a program in drinking moderation.

Further Options

Keeping on top of the rapid pace of change and increasing diversity of information technology is a concern for students and busy practitioners. Some good sources to check periodically include:

- Benton Foundation (*http://www.benton.org*)
  Organization that follows IT and community trends and impacts

- Cyber Dialogue (*http://www.cyberdialogue.com*)
  U.S. organization that tracks online health consumer trends

- NUA (*http://www.nva.org*)
  Irish organization that is the world leader in surveys of Net users

- Slash Dot (*http://www.slashdot.org*)
  Bible for all things Open Source and new technology

- Shift Magazine (*http://www.shift.com*)
  Canada's answer to Wired (good IT coverage)

- Wired (*http://www.wired.com*)
  Good old standby on technology trends
- Cell Phone Technology and Trends include:
  The Wireless World *http://www.wired.com/news/wireless/*
  Yahoo Mobile *http://mobile.yahoo.com/*
  W3C WAP Forum *http://www.w3.org/TR/NOTE-WAP*

Internet-2, NGI and Beyond

Although the Internet has generated much enthusiasm, anyone who browses the Web will experience a number of often irritating limitations, such as slow response or addresses that are no longer functional or addresses that are 'under construction' and never get finished. Over 100 U.S. member universities have formed a consortium known as Internet-2: the University Consortium for Advanced Internet Development (*http://www.ucaid.edu*). One of their goals is to promote high-speed networking of a sort that is not yet available. This increased bandwidth capability will support a number of applications in health promotion and health care. For example, practitioners will be able to prescribe special educational video programs that can be delivered directly to patients via their home television and Internet connection. This home video link will be two-way, which will allow practitioners to interact with patients on the management of chronic conditions and behavioral change. This enhanced capability will also improve the use of the Internet for professional development: distance learner modules, refresher courses, and home study for health science students (Shortliffe, 1998).

A parallel project funded by U.S. federal government, called the Next Generation Internet (NGI), has established a number of test beds for evaluating capabilities and potential health applications of the Internet (National Research Council, 2000). The NGI, through the National Library of Medicine, is supporting a range of experimental applications and demonstration projects, such as remote medical consultations, collaborations among practitioners and researchers, and access to online data bases. A profile of 24 Phase I projects and 15 Phase II projects is given in Appendix B of the *Networking Health* report (National Research Council, 2000).

Telephone and Interactive Voice Technology

The Internet is captivating public attention and is growing at an explosive rate. By 2000, more than 50% of the North American population had access to the Internet. However, those who have Internet access are often restricted in other ways (e.g., students may access the internet only at specific times and only in the school lab). By comparison, over 90% of individuals in North America have access to a touch-tone telephone. Although the telephone has reached almost complete population saturation, it is greatly underutilized as a tool for health care and health promotion. Soet and Basch (1997) recently reviewed applications of telephone technology in health education and behavior change management with patients. They provide evidence that telephone interventions are a promising strategy for effecting health behavior change.

Robert Friedman and colleagues have developed and are evaluating a comprehensive Telephone-Linked-Care (TLC) technology as both an alternative and supplement to office-based delivery of ambulatory health care (Friedman et al., 1996). The TLC system carried out automated, telephone-based health care encounters with patients. The system speaks to patients using computer-controlled digitized human speech. In turn, patients communicate with TLC either by speaking into the telephone or by pressing keys on their touch-tone phone. Usually, TLC conversations last between 2 and 15 minutes. Patients have access to TLC 24 hours a day. Friedman et al., (1997) summarizes clinical applications of TLC and their evaluation status in three domains: chronic disease management, health behavior change and care-giver support.

For example, as part of the management of hypertension, patients monitor their blood pressure weekly and report values to TLC (Friedman et al., 1996). The system in turn displays this information in a graphical format to clinicians. The TLC hypertension application was evaluated in a randomized clinical trial involving 29 community-based practices and 267 elderly hypertensive patients cared for by 132 physicians. Subjects were randomly assigned to either the TLC group, in which TLC supplemented, once weekly, their usual care, or the group that received usual medical care alone. The follow-up period was 6 months. Friedman et al. (1996) found a mean medication adherence improvement of 18% for the TLC users versus 12% for usual care. Moreover, of patients at baseline who were non-adherent to their anti-hypertensive medication protocol, the practical effect of TLC was greater, yielding 36% adherence versus 26%. Moreover, mean blood pressure decreased significantly among the TLC users compared with controls. The level of blood pressure improvement from TLC is associated with an observed 40% reduction in stroke risk and a 10–15% reduction in coronary heart disease risk. Finally, patient satisfaction with the TLC system was high. Patients found it easy to use (94%), it helped them be more aware of their hypertension (95%), and it relieved their worries regarding their disease (79%). This study provides an important demonstration of the practical application of interactive voice technology for chronic disease management and behavior change.

Telemedicine/Telehealth

When distance separates individuals and organizations, information technologies such as telemedicine (acute care) and telehealth (health promotion) can support and enhance health care. Reid (1996) provides a comprehensive primer regarding telemedicine technology. Interactive video is a common medium to date, although the rapid growth of the Internet is opening up new options. Although telemedicine programs have been used for almost 40 years, significant expansion of these programs has occurred largely in the past decade. A key question is the extent to which telemedicine represents a change in practitioner-patient access to services, or a more fundamental shift in the process of providing health care and health promotion. Both are viable options at this point. Current impediments to the growth of telemedicine include lack of reimbursement, concerns regarding liability and malpractice, and issues of confidentiality and licensure (Grigsby & Sanders, 1998).

There are considerable opportunities for cost-effectiveness; however, many studies of specific telemedicine applications have not yet been conducted (Grigsby & Sanders, 1998). Balas et al. (1997) examine evidence regarding the efficacy of distance medical technology in six areas: computerized communication, telephone follow-up and counselling, telephone reminders, interactive telephone systems, after-hours telephone access, and telephone screening. Of the 80 eligible clinical trials included in their evaluation, significantly improved patient outcomes are demonstrated with respect to preventive care, management of osteoarthritis, cardiac rehabilitation and diabetes care.

Lehoux et al. (2000) propose a framework for matching health services needs with the possibilities offered by telemedicine and telehealth. They review four mechanisms of expected benefits:

1. Decreasing patient transfers
2. Decreasing trips by providers and patients

3. Meeting the needs of underserved populations

4. Building knowledge and reducing isolation

These mechanisms provide a focus for service planning, policy development and research.

> *The very conditions which make for the maximum effectiveness of the mass media of communications operate toward the maintenance of the ongoing social and cultural structure rather than toward its change.*

> —Lazarsfield and Merton (1971, p.578)

Moving On

Chapter 16 reviews the use of expert systems, especially the *Pathways To Change* (PTC) program, for tailoring interventions to the person's readiness for change. This chapter describes how an individual-based intervention for smoking cessation can be delivered to a whole population using information technology.

Computer Systems that Motivate Behavioral Change

WAYNE VELICER, RICHARD BOTELHO, JAMES PROCHASKA AND HARVEY SKINNER

The biggest single need in computer technology is not for improved circuitry or enlarged capacity or prolonged memory or miniaturized containers, but for better questions and better use of the answers.

—Norman Cousins (1966)

Overview

Expert systems are computer-based programs that build upon the decision making and problem solving capabilities of human experts. This chapter describes the development of such systems, and includes an in-depth look at the Pathways To Change program for smoking cessation. Research demonstrates that these systems are effective with a range of behaviors (e.g., smoking cessation, reducing dietary fat, reducing ultraviolet light (UV) exposure, protection from sexually transmitted diseases, risk alcohol use, drug abuse, and adherence to medical protocols) and in a variety of settings (e.g., health care and work place health promotion). Expert systems can assess and provide intervention strategies for large numbers of patients with risk behaviors, and thereby complement the use of behavioral health care in clinical practice. Unfortunately, these systems are not used as widely as they could be.

Growth of Expert Systems

During the last two decades, advances in behavioral science and information technology have led to the development of expert systems. These sys-

Table 16.1   Characteristics of Expert Systems
for Promoting Behavior Change

Efficient use of practitioner and patient time: Patients can work with expert systems on their own, without an increased time demand on practitioners' time.

Convenient contact: Patients can use different methods to interact repeatedly over time with expert systems to gain assistance in the change process.

Population-based applications: Healthcare organizations can use expert systems in a population-based manner, providing an efficient means of community-based screening and case identification.

Multiple risk factors: Patients have often multiple risk factors that require interventions at different stages-of-change. Expert systems provide such interventions either simultaneously or sequentially over time to accommodate patient preferences.

Comprehensive assessments: Expert systems conduct comprehensive assessments. Interactive systems can immediately branch to an in-depth assessment when a problem area exists.

Individualized interventions: Expert systems can provide tailored interventions matched to the patient's stage of change. For example, interventions can range from motivational counselling for patients in the early stages to detailed advice and support for those preparing to take action

Complete data base: Expert systems automatically record data to monitor both progress and regression of patients. This provides an extensive empirical data base to serve patients' needs and to evaluate the effectiveness of the system in an ongoing way.

Cost-Benefits: Prevention is expensive in terms of the personnel needed to provide population-based interventions. Expert systems are potentially a less costly alternative, taking a long-term perspective on the cost-benefits of improved outcomes.

Integration into existing interventions: Expert systems can complement practitioner interventions delivered during patient encounters. These systems can be integrated into a stepped approach to promoting behavior change.

---

tems can motivate patients to change behavior by providing assessments, personalized feedback and individualized interventions. An expert system is a computer program that simulates the reasoning and problem solving of human experts. Expert systems are an emerging technology that can be usefully integrated into existing health care and health information systems (e.g., computerized medical records). They can overcome barriers that prevent the adoption of population-based behavioral change programs into health care settings.

Characteristics of expert systems are summarized in Table 16.1. They include specific types of patient information, individualized interventions, and ways of tracking the progress of individuals and populations. Early versions of expert systems implemented the expertise of a single individual and involved no empirical data base (Negotia,1985). These systems were only as good as the expert and were updated episodically. Advanced expert systems use empirically validated theories and data systems that include both deep and surface knowledge (Harman & King, 1985; Waterman,1986). Deep knowledge refers to theoretical principles and decision structures. Expert systems use theoretical models as a basis for assessing patients and developing appropriate interventions. Surface knowledge involves heuristics, data collection, scoring systems for input variables, and use of decision rules. Data analyses are carried out to evaluate effectiveness of the system and to obtain feedback for continuous improvement.

This chapter describes a basic expert system, *Pathways To Change*; it discusses its application to a specific risk behavior, smoking cessation; it reviews outcome studies demonstrating its effectiveness; and it assesses the potential for the wider dissemination of such systems in health care and other settings.

Pathways To Change (PTC) System

Case Study

The following example illustrates features of the PTC system. Mr. S., a 34-year-old man with a 17-year history of smoking about a pack a day, went to his physician at the Lakeside Family Practice Center for a pre-employment physical. Prior to meeting with his doctor, he was invited to work with the PTC system. He spent about 15 minutes giving information to the computer. Highlights of his report are as follows:

"With regard to your current stage of change, you're not thinking about quitting smoking anytime in the near future. To make some progress, you can weigh the pros and cons of smoking, learn more about quitting, and keep thinking of how you're doing. Even though you are not thinking about quitting in the near future, you are using some useful strategies to help you consider quitting: becoming more informed, getting support, beginning to think about your smoking, and noticing how your smoking affects others. You can use additional strategies to move onto contemplation, such as addressing fears of failure and thinking about high-risk smoking situations in different ways."

After the physical examination, the patient expressed an interest in using the PTC system at a later time to re-evaluate his smoking habit. Four months later, Mr. S. completed the PTC assessment, and the following report was generated:

"You are now planning to quit smoking in the next six months. We suggest that you start by thinking about the positive features of smoking and comparing them to the negative aspects. You are already making good use of the following ideas: thinking about smoking, using substitutes instead of smoking, and noticing more about how your smoking affects others and the general public. The following ideas may help further:

- Take control in avoiding situations that tempt you to smoke, and get support from others as you plan when and how you will quit smoking.
- Put off smoking the first cigarette in the morning by 10 or 20 or 30 minutes.
- Cut back 1 or 2 or 5 cigarettes a day.
- Sometime in the next month, stop smoking for a full 24 hours.

These steps will help you get ready for your final quit day. You are at high risk of smoking when you are relaxing with friends, going to a party, restaurant, or bar. Think about how you might handle these situations."

Three months later, Mr. S. went to his family doctor about an episode of acute bronchitis. Prior to the appointment, he again interacted with the PTC computer system.

"Your answers suggest you are planning to quit smoking in the next 30 days. Congratulations. You are more aware of the negative aspects of smoking. It is important to be sure that you're ready. You are already making good use of the following strategies: getting support from others as you go through the steps of quitting; giving yourself rewards throughout the quitting process; taking more control of things that tempt you to smoke; making a commitment about using your willpower and inner strength to help yourself achieve your goal; and using other thoughts and activities when you are tempted to smoke. The following suggestions may help you:

- Set a definite quit date and come up with a detailed plan of action.
- Practice quitting by not smoking for a full 24 hours. People who do this are more successful staying smoke-free than those who do not.
- Talk to ex-smokers about how to deal with cigarette cravings, particularly, how to deal with cravings when in high-risk situations.

Mr. S. quit shortly thereafter. He stopped smoking for three weeks then relapsed. At this point he completed a re-assessment using the PTC system. Two weeks later, he quit again and relapsed again. Then, based on PTC recommendations, he decided to try a nicotine patch the next time he quit. He has been smoke-free for two years.

This case study shows how practitioners can use the PTC system to complement clinical care. It also illustrates that achieving long-term success at smoking cessation often takes several serious attempts.

How PTC Works

This expert system assesses the patient's readiness for change; a significant part of that assessment is the patient's strategies. Following the assessment, the system provides suggestions about what further strategies (processes) will help in achieving behavior change goals.

Deep Knowledge. The PTC expert system uses the Transtheoretical Model as the basis for generating interventions (Prochaska & DiClemente, 1983; Velicer et al., 1992, 1996). The key framework here is the Stages of Change, which describe how people modify a problem health behavior or acquire a positive health behavior. Five stages of change characterize patients' readiness to participate in preventive care: precontemplation, contemplation, preparation, action, and maintenance. The model includes *Processes of Change* and a series of measures including decisional balance and temptation scales. The *Processes of Change* are 10 cognitive and behavior activities that facilitate change (Prochaska et al., 1988). Cognitive processes (e.g., consciousness raising) are more critical when patients are in the precontemplation and contemplation stages. Behavioral processes (e.g., reinforcement management) are more critical when patients are in the preparation, action, and maintenance stages. The Decisional Balance tool (Prochaska et al., 1994; Velicer et al., 1985) involves weighing the pros and cons of continuing to smoke. These two scales capture cognitive processes that patients use for progress in the stages of change. The Temptation scale (Velicer et al., 1990) assesses an individual's temptation to smoke in a variety of situations. These include social situations, negative affect situations, and situations involving physical cravings. This tool is particularly useful when helping patients at later stages and in predicting relapse.

Surface Knowledge. The original data base for the PTC was constructed from a naturalistic study of more than 1000 smokers. This sample provided initial norms for making comparisons for the baseline report. After each subsequent study, the data were used to update the expert system. The control group in an intervention study provides a data base for assessment of change under natural conditions. This original system was significantly revised when the convenience sample was replaced by a representative sample appropriate for interventions targeting an entire population. A major advantage of this advanced expert system is that the data base needed for updating the system is gathered automatically during implementation.

Heuristics involve decision rules for matching the most appropriate intervention for patients at different stages of change. A series of multivariate analyses was used to verify the hypothesized relations and determine empirical cutoffs for decision rules. For each stage, the goal was to determine how much a process should be used to optimize movement to the next stage. The decisional balance and temptation scales represent intermediate outcome variables for assessing progress.

Outcome Studies

Four studies have evaluated the efficacy of the PTC system for smoking cessation. The first employed a reactively recruited sample of smokers through newspaper announcements and advertisements. Prochaska et al. (1993) compared the PTC system intervention with one of the best available self-help manuals and demonstrated that the system was more than twice as effective (25% abstinence at 18 months compared to 11%).

The second, third, and fourth studies employed proactively recruited samples to compare interventions for an entire population. Reactively recruited samples typically involve no more than 5% of the available population (Schmid et al., 1989), and tend to be disproportionally female, highly educated and in the later stages of change. In contrast, proactive procedures attempt to reach a larger proportion and a more representative sample of the at-risk population. Proactively delivered expert system interventions have the potential to provide a unique combination of materials and individualized help to a diverse population of patients.

In the second study, Prochaska et al. (in press) employed a random-digit dial phone survey was employed to recruit a representative sample of smokers. Of the identified smokers, 80% were enrolled in the study and assigned to either an expert system intervention or an assessment-only condition. At the 24-month follow-up, the point prevalence abstinence rate was 25% for the expert system, which was one-third higher than for the assessment-only condition. The difference between the two groups was larger at each assessment point, indicating that the effects of the treatment continued long after the end of treatment (six months).

The third and fourth studies shared the same recruitment. The entire population of a Health Maintenance Organization was contacted, and

85.3% of the smokers agreed to be enrolled. The third study (Velicer et al., 1999) evaluated both the impact of interactive interventions versus non-interactive interventions and the impact of different numbers of contacts. At 18 months, there was no dose response relationship. However, for each contact condition, the interactive (expert system) intervention was more effective than the non-interactive (manual-only) intervention. The point prevalence abstinence rate across the expert system was 22%. In the fourth study, Prochaska et al. (in press) compared four groups. The standard three contact conditions resulted in a point prevalence abstinence rate of 26%, which was 21% greater than the assessment-only condition.

One of the most important findings of this series of studies was the high recruitment (80% and 85.3%) and retention rates. When patients at diverse stages of, or readiness for, change are matched to an intervention system, such as the PTC, that accommodates such diversity, it is possible to intervene with the majority of all individuals, rather than only the select few who are in the preparation stage. This greatly enhances the impact of the intervention.

Adapting PTC to Other Health Behaviors

The *Pathways To Change* system has served as the prototype for development of interventions for other areas. Trials are underway for PTC systems designed to reduce the amount of dietary fat, increase the amount of regular exercise, increase the use of sun screens for protection from UV exposure, use condoms for protection from sexually transmitted diseases, and improve compliance with mammography screening. Consult the Cancer Prevention Research Center website for the latest details on the status of these interventions (*www.uri.edu/research/cprc/intervention.htm*). Outcome data for two systems, mammography screening and UV exposure, support the effectiveness of these interventions (Rakowski et al., 1998).

Multimedia interactive expert systems are undergoing clinical trials for smoking cessation (Pallonen et al., 1998), reducing dietary fat, reducing UV exposure, and protection from sexually transmitted diseases. Measure development and model testing are completed for high-risk alcohol use (Migneault et al., 1997), drug abuse, and adherence to medical protocols. Individual expert system interventions can be combined to address chronic disease management. For example, diabetes involves interventions for smoking cessation, exercise, diet, and adherence to blood glucose testing and medication protocols. Also, multiple risk factor packages could be developed for hypertension, cardiovascular health, and weight control.

Other Examples of Expert Systems

Expert systems are being developed at several research centers. Some systems rely only on expert advice, and, unlike the PTC system, do not include ongoing data collection and empirically based refinements to the system.

The TLC (Telephone-Linked-Care) System is a computer-based telecommunications system that functions as an at-home educator and counsellor for patients with hypertension (Cullinane et al., 1994). TLC communicates with patients over the telephone using computer-generated speech, and the patient communicates using either the touch-tone user pad or speech. After each contact, TLC stores the information and forwards it to the appropriate health care provider. In a clinical trial of hypertensive patients, medication adherence improved 17.7% compared to 11.7% for the controls, and mean diastolic blood pressure decreased 5.2 mm Hg compared to 0.8 for the controls.

The Nutrition for a Lifetime System is designed to reduce dietary fat and increase the consumption of fruits and vegetables. The point of contact is the supermarket purchase. Interventions consist of 10 interventions and four maintenance segments employing multimedia technology. In a clinical trial, the intervention produced an 8% decrease in percent calories from fat and a 20% increased consumption of fruits and vegetables.

The Cholesterol Lowering Intervention Program (CLIP) is an intervention for dietary change and drug treatment of hypercholesterolemia (Clark et al., 1995; DeBusk et al., 1994; Winett et al., 1991). The first component, dietary management, assesses current consumption using a food frequency questionnaire, provides a series of progress reports, and recommends drug therapy for patients who fail to achieve the targeted goals. The second component, drug therapy management, controls data collection and scheduling; reports to the attending practitioner; assists in complex decision-making; and facilitates contacts and communication among specialists, nurses, patients, and the primary care practitioner. In pilot studies, 62% of the patients showed a change on CSI (cholesterol-saturated fat index) score of one or more grades.

A research group at the University of North Carolina has demonstrated the effectiveness of addressing several risk factors by using brief tailored messages that are in accordance with the patient's stage of change. The messages are based on the health belief model. To date, the effectiveness of this approach has been demonstrated with mammography screening (Skinner et al., 1994), smoking cessation and dietary fat reduction (Campbell et al., 1994).

Your Decision to Incorporate Expert Systems

As described in Chapter 2, health care delivery is undergoing major transformation. High performance organizations take a long-term perspective on reducing the risks and harms associated with health behaviors (Chapter 9). They integrate computerized medical records with information systems to assess outcomes and utilization patterns, as well as monitor the performance of individual practitioners and the health care team. Such integrated systems could include expert systems for motivating health behavior change. Expert systems help patients achieve behavior change goals over time, and contribute toward reducing unnecessary health care utilizations, costs, morbidity and mortality.

Advantages

Table 16.2 summarizes various benefits of using expert systems. The majority of approaches to altering health behavior are designed to address immediate change, preferably by the end of the first encounter. An example is the National Cancer Institute smoking cessation program, which uses the four A's: Ask, Advise, Assist, and Arrange follow-up (National Cancer Institute, 1989; Epps & Manley, 1991). However, these programs are suitable for only about 20% of smokers who are in the preparation stage, that is, intending to quit in the next 30 days (Burns & Pierce, 1992; Kaplan et al., 1993; Velicer & DiClemente, 1993; Velicer et al., 1995). Some interventions use the concept of relapse prevention to help patients move from the action to maintenance stage. However, only a few programs are available to help practitioners deal with the majority of smokers, that is, the approximately 40% who are not thinking about change (precontemplation stage) and the 40% who are ambivalent about change (contemplation stage) (Velicer et al., 1995). Expert systems, such as *Pathways To Change*, give specific recommendations to all smokers because they tailor their recommendations to the stage of the smoker's readiness to change.

Health care settings provide ample opportunities for patients to use expert systems. In the U.S., 72–91% of adults (aged 16–65) visit a practitioner (generalist or specialist) annually (U.S. Centers for Disease Control and Prevention, 1994). In Australia and Britain, 70–80% of adults (aged 16–65) visit their general practitioner annually (Bridges-Webb, 1987). Patients regard general practitioners as highly trusted providers of health information (Richmond & Heather, 1990; Sanson-Fisher et al., 1986) and

Table 16.2   Advantages of Expert Systems

PRACTICE ISSUES	FUTURE DEVELOPMENTS
1. **Opportunity.** The vast majority of the population have a medical encounter over a two-year period, and therefore have potential access to expert systems.	1. Interactive systems are well-developed for smoking cessation and show promising results with other behaviors; future versions can implement advances based on empirical studies and advances in technology.
2. **Role.** Practitioners believe that they have a role in providing prevention and behavior health care programs. Expert systems could greatly assist practitioners in this role.	2. Practitioners have the potential of working synergistically with expert systems in ways that enhance the overall impact of prevention and behavioral health care programs.
3. **Lower costs.** Expert systems have great potential in reducing health care utilizations, avoidable costs, preventable morbidity, and mortality.	3. With rapid advances in technology, expert systems can be adapted to make them more user-friendly and accessible to patients and practitioners.
4. **Evidence-based.** Expert systems can incorporate the latest empirical data about optimum approaches to behavior change.	4. Expert systems can expedite the broad implementation and effectiveness of prevention programs. Widespread use of behavior change systems have potential of making significant contributions to achieving population health objectives.
5. **Population-based.** Expert systems can provide appropriate, population-based, prevention programs	5. Expert systems are being adapted for use on the Internet (Web), interactive voice technology and future platforms based on mobile computers (e.g., WAP: wireless application protocol). This will greatly enhance access.
6. **Feedback to practitioners.** Expert systems can provide automated feedback about patients and quality improvement reports on a regular basis.	
7. **Broad applicability.** Expert systems can be used in a variety of contexts: health, workplace and education settings.	
8. **Quality control.** Expert systems provide for a consistent, standardized and transportable intervention	
9. **Individualized.** Expert systems provide interventions that are tailored to the needs of the individual patient and practitioners.	
10. **Reinforcing progress.** Expert systems perform ongoing assessment necessary to detect and reward progress of both patients and practitioners	

counsellors about preventive care (Wallace et al., 1987; Wallace & Haines, 1984; Weinberg & Andrus 1982). In addition to primary care, hospital and community health centers are ideal sites in which to use expert systems.

Barriers

A number of factors can impede the use of information technology for behavior change programs (Table 16.3). Major barriers to introducing expert systems into health care settings include:

1. Practitioners lack training in using expert systems, are often sceptical about the usefulness of preventive interventions, and are suspicious of computer systems that lack a human touch.

2. Practitioners are inadequately reimbursed for delivering preventive and behavioral interventions.

3. Significant personnel and infrastructure resources are needed to support the use, maintenance and upgrading of expert systems.

4. Large, initial capital investments are needed to support and manage information systems.

Integrated Approach

Health care organizations can arrange for patients to interact with expert systems in three ways: reactive, proactive, and a combination of both strategies. In a reactive organization (see Chapter 9), patients interact with an expert system only when they enter hospitals or primary care settings. This approach integrates prevention into existing contacts with the health care system.

In a proactive organization, practitioners contact patients for a health status assessment and intervene on a periodic basis, depending on the risk status of the patient. This overcomes two drawbacks of a case-finding approach. First, practitioners are not limited to time-pressured, brief interventions for health behavior change, particularly when dealing with multiple complaints. Second, the strategy is not dependent on the irregular timing of patient contacts with the health care system.

High performing organizations combine both the reactive and proactive approaches: screening patients as they enter the health care setting, actively contacting patients at regular intervals, and contacting patients for followup. In this way, health care organizations can shift their approach to health behavior change from an episodic, individual-based approach (case-finding) toward a systematic, population-based approach.

Patients can use expert systems prior to, or independent of, a practitioner encounter. Expert systems conduct detailed assessments and provide patients with behavioral recommendations that are appropriate to their stage of change and individual need. Patients control the initiation and process of change. Patients can initiate contact periodically to reassess their health behaviors, access the next stage-specific interventions when they have progressed, and/or monitor their own progress over time. In effect, patients take responsibility for behavior change. However, to ensure participation, a means of contacting patients who fail to initiate contact needs to

Table 16.3   Concerns About Expert Systems

TRAINING AND PRACTICE	RESEARCH AND DEVELOPMENT
1. Lack of knowledge and skills in using expert systems (role conflict)	1. Expert systems for the different health behaviors are at various stages of development, and the impact of these systems still needs further evaluation.
2. Skepticism about practitioner's ability to influence patient behavior.	2. Systems need to be adapted for implementation and maintenance in different types of settings.
3. Concern over loss of 'human touch' when using expert systems.	3. Versions of the expert systems must be developed for different languages and tailoring of materials for needs of special populations.
4. Inadequate reimbursement for using expert systems.	4. Ongoing research is needed to evaluate and improve large-scale implementation and evaluation of expert systems.
5. Lack of personnel and infrastructure to support expert systems in practice.	
6. Large capital investment needed to implement and maintain these systems.	
7. Concern about large short-term expense needed for potential long-term gains in health care utilization and prevention of morbidity and mortality.	

be in place. Here, the patient and the health care setting share responsibility for change.

Patients and practitioners can use an expert system to complement their clinical encounters. Practitioners could receive brief updated summaries about their patients, similar to lab reports. They could use these to elaborate on and reinforce the assessment and recommendations provided. Expert systems help practitioners use their time more efficiently with patients. Thus, practitioners can use a stepped-care approach to behavior change, depending upon patients' choices and needs. Patients decide whether and when to use the expert system and whether and when to consult their practitioner.

Enhancing Impact

The impact of prevention programs on the health of a population depends on recruitment and effectiveness rates. Behavioral interventions typically are of two forms: public health approaches or clinic-based approaches (Abrams et al., 1996a, 1996b; Velicer & DiClemente, 1993). Public health approaches usually have much higher recruitment rates but lower effectiveness than clinic-based approaches. A suggested outcome measure for interventions is impact, which is the product of the recruitment rate and the effectiveness of the intervention. For example, a clinic-based intervention might result in 20% effectiveness for cessation but be able to recruit

Table 16.4 Estimated Impact of Alternative Delivery Systems
for Smoking Cessation

DELIVERY SYSTEM	RECRUITMENT smokers reached	EFFECTIVENESS quit-rate	IMPACT overall
Clinic-based	5%	20%	1%
Population-based	80%	10%	8%
Expert System: clinical & population	80%	25%	20%

only 5% of the population of smokers, resulting in low overall impact of 1% cessation (Table 16.4). In contrast, a population-based (public health) intervention that reaches 80% of the smokers but has a lower effectiveness of 10% cessation would yield much higher impact of 8% cessation.

Expert systems have the potential to enhance recruitment and effectiveness rates. In a study that used a random-digit dial recruitment, initial recruitment rates were in excess of 82.5% and effectiveness rates were more than 25%, resulting in an impact in excess of 20% cessation. Across three population-based studies, the impact of the expert system intervention was conservatively estimated at 18% cessation (Velicer & Prochaska, 1999).

Cost-benefit is a central issue with regard to implementation of expert systems. It is often difficult to estimate the extent to which technological advances will reduce the costs to implement and maintain these systems. The long-term impact of these systems depends on a combination of factors: implementation, recruitment, effectiveness, maintenance and upgrading. It may take years for an organization to achieve the major benefits accruing from such systems.

Advances in Information Technology

Ongoing developments in information technology will permit more diverse ways for patients and practitioners to use expert systems.

Integrated Systems will enable expert systems to be available not only in health care settings but also in work, school, and home settings, thus expanding the access to prevention programs. Shared data bases using Internet technology permit integration from diverse sources. Furthermore, information systems that can communicate between sites allow health care information to be more readily communicated between patients and their practitioners and among the different health care providers with whom the patient has contact. Medical records, scheduling, and expert system interventions for prevention can be integrated into a single system. The integration of the medical records and scheduling components is critical to assure regular, proactive contacts for patients who fail to initiate contact.

Voice Recognition Technology will let patients telephone and access expert systems proactively and without the need to see their practitioner. Patients enter their identification number, and a voice recognition program insures confidentiality. A computerized voice asks patients questions about their health behavior while the voice recognition technology records their responses. The expert system provides a verbal summary of the assessment, recommends changes to patients, and then sends a detailed follow-up report via the Internet or mail. Patients gain access to the system on an as-needed basis. Alternatively, the system can initiate contact in a timely and regular manner.

High-Speed Connection, high bandwidth access to the Internet, is superseding telephone (modem) connection. Thus, home contact with expert systems will have high-speed interactivity. The health status assessment can be modified interactively, and graphics, sound and animation can all be integrated into a personalized feedback report. Thus, a fully interactive contact can be scheduled at home either preceding or following contact with a health care provider, or independent of such a contact.

Applications of Information Technology

Future developments will improve the type and quality of interventions, will address the full array of risk behaviors, and will enhance the availability of expert systems to patients in different settings (health care, workplace or school).

Adapting to Diverse Populations. Expert systems using multimedia programs can pose questions simultaneously in both oral and written formats to individuals in various settings. This will permit individuals to respond to the system even if they have poor reading skills or a physical disability. For patients whose primary language is not English, the expert system will be able to switch intervention materials into the appropriate language. In areas where major subgroup differences exist, both the norms and the intervention materials could be matched to the specific culture. Input can be accomplished using either a modified keyboard, a touch screen, a hand-held device, or voice recognition. Alternative input modalities will make it easier for patients to respond to questions. Examples of such systems have been developed for schools and inner-city health clinics (Pallonen et al., 1998; Velicer et al., 1998)

Flexible Use of Technology. Health care organizations could use batch expert systems to contact patients by mail or phone at home, and use interactive expert systems when patients attend health care settings. The batch contact would involve the organization's total population and would precede the visit to the clinic. The interactive system would then be used for the follow-up contact. A prompt from the health care provider may be needed for those patients who fail to initiate contact in a timely manner. Alternatively, the interactive system could be used for the initial contact and the batch system for follow-up. Such a system could screen systematically and opportunistically for risk behavior and non-adherence to prevention or medical procedures.

Population-Based. To date, information technology has focused on the individual (patient) level. However, such systems can be extremely important at the group and population levels. Either geographic or medical communities (e.g., HMO or a managed care population) could receive summary statements about the behavioral risk status of their populations. This information could be integrated with community-based approaches to enhance the performance of primary and secondary prevention programs in health, education and workplace settings. Data from expert systems could be part of quality improvement programs to monitor the performance prevention programs in health care settings. One advantage of expert systems technology is that assessment information is gathered as a necessary part of the intervention. Information about individual patients can be aggregated and analyzed at group (e.g., all diabetic patients) or population levels. Health care organizations could use such data for ongoing quality improvement activities.

Moving On

Ultimately, the implementation of expert systems depends on whether health care organizations are willing to take a long-term perspective on improving outcomes in prevention and behavioral health care. The next chapter describes Internet websites that support health behavior change. In particular, the Smoking Zine for youth smoking prevention and cession incorporates many of the features of the *Pathways To Change* program.

CHAPTER 17

TeenNet: *Using the Internet for e-Health*

HARVEY SKINNER, OONAGH MALEY,
LOUISE SMITH, MEG MORRISON
AND EUDICE GOLDBERG

Technology is neither good nor bad … but neither is it neutral.

—Melvin Kransberg, Historian

Overview

This chapter describes e-Health opportunities for health promotion, prevention and clinical care with adolescents. The Seven Critical Functions model (Chapter 12) is applied for mapping information technology (Internet) to support both practitioners and youth in health behavior change. Practical examples are given from the TeenNet project, which has developed interactive websites for youth, including *CyberIsle, Teen Clinic Online* and *Smoking Zine*. Information is presented in an engaging, nonjudgmental and fun environment through quizzes, simulations, fact sheets, guided self-change, personalized feedback and peer discussion groups. A parallel resource for practitioners, *PractitionerNet*, provides guidelines and skill-based learning for promoting health with youth across health and educational settings. What makes TeenNet unique for organizational change is the interweaving of 'high tech' website development and community (consumer) involvement using an action research model.

Engaging Youth in Health Promotion

We face a dilemma in promoting health with adolescents. This is the developmental stage when potential health risk behaviors (e.g., smoking, alcohol and other drug use) are either initiated, or the individual passes successfully through this transition period into adulthood when the likelihood of initiation decreases substantially. However, it is often difficult to engage teens in a serious examination of health behavior and its consequences.

During middle/high school, teenagers initiate use of alcohol, tobacco and marijuana at a greater rate than at any other time. With few exceptions, health risk behaviors such as drug and alcohol use have remained steady or increased amongst youth in North America (Adlaf et al., 1999; Johnston, Bachman et al., 2000). And while youth smoking continues to show promising declines in the United States, 7% of eighth- graders, 14% of tenth- graders and 21% of twelfth-graders indicated they were daily smokers (Johnston et al., 2000). For these reasons, adolescents are a primary target for prevention and health promotion initiatives.

Youth today live in a media-orientated world. Interactive technologies (e.g., video games, computer games) captivate teens and provide enormous potential for engaging them. The increasing availability of information technology creates an innovative channel for clinical prevention and health promotion with the ability to reach a large number of young people, including those 'turned off' by traditional approaches. Health promotion programs that are interactive and involve peer led components have been shown to be the most effective (Botvin & Botvin, 1997; Dusenbury & Falco, 1997; Ellickson, 1995; Lynagh et al., 1997; Tobler & Stratton, 1997). The Web provides an ideal environment for this interactivity and peer-to-peer interaction.

Indeed, the Internet provides an extremely powerful tool for promoting health: locally, nationally and internationally. One can rapidly transmit health information via text, images, sound and video clips on a scale not dreamed of a decade ago. The Web also allows real-time communication and connectivity among multiple users that can be used to create virtual communities for self-help and mutual support. As the Web grows and matures, significant possibilities are opening up for:

1. Quickly disseminating and reaching a large number of youth locally, nationally and internationally

2. Engaging youth, especially diverse and hard-to-reach populations, through vibrant graphics and innovative effects

3. Stimulating learning through interventions that incorporate personalized feedback and tailor information to the youth's own circumstances

4. Multiple pathways or means of reaching health information from schools, local libraries, homes, community and health care settings

5. Multiple linkages to related topics such as peer-led discussion groups, lifestyle assessment and guided change, as well as specific health information and interactive games related to health issues

6. Connectivity (one-to-many) and mutual support, allowing teens to assist others and create an environment that stimulates collective action.

Drawing on work of the TeenNet Project (*www.teennetproject.org*) based at the University of Toronto, this chapter presents insights and examples of e-Health applications. The overall goal of TeenNet is to increase the number of teens engaged in positive health and social behavior. What makes this project unique is the interweaving of high tech website development and community involvement using an action research model (Skinner et al., 2001). TeenNet's websites are designed to target both youth and practitioners (health, education). The websites provide an integrated way of addressing the seven critical functions for organizational improvement in behavior change described in Chapter 12.

TeenNet e-Health Websites for Youth

The first website launched by TeenNet in 1997 was based on the concept of a teen's only island called *CyberIsle*. In 2000, the *Teen Clinic Online* and *Smoking Zine* were created. In 2001 a parallel website for health and educational practitioners *PractitionerNet*, was launched. The TeenNet websites and guiding principles are summarized in Figure 17.1.

TeenNet's Action Research Model

TeenNet works by using a participatory, community-based approach in which teens and various community organizations are involved in all stages of project design, development, implementation, evaluation and dissemination. Information technology (Internet) and community involvement are woven together through action research (Figures 17.2). TeenNet's work is guided by five principles (*PRAAA*) ensuring that its websites are:

1. **Participatory:** key involvement (ownership) at all stages by youth

2. **Relevant:** focus on health, personal and social issues identified by teens

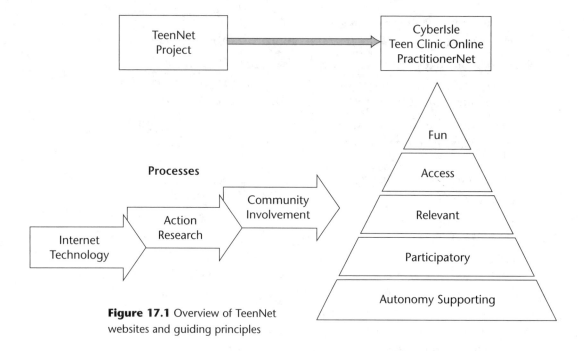

Figure 17.1 Overview of TeenNet
websites and guiding principles

3. **Autonomy-supporting:** encourages individual choice and exploration of options regarding health behavior

4. **Active Learning – Fun:** engaging, flexible and highly interactive;
   stimulates self-directed learning

5. **Accessible:** designed and adapted to be accessible and relevant to
   diverse populations of adolescents, including at risk and hard to reach
   populations

The TeenNet Action Research Model uses a spiral process (Figure 17.2)
where ideas are generated by/with community members (in particular
youth), implemented with them, evaluated by them, adjusted according to
their feedback, then re-implemented and evaluated. This iterative process is
ongoing throughout the life of the project, beginning with needs assessment and continuing through prototyping and implementation of solutions. Prototypes are designed, studied and improved using *Plan-Do-Study-
Act* (PDSA) *cycles* described in Chapter 13. Thus, evaluation and refinement
take place continuously. TeenNet's action research process not only fosters
participation, self-determination and active learning among youth from
diverse backgrounds, but also facilitates a true sense of ownership by youth.

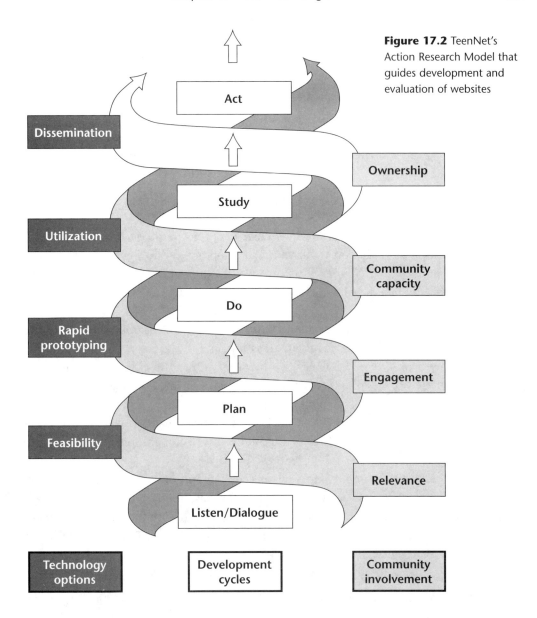

Figure 17.2 TeenNet's Action Research Model that guides development and evaluation of websites

TeenNet draws on a person-centered health promotion model described by Skinner and Bercovitz (1997) that underscores the interconnection among self-care, mutual aid and professional assistance (see Figure 3.2 in Chapter 3). Also, concepts and behavior change strategies are incorporated from Self-Determination Theory (Ryan & Deci, 2000; Deci & Ryan, 1985), Social Cognitive Theory (Bandura, 1986, 1997), Transtheoretical Model including Stages of Change (Prochaska et al., 1992), harm reduction (Erickson et al., 1997), community organization and development (Kretzmann & McKnight, 1993; McBeth & Schweer, 2000; Minkler & Wallerstein, 1996), and action research (Argyris et al., 1985). The Likelihood of Action Index described in Chapter 7 (Table 7.1 and Worksheet 7.1) is used to guide the development and evaluation of web-based interventions, including the *Smoking Zine*, for smoking prevention and cessation. Indeed, the interventions are designed to produce positive changes in likelihood of action—making the healthy choice!

The Birth of *CyberIsle*: *www.cyberisle.org*

During the summer of 1995, the TeenNet project employed high school students as teen advisors to direct the development of the TeenNet home page. The teens differed greatly with respect to their cultural background, interests, and health behaviors, such as smoking, drug use, drinking and sexual activity.

The first task undertaken by the teens was to design a home page. The teens were asked to generate ideas for how the site could be laid out and how a user would navigate within the website. In brief, the teens were asked to come up with a concept or metaphor. In the process, they surfed the net to establish a list of features, designs, graphics and content they liked. Next, they organized and conducted a discussion group with other teens to brainstorm ideas for the TeenNet website. The result was the birth of *CyberIsle*, a teens-only island.

The teens then spent weeks discussing and drawing places and activities for the island that are meaningful for youth and reflect issues youth are concerned about. The teens worked closely with both the content and technical teams to develop and bring their island to life. The following places were designed in collaboration with project staff:

1. **Beach:** both day and night beach scenes are represented

2. **Cyberia:** a nightclub that has a bar, dance floor, pool tables, DJ booth

3. **Bathrooms:** both male and female (important places for privacy, especially getting away from teachers and parents)

4. **Shuttle bus:** for moving around the island

5. **Bus pass:** this acts as a registration system, allowing the project to obtain demographic information about the users (age, sex and country of origin). Youth use their bus pass to return to *CyberIsle*. The bus pass keeps track of the number of times they visit

6. **Quizzes:** self-assessment and guided-change activities

7. **Graffiti wall:** a place for self-expression and to have fun

8. **Resource Center:** lists resources on the island, on the web and in the community. Specific resources available for special needs youth are also included (e.g., street-involved youth and youth with disabilities)

9. **HotTalk:** Online peer discussion groups, where teens gain advice and support from other teens (this quickly became the most visited area on *CyberIsle*)

CyberIsle's health information, online discussion groups, interactive lifestyle assessment programs, simulations, links and games are layered under graphics that make up the various places on the island. For example, information on eating disorders can be reached by clicking on one of the mirrors in the female washroom while facts about drugs can be reach via the jar on the boardwalk at the evening beach party.

The value of *CyberIsle*'s island metaphor is the infinite potential in what can be added to the website. In 2000, the *Teen Clinic Online* and the *Smoking Zine* were launched on the island. Currently, work is underway on the theme of youth and gambling, which will result in a *Gambling Arcade* (or similar metaphor) site where prevention of gambling problems will be addressed through interactive quizzes and simulations. The result is an ever-evolving virtual environment for youth by youth that takes a holistic approach to health. Rather than dealing with health topics like safer sex, smoking and sexual orientation in isolation, youth can access information on all or one of these topics while also having fun on *CyberIsle*'s Graffiti Wall. This approach more accurately reflects the reality of youth's life where issues interconnect and overlap.

Teen Clinic Online

From the outside, the *Teen Clinic Online* looks like a comfortable, welcoming home. Inside there are six rooms: reception, program room, hangout, pharmacy, resource room and games room. Key features include self-directed learning, developing critical thinking skills, accessing the health care system and related services in a youth's own community, and connecting to people (not just information!) on health and social issues identified by teens (e.g., body art, relationships and body image). The main objectives of the *Teen Clinic Online* are to provide youth with a forum for:

1. Where to find answers to their specific questions

2. How to evaluate the personal relevance and quality of information

3. Ways to sort through options and make decisions affecting their health

Smoking Zine (short for magazine)

The *Smoking Zine* is designed for both adolescent smokers and nonsmokers. Youth access the *Zine* from *CyberIsle*'s navigation bar or through the *Teen Clinic Online*. The *Zine* is organized into five interactive phases that provide tailored responses based on youth's feedback, and can be completed by youth over a period of time:

1. **Makin' Cents:** consciousness raising about the cost of smoking

2. **It's Your Life:** assessment of smoking status and intentions

3. **To Change or Not to Change:** looking at readiness or stages for change

4. **It's Your Decision:** weighing the pros and cons of change using a decision balance

5. **What Now?:** a summary of a youth's responses, some suggestions for next steps, and, for smokers who want to quit, a guided self-change program.

Practitioners can use the *Smoking Zine* as a component of a prevention or clinical program (e.g., link motivational counseling with feedback from the quizzes and decision balance) or provide the *Zine* to youth as a stand-alone self-directed intervention.

How TeenNet Sites Support the Seven Critical Functions

Tables 17.1 and 17.2 illustrate how Internet technology (specifically the *Teen Clinic Online* and the *Smoking Zine*) can be used for the Seven Critical Functions. Features that support practitioners and youth in health behavior change (with the corresponding functions in **bold**) are highlighted in the following 'walks' through the *Teen Clinic* and the *Smoking Zine*. You are encouraged to visit the websites and take your own tour (*www.cyberisle.org*).

A Walk Through the *Teen Clinic Online*

When youth enter the *Teen Clinic Online*, they are taken to a 'cut away' view of the clinic house (Figure 17.3). Here youth can see an image and short

Table 17.1 Teen Clinic Online and the Seven Critical Functions

	Teens	Practitioners
Professional Development	Not applicable	The **Search And Find** interactive tutorial in the **Resource Room** provides tips and techniques for searching the Web. TeenNet's criteria for evaluating Web resources can be accessed by clicking on the **Bookshelves** in the **Resource Room.**
Priming and Prompting	The *"White Board"* in the **Resource Room** links to information on health topics identified by youth (STD/STI, body image, etc.). The "why and when to see a health practitioner" for each topic can **help youth think about the different risks associated with certain health and/or social behaviors.** Links to external resources/websites on drugs can be found in the **Pharmacy**. These resources can **encourage youth to think about their own behaviors and/or attitudes towards drugs**.	The *"White Board"* in the **Resource Room** links to information on health topics identified by youth (STD/STI, body image, etc.). These resources can be used as a **starting point for conversation with youth on different risk factors/ behaviors.** Items in the **HangOut** (sofa, clock, posters, etc.) link to conversations in *CyberIsle*'s discussion board **(HotTalk).** These discussions **provide practitioners with a window on youth health interests, questions and concerns.**
Identification	The *"White Board"* in the **Resource Room** links to information on health topics identified by youth (STD/STI, body image, etc.). The "why and when to see a health practitioner" for each topic can **help youth identify their own risk factors.**	The *"White Board"* in the **Resource Room** links to information on health topics identified by youth (STD/STI, body image, etc.). The "why and when to see a health practitioner" for each topic can **assist practitioners identify risk factors.**
Continuing Care	Items in the **HangOut** (sofa, clock, posters, etc) link to conversations in *CyberIsle*'s discussion board **(HotTalk).** HotTalk peer discussion and support groups can be used to **connect youth for mutual support.** *Telephones* throughout the **Teen Clinic** link to information on **finding hotlines/crisis lines in a youth's own community as well as what to expect and deserve** when calling a hotline/crisis line.	Practitioners can track youth's use of the **Teen Clinic** and use this as a **starting point for discussions and/or assessments.** Items in the **HangOut** (sofa, clock, posters, etc.) link to conversations in *CyberIsle*'s discussion board **(HotTalk).** Through HotTalk, **practitioners can link youth with other youth for mutual support.**
Linkages and Networks	Items in the **HangOut** (sofa, clock, posters, etc) link to conversations in CyberIsle's discussion board **(HotTalk).** HotTalk peer discussion and support groups can be used to **connect youth for mutual support.** The *"White Board"* in the **Resource Room** links to information on health topics identified by youth (STD/STI, body image, etc.). Each topic provides youth with **ways to connect to people online and in their community.**	The *"White Board"* in the **Resource Room** links to information on health topics identified by youth (STD/STI, body image, etc.). Each topic provides youth with ways to connect to people online

Options for Help	
Items in the **HangOut** (sofa, clock, posters, etc.) link to conversations in *CyberIsle's* discussion board **(HotTalk).** HotTalk peer discussion and support groups can be used to **connect youth for mutual support.** *Telephones* in the **Teen Clinic** link to information on **finding phone lines (hotlines, crisis lines) in a youth's own community as well as what to expect and deserve** when calling a hotline/crisis line for help. The *"White Board"* in the **Resource Room** links to information on health topics identified by youth (STD/STI, body image, etc.). Each topic provides youth with **questions to ask health practitioners and ways to connect to others online and face-to-face to get the help they need.**	and in their community. These resources can **assist practitioners with referrals.** The *"White Board"* in the **Resource Room** links to information on health topics identified by youth (STD/STI, body image, etc.). Each topics includes "why and when to see a health practitioner— this can be **used in conjunction with motivational counselling.** Items in the **HangOut** (sofa, posters, etc.) link to conversations in CyberIsle's discussion board **(HotTalk).** Through HotTalk, **practitioners can link youth with other youth for mutual support.**
Information Management	The *Teen Clinic Online* is a vehicle for meeting and/or delivering the Seven Critical Functions in an easily accessible format that is paced to the user and available 24/7. As one teen said. "You can find it somewhere else, but this is a huge package deal."

description of each room. Starting in the *Reception* area, youth are greeted by a different receptionist depending on the time of day (Figure 17.4). In the Reception area, youth can find out a bit more about the clinic (what's there and who's behind the website). One focus of the *Teen Clinic Online* is to help youth develop skills and knowledge around connecting to resources in their own community to get the help they need and take control of their own health care (**Options for Help, Linkages and Networks** in Tables 17.1 and 17.2). In the Reception area, youth can click on the telephone to learn what to expect from a hotline and how to find one in their community. "*What you should know*" – a link from the front of the receptionist's desk – talks about what youth should expect and are entitled to when receiving health care. For practitioners, these resources can be used to facilitate an open dialogue about appropriate care (**Options for Help)**

In the Clinic's *Resource Room* (Figure 17.5), the "white board" on the back wall links to information on health topics identified by youth, including STDs (sexually transmitted disease) and STIs (sexually transmitted infections), Body Art, and HIV/AIDs (Figure 17.6). For each topic, a definition and select online resources are provided, as well as ways to connect with others on the Web, over the phone and face-to-face (**Options for**

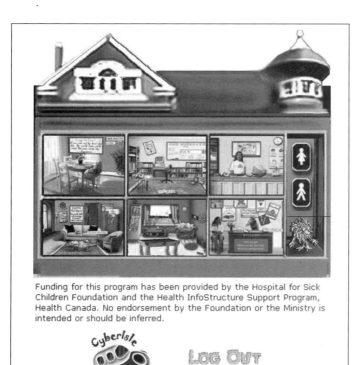

Figure 17.3 *Teen Clinic Online:* Map Page

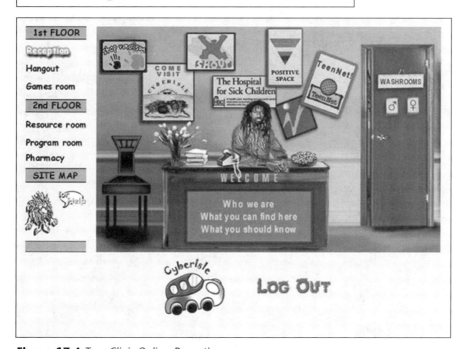

Figure 17.4 *Teen Clinic Online:* Reception

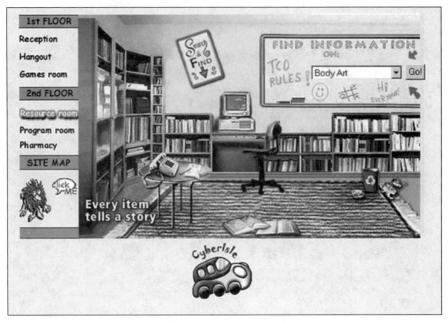

Figure 17.5 *Teen Clinic Online:* Resource Room

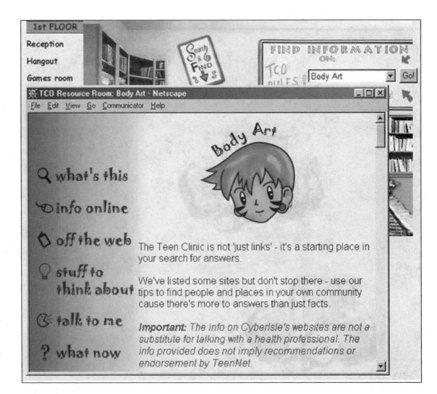

Figure 17.6 *Teen Clinic Online:* Resource Topic on Body Art

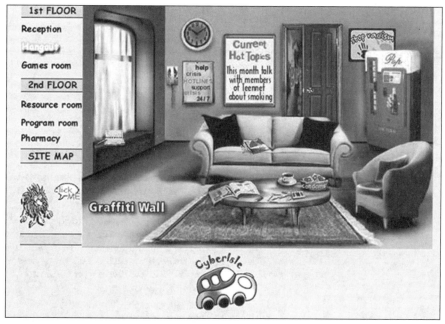

Figure 17.7 *Teen Clinic Online:* Hangout Room

Help; Linkages and Networks). Each of the topics also outlines when a youth might want to see a health practitioner, including a list of questions to ask. These features can be used by youth alone or with a practitioner when talking about different health and social issues and/or when identifying risk factors (**Priming and Prompting; Identification**). Youth and practitioners who want to improve their web searching skills can click on the *Search and Find Poster* to connect to the *Search Tutorial*. The Search Tutorial is an interactive and fun way to learn (**Professional Development**).

In the *Hangout* (Figure 17.7), youth can talk to each other about different subjects, including sex, relationships, drugs and racism. Each of the objects in the Hangout (sofa, chair, ashtray, poster, etc.) links to a different conversation topic in HotTalk, *CyberIsle's* discussion forum. For example, the sofa links to conversations on relationships and family. Through HotTalk, youth can connect with other youth who are experiencing or have experienced the same issues (**Options for Help, Continuing Care, Linkages and Networks**). By becoming familiar with the concerns of youth expressed in HotTalk, practitioners can enhance their communication and empathy with youth when engaging in motivational counseling (**Options for Help, Continuing Care**).

Table 17.2   Smoking Zine Websites for Smoking Prevention and Cessation

	Teens	Practitioners
Professional Development	Not applicable	Using the *Smoking Zine* can help practitioners understand and feel more comfortable using a technology (the Internet) that engages youth.
Priming and Prompting	**Makin' Cents (Phase 1):** interactive game where youth "go shopping with cigarette packages." Provides a **forum for youth to think about the costs of smoking.**	**Makin' Cents (Phase 1):** interactive game where youth "go shopping with cigarette packages." Makin' Cents can be **used by practitioners to discuss the financial cost of smoking with both smokers and nonsmokers.** **What Now?** (**Phase 5**) provides youth with a summary profile of their smoking behavior and attitudes. This **profile can be printed and used by practitioners to facilitate a discussion around smoking with youth.** Each Phase of the *Zine* includes a link to **HotTalk** (*CyberIsle*'s peer-to-peer discussion forum) HotTalk provides practitioners with an opportunity to **observe youth's smoking interests, questions and concerns.**
Identification	**It's My Life (Phase 2):** smoking assessment that enables youth to **self-identify as a smoker, nonsmoker, or experimenter.** **To Change or Not to Change (Phase 3):** using a graphical continuum, **youth identify their readiness to change their smoking/nonsmoking behavior.** This assessment also allows youth to identify how confident they are about the change and its importance to them. **What Now?** (**Phase 5**) provides youth with a summary profile of their smoking behavior and attitudes. This **profile can be printed for use by the youth alone or when consulting a practitioner.**	**It's My Life (Phase 2):** this smoking assessment can be used by practitioners to **identify a youth as a smoker, nonsmoker, or experimenter.** **To Change or Not to Change (Phase 3)** using a graphical continuum youth identify their readiness to change. This assessment includes a measure of a youth's confidence in the change and its importance to them. The results from this assessment **can be used by practitioners to identify the most appropriate course of action for a youth.** **What Now?** (**Phase 5**) provides youth with a summary profile of their smoking behavior and attitudes. This **profile can be printed and used when identifying options with a youth.**

Continuing Care	Each Phase of the *Zine* includes a link to **HotTalk** (*CyberIsle*'s peer-to-peer discussion forum) HotTalk peer discussion and support groups can be used to **connect youth for mutual support.** The *Smoking Zine* **Logout Feature** enables youth to **complete the 5 Phases of the Zine when they are ready.** Youth can also **return to the Zine and redo different quizzes/ assessments to see if anything has changed for them.** **Note to Self** enables youth to keep a record of personal thoughts and observations as they complete each stage of the Smoking Zine. Youth can **keep these observations private or discuss them with practitioners.**	Practitioners can track youth's use of the *Smoking Zine* and use this as a **starting point for discussions and/or assessments.** The *Smoking Zine* **Logout Feature** enables youth to complete the 5 Phases of the *Zine* in one sitting or over a period of time. Practitioners can **encourage youth to re-visit the Zine and re-do some of the Phases to see if their smoking behavior and attitudes change over time.** **Note to Self** enables youth to keep a record of personal thoughts and observations as they complete each stage of the *Smoking Zine.* **If youth feel comfortable sharing these thoughts, Note to Self can form the basis for discussion.**
Linkages and Networks	Each Phase of the *Zine* includes a link to **HotTalk** (*CyberIsle*'s peer-to-peer discussion forum) HotTalk peer discussion and support groups can be used to **connect youth.** The *Smoking Zine* is part of a total youth virtual environment (**CyberIsle**). Thus youth have access to online resources on a range of health and social topics.	The *Smoking Zine* is part of a total youth virtual environment (**CyberIsle**). Through *CyberIsle,* practitioners can connect youth to **online resources on a range of health and social topics.**
Options for Help	**What Now? (Phase 5) includes an** interactive smoking cessation resource for youth who are smokers and ready to quit. **Alone or with a practitioner, youth can create a quit plan that's right for them, including a goal, smoking triggers, ways to avoid temptation and a support network.** Each Phase of the *Zine* includes a link to **HotTalk** (*CyberIsle*'s peer-to-peer discussion forum) Through HotTalk, youth can **connect to other youth for mutual support**.	**What Now? (Phase 5) includes an** interactive smoking cessation resource for youth who are smokers and ready to quit. **Practitioners can work with youth to create a quit plan that's right for them, including a goal, smoking triggers, ways to avoid temptation and a support network.** Each Phase of the *Zine* includes a link to **HotTalk** (*CyberIsle*'s peer-to-peer discussion forum) HotTalk can be used to **connect youth for mutual support**.
Information Management	All the TeenNet websites provide ways of delivering Seven Critical Functions is easily accessible 24/7 hours, paced at user speed and allows for interaction among practitioners.	

A Walk Through the Smoking Zine

The *Smoking Zine* is an interactive 5-phase approach to smoking prevention and cessation that can be completed by youth in one sitting or over a period of time. Youth receive personalized responses for each stage of the *Zine* and a tailored response when all five stages are complete.

The *Zine* opens with an image of a billboard showing the five phases of the *Zine* and a cigarette (Figure 17.8). As youth work through the *Zine*, the different phases light up and the cigarette 'burns down'. The *Zine* begins at Phase 1 with a consciousness raising game called Makin' Cents (Figure 17.9). In "Makin' Cents", youth go shopping at a mall where all the items are priced in cigarette packs. The number of cigarette packs youth have to go shopping with is based on how much they currently smoke or think they could smoke. Makin' Cents is a powerful tool for showing youth how expensive smoking is and what they could buy if they didn't spend their money on cigarettes. Practitioners can use Makin' Cents as a way to start youth thinking about the monetary cost of smoking (**Priming and Prompting**).

Phases 2, 3 and 4 of the *Zine* provide a number of assessments that allow youth to assess their behavior, attitudes and beliefs around smoking, quitting and/or being smoke-free. In particular, Phase 3 (Figure 17.10) allows youth

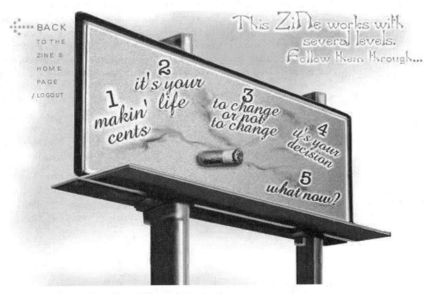

Figure 17.8 *Smoking Zine:* Billboard Navigation

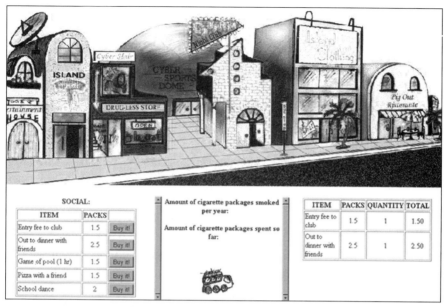

Figure 17.9 *Smoking Zine:* Makin' Cents for consciousness raising

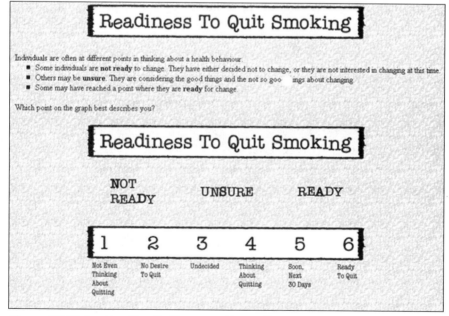

Figure 17.10 *Smoking Zine:* To Change or Not to Change
for matching interventions to readiness for change

to think about whether they are ready to change their smoking behavior (including starting to smoke), as well as how confident they feel about this decision and how important it is to them. This phase draws on the Stages of Change Model described in Chapter 9 (Worksheet 9.1). The next phase (Phase 4) presents questions reflecting the pros and cons of change regarding the youth's smoking status using a decision balance (Worksheet 9.2). In Phase 5, youth are presented with a summary of their quiz and/or assessment scores as well as some suggested next steps. This summary can be printed and is an ideal focus for practitioners discussing smoking with youth (**Options for Help**). For example, from the summary, practitioners can determine whether a youth is a smoker or nonsmoker, and how important quitting or remaining smoke-free is to the youth (**Identification**).

Youth interested in quitting are presented with a comprehensive, interactive 'Quit Program'. Alone or with a practitioner, youth can create a quit plan that's right for them, including a goal, smoking triggers, ways to avoid temptation and a support network (**Options for Help**). At every stage of the *Zine*, youth can link into HotTalk (*CyberIsle*'s discussion forum). In HotTalk, for example, youth trying to quit smoking can connect to other youth for mutual support and care (**Linkages and Networks**). If a youth isn't ready to quit, practitioners can ask the youth to return to the Zine at a later date, re-do one or more of the phases and discuss any changes in results (**Continuing Care**).

Evaluation

Process and Implementation Evaluation

TeenNet is conducting process evaluations in four key areas:

1. **Community Involvement:** Teens have been integrally involved in TeenNet from the onset. Between 1995 and 1997, TeenNet employed 14 youth, including two street-involved youth, and used 20 youth in a Teen Advisory Group on the development of *CyberIsle*. Between 1998 and 2000, TeenNet employed six youth, and used three Teen Advisory Groups to develop the *Teen Clinic Online*. In 1999–2000, eleven youth worked to develop the *Smoking Zine*. School personnel, community organizations and health professionals were also consulted.

2. **Reality Checks (Formative Evaluation):** Before converting components into web formats, TeenNet conducts *Reality Checks* with groups of teens. In these pilots, teens reword questions, delete inappropriate comments, and comment on design, graphics and navigation.

3. **Quality Review Committee:** Groups consisting of teens, teachers, health workers, parents, school administrators assess the quality of hotlinks on *CyberIsle* using TeenNet's checklist for quality assurance.

4. **Qualitative Evaluation:** *CyberIsle*, the *Teen Clinic* and the *Smoking Zine* have all been evaluated by different sets of teens using short answer questionnaires, one-on-one interviews and/or focus groups. Comments from the teens are collated and fed back to the technical team, who then incorporate the teens' suggestions and reconstruct parts of the websites according to evaluation results.

What Do Youth Think About *CyberIsle*?

Youth feel *CyberIsle* is innovative—*"Very different than what I've seen before"*; that the site is graphically appealing—*"Pretty cool. I like it."*; that it is accessible *"Easy to access"*; and that *CyberIsle* is relevant to youth—*"Interesting, something [teens] could relate to."* Teens liked *CyberIsle*'s approach to smoking (*the Smoking Zine*)—*"It didn't force morals and opinions on me. It just helped me to realize how much time and money I was spending on smoking." "I liked the activities … I always love filling out surveys and learning more about myself. I think the notepad for yourself is an excellent idea too. I liked how the program takes you step by step."* Teens find the comprehensiveness of *CyberIsle* particularly appealing; *"It's just good, you could find it somewhere else but this is a huge package deal".* Teens also feel that *CyberIsle* is a more interactive and fun way to learn compared to traditional health promotion approaches; *"You don't want to ask the teacher because everyone will (ask) why do you want to know that. So when you go into CyberIsle you can read … what you want to know about … you can be embarrassed at school."*

HotTalk – Analysis of Peer Discussion Groups

HotTalk is a communication platform that facilitates discussion among teens about relevant health and social issues, via computer networking. HotTalk is the most popular place on *CyberIsle*. Almost every visit to *CyberIsle* includes a visit to HotTalk, where teens talk to other teens about such issues as depression, suicide, sexual activity, drug legalization, teen pregnancy, eating disorders and date rape. Teens use HotTalk to share mutual experiences, ask and give advice, refer each other to community and web-based resources, discuss current affairs, and debate ideas.

Teens identified that they wanted HotTalk to be a self-regulated or a teen-moderated discussion forum. To respect this decision, project team members read HotTalk conversations on a daily basis but only respond to ensure that HotTalk remains a safe environment for youth to exchange thoughts and ideas. TeenNet project team members also direct users who are struggling with serious issues (e.g., suicide or date rape) to contact a professional. For example, if the user identifies that they live in Canada, project team members direct them to Kids Help Phone.

The following is a list of some of the discussion topics:

- **Smoking:** Butt Out, Teenage smoking, To Quit or Not to Quit
- **Sex:** sex and age, gay teens, I just had a baby, I need a friend!, date rape, Damit why me (being pregnant)
- **Alcohol and drug use:** Drugs What do you do and What do you think?, Alcohol, my friends and weed, Be Wise—Legalize, pot smokin, flower children
- **Depression and suicide:** tHe sUN sHInEs~but i don't, I Feel Like Tearing Out My Spleen 'Cause I'm a teen, My so called life, Anyone ever been through this
- **Body image and dieting:** Beauty Is Only Skin-Deep, Being Overweight Ain't That Fun.

Quantitative Results

CyberIsle was officially launched at the end of February 1997. As of February 2001 there are over **32,000 registered users** and there have been over **340,000 visits** to *CyberIsle* (including the *Teen Clinic* and the *Smoking Zine*)

- **65%** are female, **35%** are male
- Average age of users is **15.74 years** old
- Most visited place: **HotTalk** (peer discussion groups)
- Registered visitors spend an average of **15 minutes** per visit to *CyberIsle*
- Visitors have come from: Canada, U.S., Australia, Bahamas, Estonia, Kuwait, Poland, Thailand, Iceland, Israel, etc.

Engaging Hard to Reach Populations: Street-Involved Youth

Without technological equity, the academic achievement gap between groups can only widen, and that gap will threaten the prospects for employment, community inclusiveness, and ultimately, health in the future.

—Nancy Milio (1996, p.113)

TeenNet has explored the possibility of using the Web for drug educa-tion with street-involved and low socioeconomic youth. 'Street-involved' or 'street-connected' youth refers to people under the age of 25 who par-ticipate in street life. Many are homeless, some may live in shelters, hostels, with friends or relatives, and some may still live at home, but all participate in street life.

In 1998, 20 youth (13 female, 5 male, 2 transgender) who attended Shout Clinic (a downtown Toronto clinic that provides comprehensive health services to street-involved youth) were interviewed for approxi-mately 15 minutes and asked questions related to what drugs they take (both medical and recreational), what specific information they want to know about those drugs, where they currently obtain drug information, and questions related to Internet usage. Even though this was a small sam-ple, the study showed a willingness to use the Internet for accessing drug information:

- 95% of youth were currently receiving drug information
- 70% disliked the information they received
- 90% were willing to use the Internet for accessing drug information
- 75% currently had Internet access through friends, cafés, schools, home, and public libraries
- 41% of those with access used the Internet two to three times per week.

In 1998, as part of the development of the *Teen Clinic Online*, the Teen-Net project conducted nine focus groups with youth. Two focus groups were run with street-involved youth at Shout Clinic and Beat the Street (a literacy agency focusing on street-involved youth in Toronto). Compared with the other youth studied, the street-involved youth had among the highest Internet access away from school (67% and 75%), and were the most frequent users of the Internet with 'EVERYDAY USE' being 17% and 25%. As one youth said *"access isn't a problem its education … from this point I can walk probably six or seven places where I can use the Internet."*

In the focus groups, youth were asked to reflect on how their health issues and needs were or were not met. In particular, youth were asked how and why they used or did not use various technologies. In contrast to the other youth studied, the street-involved youth indicated no lack of information, but a real difficulty in assessing quality when sorting through an overwhelming amount of information.

Quantity Overwhelming: *"...ya and it can get just overwhelming on just the number of sites that have nothing really to do with what your looking for."*

Quality of Information: *"Yep, I umm, don't consider most of it reliable cause there's just too much crap and anybody can go out and put a site out like health.com and say you know like, HIV has been found in Coca-Cola. You know they can do that ... umm, you just don't know where you can go for actual information ..."*

Conclusion

We began this chapter with the dilemma: How do we engage teens in health promotion? The Internet offers an exciting and versatile way of attracting their attention—even hard-to-reach and high-risk populations such as street-involved youth. But information technology by itself is insufficient. Our experience on the TeenNet project underscores the value of having youth participation 'from day one'. Indeed, two teens involved in developing *CyberIsle* expressed their sense of ownership and pride in what they were creating:

> It makes me as a teen feel good that people care about what teens think and what they have to say. Most of the time we are overlooked. Not many teens get the chance to actually be heard ... thank you.

These reflections capture the essence of promoting health by blending community participation with information technology.

Moving On

The TeenNet website provide examples of a rapidly emerging new site for health care and health promotion made possible by information technology. Termed 'e-health', this new approach is transforming how consumers (patients) access health information and how they interact with practitioners and the health care system. The next chapter examines basic questions about e-health from a consumers' perspective.

CHAPTER 18

Consumer Perspectives on e-Health

CAMERON D. NORMAN, SHAWN CHIRREY AND HARVEY SKINNER

People almost always want as much information as possible.

—H. Waitzkin (1984)

Overview

Information technology is revolutionizing the way consumers and practitioners interact with the health care system. Through personal computers, hand-held and wireless technologies, we now have access to more health information than ever before. But the question remains about whether this enhanced access to information will result in more informed decisions and better health outcomes. This chapter examines basic questions about e-Health from the consumers' perspective: will e-Health help answer consumer's health questions or create confusion and anxiety; how can e-Health be used for mutual aid, support and self-care; and in what ways (positive and negative) is e-Health transforming the consumer-practitioner interaction and quality of the therapeutic relationship? Many e-Health applications have developed in diverse and rather chaotic ways. An integrative model is needed for ensuring that e-Health applications are: 1) accessible, 2) responsive and 3) empowering for patients and practitioners alike.

Rise of e-Health Consumers

The explosive growth of health information via the Internet has been referred to as a "revolution of unprecedented magnitude" (Jadad & Gagliardi, 1998, p.611), while others liken it to a disease for which we do not yet have a treatment (Coiera, 1998). Currently, the three top uses of the

Internet are for news, shopping (either for purchasing or 'online window shopping') and travel, in that order. While health information falls in fourth place, it is the fastest growing content category for online users with a growth rate of 34% per year, greater than the actual growth rate of the Internet itself (Cyber Dialogue, 2000a). In the U.S. 48% of those online use the Internet for health information, the rates in Canada are comparable with over 50% of consumers and 73% of physicians currently using health resources on the Internet—rates that are predicted to increase in the coming years (Canadian Medical Association Journal, 2000; Cyber Dialogue, 2000b; Medical Post, 2000).

Although health practitioners and consumers may differ in the detail and types of information used, they face similar issues integrating this information into health promotion and health care. In this chapter, we focus on these challenges regarding how e-Health influences consumers and practitioners in what is commonly referred to as 'interactive health communications' or IHC (Robinson et al., 1998).

Traditionally, health information was designed for and available to health practitioners (Inlander, 1991). Prior to the 1970s, practitioners maintained a key role as gatekeepers of health information for patients. With the rise of the consumer health movement in the 1970s came a shift from patients being passive recipients of information to patients as consumers. This shift emphasized greater responsibility on the part of the consumer for self-care, preventive measures and shared decision-making. These changes coincided with a decrease in the actual amount of time that physicians had available to spend with individual patients (Gilbert et al., 1997).

The growth of Consumer Health Information Services (CHIS) across North America in the 1980s and 1990s contributed to the evolution of the consumer health movement. CHIS centres were developed, in part, to address the growing desire for information among consumers (Patrick & Koss, 1995). Not only was health information seen as a public service to be offered to patients, but also its commercial potential exploded, resulting in a new marketplace for magazines and books targeted at information-hungry consumers. In both cases, the information being offered ranged widely in its authorship (patients, doctors and other forms of health practitioners), content (from basic allopathic and naturopathic medicine to that of untested alternatives) and overall quality. It was at this time that the phrase 'medical consumer' emerged, referring to individuals who took it upon themselves to have a dialogue and negotiation process with their doctor, as

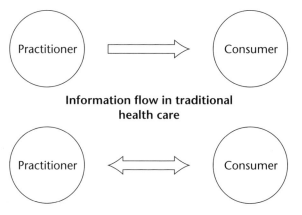

Information flow in traditional health care

Information flow in e-Health

Figure 18.1 Comparing information flow in traditional health care and e-Health.

opposed to passively consuming information provided by their physician (Reeder, 1972). Since then others have described health information consumers as active and responsible health consumers (Ferguson, 1991).

With the emergence of new technologies (i.e., the Internet, especially the World Wide Web; cell phones and wireless Web access; interactive voice response systems and phone-based counselling services), the availability of health information has grown rapidly. Electronic-Health (e-Health) based information has added dramatically to the ease of accessibility and availability of previously hard to reach information, as well as to the sheer volume and types of resources made available.

Traditionally, health information has been transmitted in a unidirectional manner from practitioner (or information provider) to consumer (Figure 18.1). This practitioner-oriented approach emphasized the practitioner as possessor of information while the patient consumes the information. However, with e-Health systems information, transmission becomes bidirectional (Figure 18.1). Both practitioner and consumer learn from one another, and each becomes what Wurman (2001) calls 'prosumers' or creators *and* consumers of information. Although practitioner-oriented, or top-down, approaches remain the dominant position in the health sector, the communication balance is changing with e-Health.

A consumer-oriented approach to e-Health recognizes that health information is co-created by practitioners and consumers. This underscores the influences that prior health knowledge, experience, cultural background and social position can play in the transmission of information from sender to receiver. Many nontechnical factors influence a consumer's appraisal and use of health information found on the Internet. Tacit understanding, for example, has been an important component of human information processing and decision-making for centuries. Yet, health professionals often disregard this when analyzing consumer decision-making behaviors (Jadad & Enkin, 2000).

The rise of evidence-based medicine has emphasized rational decision-making and empirical evidence, which contrasts with the more tacit and experiential approaches of consumers to health information. This is widening the gap between consumer and practitioner perspectives (Lewis, 1999). The implication for e-Health is not that evidence should be disregarded, but rather that sociocultural factors be considered when providing health information and appraising the consumer's decision-making process. These 'softer', or nontechnical, factors need to be integrated into a consumer-oriented approach to e-Health.

Information alone rarely produces change (see Chapter 7). Rather, information is part of a continuum of understanding and processes of change (Shedroff, 1999). For information to actually inform, it must have relevance to the user (Thayer, 1988). To accomplish this, information must fit with the values, circumstances and needs of the consumer—the context of one's life. Seely-Brown and Duguid (2000) refer to these contextual factors as being part of the 'social life of information.' They contend that much of the information generated occurs within social interactions irrespective of whether it is electronically mediated. Data are generated everywhere—information is the meaning given to data by people who see it's relevance to their lives. Wurman (2001) echoes this by pointing to the abundance of means available to generate streams of data (e.g., Internet) and the paucity of tools to help people interpret these data. Thus, one of the principal challenges affecting e-Health is creating effective methods to help people derive meaning from data and turn information into knowledge (Jadad & Enkin, 2000). It is at this juncture between data, information and knowledge that e-Health applications can have the greatest impact (Figure 18.2).

Will enhanced access to health information unnecessarily increase health services utilization, cause confusion, and lead to self-diagnosis and misdiagnosis? Research on consumer uses of health information, both online and paper forms, suggests otherwise. For example, it has been proposed that enhanced access to health information will result in more frequent doctors visits. However, Pifalo et al. (1997) found the inverse resulting, in part, from decreased patient anxiety. Studies show that informed consumers make bet-

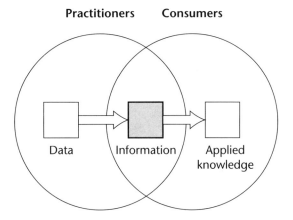

Figure 18.2 The spectrum of understanding in e-Health.

ter overall decisions about their health and treatment options (Marcus & Tuchfeld, 1993), and are more likely to follow the required instructions and adopt health-promoting behaviors (Pifalo et al., 1997). Gilbert et al. (1997) found that informed patients are less susceptible to false or misleading health product advertisements and are more likely to have a better relationship with their physician. Others have found that knowledgeable patients typically have better health and medical outcomes, such as improved diabetes control, better postoperative recovery times and fewer incidences of postoperative infections (Boore, 1978; Greenfield et al., 1988).

Given the increasing abundance of health information available via e-Health applications, how can consumers evaluate its relevance and quality?

Information Quality: Different Stakeholders, Different Needs

A 1999 study on Web indexing suggested that search engines such as Yahoo! Alta Vista, Google and Northern Light individually cover no more than 16% of the World Wide Web and only 38.3% in combined coverage (Lawrence & Giles, 1999). Entering 'health' as a search word in Google, the largest index of the Web, produced over 45,100,000 web pages from the 1,396,920,000 total pages indexed (as of January 28, 2001). This illustrates that the Internet alone provides more information than any individual consumer can possibly use or comprehend. These millions of web pages contain information of varying quality, with few obvious means of distinguishing between high- and low-quality sources.

Quality is a concern for both health practitioners and consumers who take advantage of e-Health (Canadian Medical Association Journal, 2000). Unlike traditional media sources that use editors and producers to vet information prior to transmission to the public, the Internet allows anyone to distribute information to the world. Indeed, the ability for any individual to reach a global audience has allowed the Internet to become a very powerful force for delivering information. While such democratization of information allows for a diversity of voices and perspectives, it also brings forward issues of legitimacy with respect to source. To that end, information quality remains a major challenge for e-Health.

Not only is quality of information a challenge in online health, but so too are the issues of confidentiality and privacy. In many respects this is tied to the issue of complete and clear disclosure, which is a key criterion to many of the e-Health quality checklists. E-Health consumers are very concerned about the issue of confidentiality and privacy of health information on the Internet. A recent study (Cyber Dialogue, 2000a) revealed that health information consumers are more concerned about sites sharing their information without permission to third parties than they are about having their health information 'hacked' into (75% versus 59% amongst general users and 85% versus 73% amongst online users with poor health). At issue is the desire to get personalized content by providing personal information and preferences to websites, while having one's privacy respected. While consumers are concerned about privacy, they typically fail to take the steps required to ensure it (e.g., by reading about policies on websites or ticking the right boxes on the online forms to optout).

Studies have examined the quality of health information on such topics ranging from cancer (Biermann et al., 1999; Hoffman-Goetz & Clark, 2000), fever management in children (Impicciatore et al., 1997), to female urinary incontinence (Sandvik, 1999). In many cases, information quality was highly suspect. While documented cases of harm arising from poor information on the Internet are few, there is concern about the potential harm that poor quality or misleading information can engender.

Approaches to addressing quality in consumer health information fall largely within two major theoretical frameworks: a **consequentialist** (or moralistic) framework and a **deontological** (or common morality) framework. The former emphasizes 'right' and 'wrong' decisions based upon their health consequences, while the latter emphasizes consumer autonomy and the need for consumers to make informed choices based on the information alone (Entwistle et al., 1996). These frameworks underlie two approaches to promoting quality assurance in consumer health information: credentialing and critical appraisal skill development.

Third-Party Credentialing. Third party credentialing typically involves reports from expert reviewers or 'seals of approval'. An example of this kind of approach is the Health on the Net (HON) code for health websites (*http://www.hon.ch*). The HON code is placed on websites that adhere to a set of quality criteria deemed to indicate quality health information. Another form of credentialing comes in the form of health meta-sites, websites that consolidate health information on a wide variety of issues and offer many different ways to connect people to health information. Examples of meta-sites include *Healthfinder* (*http://www.healthfinder.org*) and the *Canadian Health Network* (*http://www.canadian-health-network.ca*). They feature a range of proprietorship from for-profit commercial sites to government-sponsored programs. To filter content, these sites typically use panels of experts and consumers to select the most credible and reliable sources available on the Web for any given topic and provide links to these services on their site. Meta-sites frequently offer users a variety of different features besides links, including original content, e-mail lists, discussion forums, real-time webcasts and daily health tips.

The key to the success of a third party approach is to have the site's authority recognized. In the case of seals of approval, the public must be aware of what the seal of approval stands for, what its criteria of inclusion and exclusion are, and the means by which websites obtain such seals. Without a clearly recognized process of filtering, such seals of approval are unlikely to have significant impact in reducing information quality perception problems. Similar problems of legitimacy exist with health meta-sites. For meta-sites to be credible, they must represent some form of trusted authority on health. In the case of the *Canadian Health Network* (CHN), the credibility arises from a network of recognized leaders in health research and services across the country.

Without public recognition of the authority of a site, third party credential approaches will not work. This matter has been particularly relevant to the commercial meta-sites. A case in point is *DrKoop.com*, a revenue-generating e-commerce and health information site that relies on the trusted name of former U.S. Surgeon General C. Everett Koop, a primary investor in the website. While Dr. Koop himself was viewed as a venerable and respected source of health information, incomplete disclosure around funding sources led to criticism, from medical ethicists and the public alike, who challenged the objectivity and reliability of the information on *DrKoop.com* (British Medical Journal, 1999b; Noble, 1999). By not disclosing financial arrangements that many recommended health sources had paid to be profiled on the site, *DrKoop.com* effectively undermined the credibility of the site and its high-profile proprietor (British Medical Journal, 1999a). Another issue affecting the third party approach is that it requires meta-sites to stay abreast of a field of scientific literature that expands at a rate of more than 12,000 articles per year, while simultaneously delivering information to people in a timely manner (Jadad, 2001).

Critical Appraisal. Critical appraisal involves a consumer-centered strategy whereby consumers are taught critical appraisal skills. This approach focuses on teaching users to recognize the best practices of e-Health in order to make informed decisions about online health information. These can be transmitted through specific courses (e.g., Sheppard et al., 1999), professional guidelines (e.g., Gustafson, et al., 1999; Winkler, et al., 2000), or online and interactive checklists (e.g., Mitretek Systems, 2001). This consumer-centered approach typically employs rating tools to emphasize specific criteria that have been identified as the best practices for online health information. These criteria typically include accuracy, reliability, currency, author affiliation and authority and some design factors in their assessment of a particular website (Kim et al., 1999).

Norman and Skinner (2000) examined these criteria against the best practice criteria identified by youth consumers and found that few available rating scales addressed quality from perspectives other than the professional's point of view. In their review of 25 guideline documents and rating tools for critically appraising health information on the Internet (both online and offline), Norman and Skinner found that criteria such as the values and beliefs emphasized, skill development opportunities, respectful language tone, emphasis on individual choice and the involvement of consumers in developing the site were largely absent (Table 18.1).

The best practice criteria identified by youth consumers were obtained through focus groups in which youth were asked to critically appraise health websites using conventional criteria. To gain trust with youth, sites had to present information in ways that were respectful of their interests and needs as well as present information in a manner that was accessible—both in content and in style.

Table 18.1   A Consumer's Guide to Online Health Information

1. Accessibility

a. Is the site's purpose clearly evident?

b. Do I encounter a lot of errors or missing links while navigating?

c. Are there tools to assist me in searching the sites? (e.g., search engine)

d. Is the information on the website easy to download or does it take a long time?

e. Is the information on the website easy to download or does it take a long time to require plug-ins or software?

f. Does the site provide me with the level of depth of information I need?

g. Is the site easy to navigate (can I find what I am looking for)?

Credibility

a. Are the authors qualified to make the statements they do and can I tell?

b. Is the site or author recognized as an authority by people I trust?

c. Is the site owners name and contact information clearly posted on the site, and can I contact them easily?

d. Do the site owners encourage users to seek *independent* second opinions?

e. Are conflicts of interest clearly stated (e.g., advertising revenue)?

f. Are the links to other *quality* health sources available on the site?

g. Is the information on the site currentl and up-to-date with posted dates indicating the date information was created, posted and last updated?

h. Do the site owners have a clear statement of disclosure visible to inform me about their information-use policies and security?

3. Personal Fit

a. Does the content fit with my personal values?

b. Does the information meet my needs (i.e., does it answer my questions) or can it help me find my answers elsewhere?

c. Was the website designed with me in mind?

d. Does the site encourage me to make healthy decisions? (e.g., self-assessments, decision aids)

e. Is the language respectful of me as a consumer or more paternal?

f. Is the site interesting and enjoyable to use?

4. Interactivity and Active Learning

a. Is the site interactive?

b. Are the tools to help me make healthy decisions? (e.g., self-assessment, decision aids)

c. Does the site offer me opportunities to connect to others (e.g., chat rooms, bulletin boards, links to self-help resources)

d. Are there opportunities to learn new skills via the website?

The key challenge facing this approach to quality is ensuring the reliability and validity of critical appraisal tools. A review of such tools by Jadad and Gagliardi (1998) indicated that most tools did not disclose the results of reliability and validity testing of their instruments (if such testing was done at all), and the authors questioned whether such tools assess what they claim to measure. Furthermore, little published evidence exists regarding the effectiveness of such tools in affecting health knowledge or behavior.

There is no common agreement on what is the best approach to assessing the quality of websites, or indeed whether it can be done at all. Some suggest that rating health information is a step toward empowering consumers (Eysenbach & Diepgen, 1999) while others suggest that rating the quality of health websites effectively may be impossible given the Web's unique characteristics (Delamothe, 2000). There is, however, nearly universal agreement among practitioners and consumers alike that ensuring quality is critical to the future of e-Health.

Self-Help Online

No matter how well-informed patients are about their medical conditions, most need the reassurance of talking to others who have been in similar situations, who can demystify the health delivery system, and who can provide emotional and social support when things are not going well.

—Alemi, et al. (1996)

One area of e-Health that has received extensive research is in its support of self-help activities. Self-Help/Mutual-Aid as a movement has been fundamentally supportive of consumer's drive for health and mental health information. Self-help goes beyond simply providing information to include the provision of practical and emotional support for people navigating through health information and the health care system.

Brief History

Self-help first appeared formally in North America with the advent of Alcoholics Anonymous in 1935 (Borkman, 1999). However, it truly came of age in the 1970s, coinciding with the rise in the consumer health movement. Interest in self-help grew, in part, from the support of researchers and social scientists that began to tout the effectiveness and impact of 'small grassroots groups'. Self-help continued to grow through the 1980s with the founding of Self-Help clearinghouses across North America, Europe and worldwide. These clearinghouses provided a self-support system to the self-help community and the public at large by providing information and referral services to existing groups while helping to assist new groups to develop. Self-help has continued to bloom with the growth of information technologies in the late 1980s which enable online support groups (Oka & Borkman, 2000).

Self-help as a concept is frequently confused and misunderstood. Self-help is often equated with books you find in that ever-popular section of your local bookstore. It is often mistaken to be the same thing as self-care (i.e., caring for one's own health or that of a loved one through maintenance and self-administering of treatment for one's condition). But while self-help and self-care share common elements and at times overlap, they are not equatable (Health Canada, 1998).

Self-help is a process of voluntarily sharing mutual support and information around a common concern. Examples of self-help topics range from living with breast cancer, or maintaining alcohol sobriety, to parenting twins, or being single women in a new city. Traditionally self-help occurs in the format of face-to-face support groups that meet on a regular basis. Self-help is no stranger to technology. There are many examples of self-help groups utilizing technology (i.e., teleconferences, peer-support phone lines, online groups through computer bulletin board systems, pen-pal networks), all in the name of supporting peers that share a common issue. Self-help groups were using technologies prior to the spread of the Internet.

Chirrey and McGowen (1999) describe self-help as a process of sharing common experiences, issues and/or problems. Self-help groups share some common characteristics including being participatory in nature (i.e., getting help, giving help, and learning to help yourself) as well as sharing (i.e., knowledge, experience, information, practical and emotional support). Self-help groups do not charge fees to participants, although a nominal donation to cover expenses is sometimes requested, but never required. Groups typically run either within a pre-established structure (e.g., 12-step model of anonymous groups) or develop their own explicit processes regarding the running of meetings (i.e., rotating or regular facilitation). Self-help initiatives continue on an ongoing basis, are voluntary in nature rather than mandatory, and are open to new members. Self-help activities are run by and for the participants, as distinct from professional facilitators common to therapy-based support groups.

Migration Online

Self-help has stepped onto the information highway through two main ramps. First, many groups, organizations, networks and clearinghouses have developed an online presence to promote their face-to-face activities. At last count, over 60% of national and international self-help associations and organizations were accessible over the Internet (Madara & White, 1997, p.93). Many self-help organizations and clearinghouses offer information and referral services to face-to-face support groups through online databases such as the American Self-Help Clearinghouse (*www.selfhelpgroups.org*) and the Self-Help Resource Centre of Greater Toronto (*www.selfhelp.on.ca*). According to Madara et al. (1988), such computerized services have used 'high tech' solutions to promote 'high touch' support networks.

The most interesting foray into the technology world for self-help has been through the explosive growth of online support groups. Existing online groups have grown dramatically in size, as exemplified by CompuServ's Diabetes Forum, which had 40,000 members involved between 1990–1996 and grew to 65,000 in 1997 (one year)—growth coinciding with the Internet's initial growth spurt (Madara, 1997). The actual number of active online self-help groups in the forms of both e-mail-based listservs and web-based discussion groups (e.g., asynchronous bulletin board posting systems and real-time chat groups) has grown in leaps and bounds and is now estimated to number in the hundreds of thousands.

Online self-help groups provide people with several advantages over its face-to-face counterpart, including ease and convenience in terms of 'attending a meeting'; complete anonymity; increased access to support groups for rare conditions; and helping to overcome physical barriers or restrictions to travel to groups. Arguably the most significant advantage is the shift of consumers from passive information recipients to actual producers of knowledge and information. Online self-help provides its users with a means of support, a source of practical and technical information, a way to share experiences and ideas, and a potential source of empowerment. Online self-help efforts, like its face-to-face counterpart, sometimes lead to real world advocacy efforts. While it is evident self-help online has advantages, whether it provides the same 'high touch' qualities of its real-world counterpart remains to be seen.

Another significant difference with online self-help is the increased blurring and mixing with the area of self-care. Many individuals go online seeking health information related to a particular issue or condition that they are faced with and often stumble upon self-help as an adjunct or clarification point for their health issue. In contrast, many individuals end up in face-to-face self-help groups as a result of frustration with a health care system that failed to serve them adequately. People often go online to find a solution to their health concerns. Then, they stay after the initial information hunt because of the mutual support and 24-hours per day connections that online self-help offers.

The Internet has probably had it greatest impact on self-help as it relates to rare disorders and orphan diseases. Organizations such as the National Organization for Rare Disorders (NORD) in the United States (*www.rarediseases.org*) and its Canadian counterpart, the Canadian Organization for Rare Disorders (CORD) (*www.cord.ca*), are examples of self-help networks using emerging technologies to provide assistance to people affected by rare and orphan diseases. The distance between once-isolated small groups of rare condition patients, scattered throughout a given country or the world has been narrowed through online communities and discussion forums. In several instances, online communities have greatly helped both patients and practitioners understand the illness that they face, leading to improved care and outcomes.

One example is that of the American Self-Help Clearinghouse helping persons with Ehlers Danlos Syndrome (EDS) to form an online presence through web-based conferences (Madara, 1995). This led to the creation of a national organizations for EDS, that attracted so many new members that the national incidence rate was now estimated at 1% of 5,000 instead of the inaccurate rate of 1% per 750,000 that had been previously estimated. Examples such as this show the real benefit of online self-help groups, not only to those that suffer from the condition but also to practitioners and researchers.

Transforming the Patient-Practitioner Relationship

Perhaps the most noticeable way in which e-Health is affecting health care is by changes in the patient-practitioner relationship. Within this relationship, it is the patient who is most commonly regarded as the consumer. However, the role of practitioner-as-consumer is increasingly being recognized, as the transfer of information becomes bidirectional in the e-Health environment. Indeed, the way this information is communicated should heighten attention on ways in which the patient-practitioner relationship is changing. How can e-Health applications be designed to effect positive a transformation?

Roles and responsibilities for health have undergone significant change over the past 30 years. This has put a burden on the patient and family to engage in greater self-care (Waitzkin, 1991). There is now an expectation that people will seek information about illness prevention and treatment outside of the medical encounter. Indeed, to be uninformed is to violate the new 'sick role' for consumers. This shift has led many to the Internet for health information in order to complement the care they receive from health practitioners. As such, 84% of Canadian physicians reported having patients present them with medical information from the Internet (Canadian Medical Association Journal, 2000), and over 70% of physicians reported having had a patient bring web-based information to a consult in the past month (Medical Post, 2000).

A PriceWaterhouseCoopers (2000) study found that of the 22% of Canadians who use the Internet for health information, only 33% discussed the information they found with their physician. The lack of control that practitioners have over what their patients find on the Internet coupled with their desire to use the Internet has prompted many physicians to go online themselves. In the U.S. consumers are not only going online for health information to bring to their doctor, but also using the Internet for comparative data on doctors and health services. American e-Health consumers are going online to seek evaluations about doctors (76%) and hospitals (72%) to help them determine who is selected to fulfill their health needs (Cyber Dialogue, 2000b).

Several Health Maintenance Organizations (HMOs) have explored or now turned to providing 'infoscriptions' (approved health information sources online) to their insured patients, to ensure that they are receiving information that is of good quality and reliable (Goedert, 1997; Morrissey, 1997). Others have explored providing their insured patients with e-mail access to a physician to ask non-emergency medical questions.

To address consumer interest in e-Health service provision, a variety of online services have emerged in recent years. An example of such a service is E-Salveo (*http://www.esalveo.com*), an online facilitator that matches consumers with local practitioners who are interested in engaging in interactive health communication. For a fee, E-Salveo facilitates an online relationship between the patient and practitioner and ensures that all the appropriate health billing is recorded. This service allows patients and physicians to consult around non-urgent health matters including basic health questions, providing sick notes and renewing prescriptions—services that can be provided quickly and efficiently without the need for a face-to-face appointment. In mediating the physician-patient relationship in a virtual environment, E-Salveo is offering a means of connecting people rather than providing an actual health service in itself. In doing so, 'matchmaker' services like this make the health system more responsive to the needs of consumers using e-Health.

Services like the one just described exist partially because of barriers to sharing information among people within the traditional health care model. e-Health has the potential to reduce these barriers through either real time or asynchronous uses of technology. The most popular means of providing physician-patient communication using e-Health is via e-mail. Despite the advances in technology available through the World Wide Web, e-mail is still widely regarded as the most popular Internet application. The number of e-mails transmitted per year has risen above letters, phone calls and faxes and is poised to become one of the most important means of communication in the coming years (IDC, 2000) Recognizing this trend, many physicians have begun using e-mail to contact their patients (and vice versa). The 2000 National Survey of Doctors in Canada found that 23% of physicians currently use e-mail to communicate with their patients and 51% expressed interest in doing so in the coming months. While the specific numbers of e-mails sent between patients and physicians is unknown, it is evident from surveying trends in the medical informatics literature that e-mail use in health encounters has increased.

Electronic communication has unique challenges that may not always be evident to practitioners or consumers. 'Netiquette' involves informal guidelines for e-mail communication; these include cautions on the use of capital letters (indicated as yelling) and the use of sarcasm online (it may be misinterpreted). Indeed, using text-based communication such as e-mail opens up the possibility that information may be misunderstood due to the lack of social cues involved in the encounter. Recognizing these concerns, the American Medical Informatics Association (AMIA) drafted guidelines for the clinical use of e-mail with patients in 1997 (Kane & Sands, 1998) in anticipation of the widespread adoption of e-mail use in primary care. The AMIA's guidelines were designed to improve communication between patient and practitioner and to manage the medical-legal aspects of patient care that are unique to e-mail communication.

The assumption guiding the AMIA's guidelines is that e-mail communication will be engaged by means of mutual agreement. However, this is not always the case in everyday practice. Eysenbach & Deipgen (1999) examined the motivation, expectations and beliefs of patients seeking medical information by analyzing 209 unsolicited e-mail received by physicians at a hospital dermatology department. It was found that 40% of inquiries could have been answered by a librarian, 27% of the cases had questions that were unanswerable without a face-to-face clinical encounter, and only 28% of the questions were answerable via e-mail alone. These findings point to problem inherent in providing essentially unlimited patient access to physicians. Appropriate boundaries need to be established regarding how the Internet can and should be used in health care.

An Integrated Model for e-Health

For e-Health to have broad impact it requires integration with traditional health promotion and health care approaches. In order to accomplish this, an integrated model of e-Health is needed. To be successful in meeting the challenges discussed in this chapter, an integrated e-Health model must work within the dynamic relationships among consumers, practitioners and health organizations. Jadad (1999) argues that, for e-Health to be successful and purposeful, partnerships between stakeholders must exist at all levels. Also, e-Health needs to build on organizational models, such as the Seven Critical Functions described in Chapter 12 for supporting consumers and practitioners in health behavior change. Examples of integrated e-Health applications that support the Critical Functions are given in Chapters 15, 16 and 17.

As the examples presented in this chapter illustrate, e-Health traverses the boundaries between health care and health promotion by creating a new arena within the health sector. e-Health bridges between traditional health care, which is largely top-down, emphasizes clinical and experimental research information, is institution-based and practitioner-centered; and health promotion, which is typically bottom-up, emphasizes community experience, is community-based and consumer-centered. e-Health is both and neither of these two models; rather it is a new model in itself, uniquely positioned between each of these complementary approaches to addressing health issues (Figure 18.3).

An integrated model of e-Health needs to be: 1) accessible, 2) responsive, and 3) empowering (Figure 18.4). While such qualities may be seen

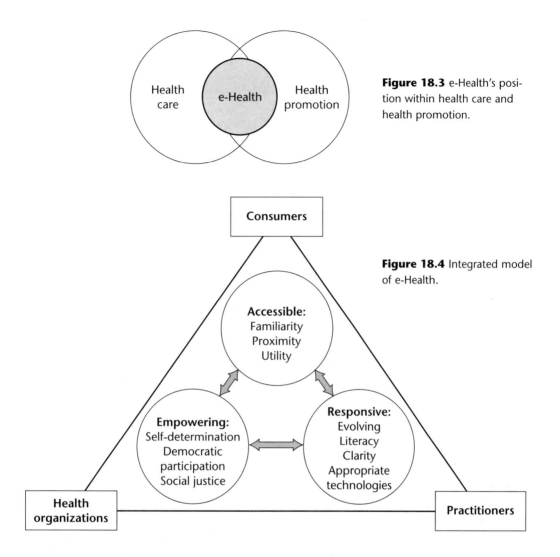

Figure 18.3 e-Health's position within health care and health promotion.

Figure 18.4 Integrated model of e-Health.

as necessary in any health care model, there are specific issues and challenges for e-Health applications. This model must not only serve to enhance health but also address the systemic issues that prevent e-Health from providing benefit to *the population as a whole*—not just those who have the appropriate resources. In essence, e-Health must address the digital divide in terms of increasing access to health resources and improving health information quality.

Accessibility. Accessibility encompasses design features that allow individuals and special populations to take full advantage of e-Health benefits. This involves availability and familiarity with the technology. People need to know how to use it effectively: what e-Health can and cannot do in the promotion of health and provision of care. Akin to this is the issue of proximal distance, ensuring that people can literally access the technology they need. This requires policy to ensure that all members of society have access to emerging technology on some level. While it is not reasonable to assume that everyone will always have equal access to technology, it is possible through policy and practice to ensure some form of equity in information access, especially for disadvantaged populations.

Responsiveness. Responsiveness means creating services and infrastructures that are consumer-driven rather than technology-driven. This includes the development of search tools that allow consumers to get their questions answered in a timely manner by providing information and resources that are helpful and relevant. Responsiveness also includes means of determining the most reasonable and cost-effective resource for answering different questions at different times. Such responsiveness must include means of reducing 'data smog' (or non-useful information clutter) rather than contributing to it (Shenk, 1997).

Literacy is the key feature of responsiveness. Effective e-Health is not possible if consumers and practitioners lack the skills to understand or appraise online health information. Norman and Skinner (2000) introduced the term 'digital health literacy' (DHL) to describe the unique set of literacy skills required to navigate through health information on the Internet. DHL encompasses skills from basic reading literacy, health literacy, computer literacy and media literacy that individuals must possess to adequately appraise online health information. DHL also allows consumers to determine who and what they can trust on the Internet.

A final component of responsiveness is evolution. In an ever-changing health and technological environment, e-Health must continually evolve to meet the needs of consumers and practitioners alike. This means undertaking continual needs assessments and evaluations of practices and policies related to e-Health. These evaluative activities will determine the degree to which e-Health is contributing to or preventing positive changes in health and increase our understanding of how it may be done differently.

Empowerment. Empowerment involves collaborative and democratic participation, distributive justice and self-determination (Prilleltensky, 1994). This feature of the e-Health model emphasizes the need for all stakeholders in the health sector to work together to purposefully shape e-Health's evolution and to ensure that it addresses the needs of the entire population. Empowerment includes consumer participation in the development of e-Health materials and services along with shared decision-making regarding how e-Health is used in each practitioner-consumer relationship. By ensuring that the use of e-Health in each health encounter is negotiated, both practitioners and consumers will be in a position to best use information technology effectively to address the needs of both consumers and the health system in general.

Conclusion

This chapter has illustrated ways in which e-Health is growing and affecting health care and health promotion. Much of this growth has been haphazard—emergent rather than directive. One of the by-products of this unguided growth is the digital divide, the gap between the information 'haves' and 'have-nots' (Milio, 1996). As with many technological innovations, Internet use is largely distributed along economic, geopolitical and educational lines, and, to a lesser degree, by gender and ethnoracial identity (Lazarus & Lipper, 2000; NTIA, 1999). Another product of this rapid growth is that e-Health is largely technology-driven. That is, existing technology is applied to the health system, rather than designing technology for significant needs of the health system. Too often we fit people to technology, rather than technology to people's needs. Some have suggested that society has entered a period where the discussion of technology shifts from 'what it can do for me' to 'what does it do to me' (Vicente, 2001).

None of this is inevitable. Through active and purposeful collaboration between consumers and practitioners, an e-Health system can be developed that promotes health, helps prevent disease and enhances care while building community capacity and fostering community mobilization around health issues (Milio, 1996; Minkler, 1997). E-Health is uniquely positioned to accomplish these goals—if it evolves purposefully and in the service of *all* stakeholder groups, not just practitioners and organizations. E-Health should not be seen as a panacea for health reform. Rather, it should be regarded as a useful means of providing integration to health care and health promotion efforts while responding to a rapidly changing environment. As e-Health becomes normalized, unguided growth may prove to be more harmful than helpful. The question for practitioners and consumers alike is: How can we ensure that e-Health systems provide effective, efficient and equitable health services?

Moving On

The last chapter in this book provides a framework (*Your Personal Learning Plan*) and web-based tools for your ongoing development in personal and organizational change.

Afterword

I do not mind learning. I just don't like being taught.

—Winston Churchill

CHAPTER 19

Your Personal and Organizational Learning Plan

I had lived past the first rush of arrival, when raw talent can carry you across most barriers. Now I had to learn enough to last a lifetime. I am still learning.

—Pete Hamill (1994, p.265)

Overview

Experience teaches that if learning is to be effective, you need to get beyond good intentions and develop a realistic action plan, *starting now*. Education 'sticks' when it is interactive and challenging and when it includes sequential activities you can practice and by which you can hone your skills (Davis et al., 1999). Parker Palmer (1998) underscores the need to begin with ourselves by integrating the intellectual, emotional and spiritual dimensions of learning. His book, *The Courage to Teach*, raises questions that often go unasked and celebrates reconnecting students and teachers alike with a deeply engaging passion for learning.

Worksheet 19.1 helps you to develop such a plan, one aimed at improving both your personal learning and your organization's effectiveness. Some key supports and ideas to stimulate your learning are described in this chapter, including the outline for my Health Behavior Change course, a comprehensive website with interactive learning components designed to complement this book (*www.HealthBehaviorChange.org*), and a profile of five additional books on organizational improvement.

Health Behavior Change Course

I teach this graduate level course (CHL 5804S) at the University of Toronto with my colleagues Curtis Breslin and Joan Brewster. It has proven to be a fruitful testing ground for the ideas and practical tools described in this book. The goal of this course is to provide the necessary knowledge and skill-based learning for changing health behavior in individuals and health organizations. Details are available at the course website (*www.HealthBehaviorChange.org*). *Promoting Health* is used as the key text.

The course provides a critical examination of the need for health care reform, especially the need for putting prevention and health promotion into practice, and the key role that health organizations play in this transformation. Psychological processes underlying motivation and the social context of behavior change are studied. Understanding readiness for change, as well as effective ways of reducing resistance and enhancing motivation are addressed. In particular we teach a Five-Step Model that emphasises concepts and practical tools for organizational improvement. Thus, the course focuses on understanding and integrating behavior change at multiple levels: individual (patient, practitioner), organization and community.

Course Objectives

- To develop an understanding of current theories and concepts of health behavior change in individuals, practitioners and organizations
- To review strategies for integrating health behavior change at different levels: microlevel (individual, practitioner) and macrolevel (organization, community)
- To integrate concepts and relevant research with skill-based learning exercises and practical tools
- To stimulate lifelong learning and self-improvement regarding one's own health behavior.

Table 19.1. gives an outline of the course sessions.

Organizational Analysis Assignment

The following assignment on organizational change has proven to be a particularly valuable learning experience for students. Try it at your setting.

1. Select a health care setting for analysis. Settings that students have used range from family practice clinics, specialist medical clinics, community health centeres, comprehensive health organizations (Health Maintenance Organization), special population clinics (e.g., women's health; HIV), dental practices, student health services, occupational medicine health clinic, to fitness clubs.

Table 19.1   Health Behavior Change: Course Outline

Harvey Skinner, Curtis Breslin and Joan Brewster
University of Toronto

Session Outline
1. The Challenge: Demystifying Health Behavior Change
2. Readiness for Change: Transtheoretical Model
3. Motivational Interventions. When do they work and why? Self-Determination Theory, Motivational Interviewing
4. Theories of Health-Protective Behavior: Health Belief Model; Theory of Reasoned Action/Planned Behavior
5. Social Cognitive Theory: Self-Efficacy and Beyond
6. Skill Development Workshop in Motivational Enhancement
7. New Frontiers: Role of Information Technology in Behavior Change
8. Changing Practitioner Behavior
9. Organizational Change: Five-Step Model for Improving Performance
10. Organizational Change: Seven Critical Functions
11. Organizational Change: Improve Using Rapid Change PDSA Cycles
12. Organizational Change: Student Reports on Organizational Analysis
13 'Tying It All Together': Multi-Level Interventions Individual, Organization, Community

Further details on this course are given at the web site: *www.HealthBehaviorChange.org*

2. Select a health issue/behavior(s) that you want to assess.

3. Visit the setting and conduct an analysis of the setting's performance with respect to the selected issue. You might begin by completing *Your Organizational Prototype* (Worksheet 9.1) and *ACTSS* analysis of the capacities for improvement (Chapter 10). Then, deepen your evaluation using the *Critical Functions Analysis* CFA (Chapter 12) to identify key opportunities for improvement.

4. Write up your analysis, and include a plan for rapid cycle improvement drawing upon Worksheet 13.1. If you like, use the Lakeside case study in Chapter 12 as a model.

Websites

To complement this book and your continued learning, visit my Internet website at *http://www.HealthBehaviorChange.org*. This website provides continuing education modules and self-directed learning using material from

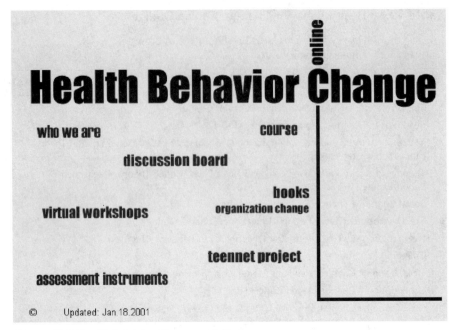

Figure 19.1 Health Behavior Change website homepage.

the book, skill development exercises, updates on key resources, hotlinks to related sites, and a Discussion Forum for interaction with the author and others engaged in organizational and individual behavior change (Figure 19.1). The website is geared to serve as a timely way to build upon and learn from others using the concepts and tools described in this book.

Also, visit the comprehensive website of the Institute for Healthcare Improvement at *http://www.IHI.org*. The IHI is a leading force in developing and disseminating new knowledge for health system improvement. As well, for interesting information and resources on behavior change, see Peter Senge's *The Dance of Change* and *The Fifth Discipline Fieldbook* at *http://www.fieldbook.com*.

Other Recommended Books

Building a high performance organization certainly qualifies as a major voyage; indeed, it entails lifelong individual and organizational learning. Suppose that you have just been offered your dream position as a change agent at a premier health care organization. They need you immediately;

pack lightly but take the things most beneficial for your journey. In addition to *Promoting Health*, you can take five other books.

These are books I would take as aids to navigation in organizational change. Note: I have arranged the books beginning with the micro- and progressing to the macro- approaches to organizational change.

1. Langley, G.J., Nolan, K.M., Nolan, T.W., Norman, G.L. and Provest, L.P. **The Improvement Guide: A practical approach to enhance organizational performance.** San Francisco, Jossey-Bass, 1996.

> Langley and colleagues provide an incredibly direct and practical approach for 'making it so' (for fans of *Star Trek*). This book provides a basic PDSA model (Plan-Do-Study-Act cycles) for continuous improvement. The authors apply the model to develop, test and implement change that produces significant improvement. This book is short on rhetoric, high on practical guidance.

2. Bryson, J.M. **Strategic Planning for Public and Non-profit Organizations**: **A guide to strengthening and sustaining organizational achievement.** Revised edition. San Francisco: Jossey-Bass, 1995. A workbook is also available from Jossey-Bass, 1996.

> This superbly clear and practical book describes a 10-step strategic planning process that includes concepts, techniques and process guidelines. This is 'one stop shopping' for strategic planning and action steps that address the organization's external and internal environments.

3. Kotter, J.P. **Leading Change**. Boston, MA: Harvard Business School Press, 1996. This book is an extension of his article in the **Harvard Business Review**, March–April, 1995.

> Once you have the basics on improving performance (Langley and colleagues) and strategic planning (Bryson), then Kotter's book provides both inspirational and practical advice on organizational transformation. He begins by making a fundamental distinction between managing versus leading change. Only leadership can motivate significant shifts in the way things are done, blast through inertia, and anchor change in the organizational culture. Kotter presents an Eight-Stage Process for successful transformations that will enable your organization to develop a future vision and effective strategies for getting there.

4. Senge, P. **The Fifth Discipline: The Art and Practice of the Learning Organization.** New York: Doubleday/Currency, 1990.

> This book is a classic on applying systems theory to organizational renewal and improvement. Senge describes five disciplines for building learning capacities in organizations: personal mastery, mental methods, shared vision, team learning and systems thinking. In 1994, Senge added **The Fifth Discipline Fieldbook** to provide a compendium of practice guides and resources for implementing the five learning disciplines. Recently, Senge and colleagues extended the series to include **The Dance of Change** (1999), which addresses the forces that create (growth) and impede (limit) change throughout the life cycle of a change initiative. All three books are incredibly rich sources of ideas and tools for leading and sustaining organizational change.

5. Stacey, R.D. **Complexity and Creativity in Organizations**. San Francisco, CA: Berrett-Koehler Publishers, 1966.

> This book is most helpful when you have one of those days where you feel stuck, confused, or even overwhelmed. In this circumstance, the only sensible thing to do is go home and read Stacey's book! Drawing upon chaos theory, Stacey helps us understand the unpredictable, hidden and nonlinear ways in which organizations function. Using psychodynamic theory he underscores the affective component of organizations, that is, the powerful anxieties and fears about change that are often left unspoken and unattended. To be successful, you need to understand and address them.

These five books span the gamut between the rational, predictable and long-term vision from the tower. They help you awaken from the interpersonal entanglements, foggy vision, and chaos of what often feels like the swamp of day-to-day activities; they help you plan and carry out the day-to-day actions of organizational change.

And if you could pack only one book on leadership? Here is our suggestion: Header, J. **The Tao of Leadership**. New York: Bantam Books, 1995. In the final analysis, achieving a high performing organization comes down to two vital components, leadership (vision) and management (attention to detail). Leadership is fundamentally based on wisdom and direction. Lao Tzu's book, *Tao Te Ching*, is one of the oldest and best collections of sage advice. Header has used the insights of the *Tao Te Ching* to create an inspirational book that describes the elements of effective leadership. Insights of this nature require a lifetime to absorb and put into practice.

Closing Word

I wrote this book while deeply immersed in leading a merger of three academic departments (Behavioural Science; Preventive Medicine and Biostatistics; Community Health) to form the new Department of Public Health Sciences at the University of Toronto. This experience convinced me that it is one thing to read about organizational change, and yet another to make it happen successfully.

In writing this book I have drawn upon these experiences and those of others who are leading change. A clear view from the 'tower' often gets mired in the 'swamp' of implementation, endless details and politics. Here are three pieces of wisdom that helped me and may help you lead successful organizational change on the shop floor.

1. **Stick to Your Vision and Core Values:** It is critical that you have a clear and compelling vision and that you articulate the core values that guide your decisions. Time and again, when faced with a crisis, an unbelievable opportunity, or an intransigent resistance, referring to your vision and core values will help you steer a proper course.

2. **Share the Limelight:** Go out of your way to engage others in a shared vision. Find out what they want and need; help them to make their own valuable and unique contributions. A wise colleague of mine, Fred Glaser, once told me that "you can accomplish a lot of good as long as you don't want to take all the credit."

3. **Some Days, Just Go Home:** Sooner or later you will have a day when the obstacles for change seem too daunting, the fog has rolled in, you feel confused or just too tired, angry, or frustrated to make sound judgments. At these times, the best thing you can do is go home. Tomorrow, the sun will rise, the confusion will have lifted somewhat, and you will have regained your energy and direction.

Promoting Health Through Organizational Change offers enough challenges to last a lifetime. Perhaps we will meet sometime on this journey, share our accomplishments and frustrations, debate the merits of a new approach, or simply enjoy the pleasure of each other's company.

May you emerge victorious from the organizational maze in which you've been travelling.

Worksheet 19.1 My Learning Plan

	Personal Change	**Organizational Change**
WHAT **aim**	I will personally ...	My organization will ...
HOW **options**	Site visits, Mentoring, Courses, Conferences, Books/Articles, Distance learning (Internet)	Ideas/Tools for discussion at next meeting of senior management, committee and/or team
WHEN **rewards**	Set specific targets and reward yourself for success.	Set specific targets and reward the team for success.

Appendix

Your Organizational Prototype

Instructions: Circle the number in each row that best describes your organizations's current functioning (focus on a particular level: unit, department, program or site).

	Reactive	Proactive	High performing
Focus	Primarily clinical 1 2 3	Prevention and clinical care 4 5 6	Clinical, prevention and health promotion 7 8 9
Level	Individual 1 2 3	Individual, some outreach 4 5 6	Individual, community and population 7 8 9
Time frame	Present "Fight fires" 1 2 3	Short/Medium term 4 5 6	Short/long, investing in future 7 8 9
Leadership	Minimal or autocratic 1 2 3	Constructive 4 5 6	Visionary, inspiring 7 8 9
Influence mode	Controlling or laissez faire 1 2 3	Coaching 4 5 6	Empowering 7 8 9
Quality orientation	Informal Self-proclaimed 1 2 3	Quality assurance 4 5 6	Continuous improvement 7 8 9
Accountability mainly to	Professionals 1 2 3	Patients/ Clients 4 5 6	Patients, professionals and public 7 8 9
Management style	Disorganized or rigid 1 2 3	Flexible 4 5 6	Synergistic, participatory 7 8 9
Communication	One-way, sporadic 1 2 3	Two-way 4 5 6	Multi-directional, continual 7 8 9
Professional development	Low priority 1 2 3	Optional, opportunistic 4 5 6	High priority, ongoing 7 8 9
Morale	Complacency, discouraged 1 2 3	Supportive, encouraging 4 5 6	High, self-sustaining 7 8 9

ACTSS:
Success Factors for Organizational Improvement

- ■ **Affective**

- ■ **Cultural**

- ■ **Technical**

- ■ **Structural**

- ■ **Strategic**

Harvey Skinner Ph.D.
and
Richard Botelho M.D.

Instructions

Ratings:

To what degree are Affective, Cultural, Technical, Strategic and Structural (ACTSS) critical success factors present in the organization?

1. Use the five-point scale in the following tables to record your evaluation of each success factor as either an organizational support or barrier.

2. Sum and then plot on the profile sheet the total score for each factor (ACTSS) as well as the overall score (average of all ACTSS factors).

Specific Supports and Barriers:

1. List (brainstorm) specific organizational supports and barriers for each ACTSS factor.

2. What is their relative importance and need of attention in order to maintain a strength or address a barrier?

3. Record the top three supports and barriers.

Level of Analysis:

For larger and/or complex organizations, focus first on distinct areas (e.g. departments, programs, divisions, sites) and then create a composite profile of the organization's capacity for improvement as a whole.

1. AFFECTIVE FACTOR

−2 = major barrier −1 = barrier 0 = neither 1 = support 2 = major support	
Success Items	**Rating**
1. Staff feel secure about their positions	-2 -1 0 1 2
2. Individuals have a sense of personal control over their work (lower stress levels)	-2 -1 0 1 2
3. Staff feel part of the team, yet appreciated for their individual contributions	-2 -1 0 1 2
4. On most days staff look forward to coming to work (little signs of 'burn out')	-2 -1 0 1 2
5. There is confidence that the organization can adapt successfully to change	-2 -1 0 1 2
6. Staff at all levels feel a sense of pride and trust about the organization ("we are all in this together")	-2 -1 0 1 2
Total	

Top Three Supports	**Top Three Barriers**
1.	1.
2.	2.
3.	3.

2. CULTURAL FACTOR

−2 = major barrier −1 = barrier 0 = neither 1 = support 2 = major support	
Success Items	**Rating**
1. Leadership style based on participation, creating trust and empowerment (nonblaming)	-2 -1 0 1 2
2. Leaders and managers have an understanding and long-term commitment to improving performance	-2 -1 0 1 2
3. Practitioners and staff have an understanding and support initiatives for improving performance	-2 -1 0 1 2
4. Openness to innovation and improvement fostered at all levels of the organization	-2 -1 0 1 2
5. Low level of resistance to improvement initiatives (e.g., not seen as threats to change/eliminate positions or power)	-2 -1 0 1 2
6. Outward-, forward-looking emphasis on meeting the needs of patients/clients and other stakeholders (versus inward or insular focus)	-2 -1 0 1 2
Total	

Top Three Supports	**Top Three Barriers**
1.	1.
2.	2.
3.	3.

3. TECHNICAL FACTOR

−2 = major barrier −1 = barrier 0 = neither 1 = support 2 = major support	
Success Items	**Rating**
1. Professional development of staff regarding knowledge and skills in quality improvement	-2 -1 0 1 2
2. Team building and problem-focused training available	-2 -1 0 1 2
3. Capability across the continuum of patient care for data collection regarding improvement needs and outcomes	-2 -1 0 1 2
4. Understanding of integrated systems and interconnected steps in providing services (e.g., work process flow diagram)	-2 -1 0 1 2
5. Practitioners and staff are clear about how their work fits into the broader picture of the organization	-2 -1 0 1 2
6. Quality improvement tools, project management and decision support systems available	-2 -1 0 1 2
Total	

Top Three Supports	Top Three Barriers
1.	1.
2.	2.
3.	3.

4. STRUCTURAL FACTOR

−2 = major barrier −1 = barrier 0 = neither 1 = support 2 = major support	
Success Items	**Rating**
1. Flexible, nonbureaucratic climate that stimulates personal initiative and achievement	-2 -1 0 1 2
2. Mechanisms for evaluating progress and keeping improvement projects focussed on achieving goals	-2 -1 0 1 2
3. Resources, budget and planning systems in place to support continuous improvement work	-2 -1 0 1 2
4. Performance appraisal and reward systems aligned to support quality improvement	-2 -1 0 1 2
5. Mechanisms for fostering departmental support for team involvement and conflict resolution (e.g. 'turf 'protection)	-2 -1 0 1 2
6. Integration of formally separate functions, such as utilization review, risk management and quality assurance	-2 -1 0 1 2
Total	

Top Three Supports	**Top Three Barriers**
1.	1.
2.	2.
3.	3.

5. STRATEGIC FACTOR

−2 = major barrier −1 = barrier 0 = neither 1 = support 2 = major support	
Success Items	**Rating**
1. Organizational priorities and strategic directions identified (e.g., for prevention and behavioral health care)	-2 -1 0 1 2
2. Quality improvement initiatives directly linked to strategic directions of the organization	-2 -1 0 1 2
3. Active involvement and 'buy in' of physicians and other key groups (or individuals)	-2 -1 0 1 2
4. Work of different teams coordinated to focus efficiently and effectively on improvement priorities	-2 -1 0 1 2
5. Learning gets transferred from one set of projects to another, so that synergies are captured	-2 -1 0 1 2
6. Sharing of quality improvement data and results with staff at all levels to keep the improvement process highly visible throughout the organization	-2 -1 0 1 2
Total	

Top Three Supports	Top Three Barriers
1.	1.
2.	2.
3.	3.

CFA: Critical Functions Analysis

Organizational Supports for Health Behavior Change

Harvey Skinner. Ph.D.

Richard Botelho. M.D.

Shawna Mercer. Ph.D.

Eileen de Villa. M.D.

Date: _____   Setting: _____

Health Issues/Programs Assessed:

1. _____   2. _____

Analysis Conducted By: _____

The principal aim of a *Critical Functions Analysis* (CFA) is to analyze an organization's status on essential supports for practitioners and patients in health behavior change. Completion of the CFA will provide an internal data base, including a baseline measure for continuous improvement cycles (Steps 2 and 3 in Figure 1). This booklet is designed so that you can record your ratings for two health issues/programs.

Completing the CFA Quantitative Ratings

Status: For each item, circle the number which best reflects the current status of that activity or process in the health setting:

0 =   **Absent** (or **Minimal**): major improvement needed in all areas

1 =   **Fair:** some processes in place but improvement clearly needed in a number of areas

2 =   **Good:** organization does very well in all areas, or is extremely strong in some but not as strong in others

3 =   **Excellent:** in all aspects

   N/A = not applicable to this setting (write this in if appropriate but use sparingly).

   Observations: Make notes about any important features, missing elements, strengths, or weaknesses. These can be embellished upon in the **Points of Pride, Areas Needing Improvement** or **Suggestions for Improvement** sections.

   Scoring: Use the *Scoring Template* and *Profile Template*

a) Compute: Total Score Received / Total Possible Score x 100 = % Score

b) Plot the % Scores for the seven critical functions on the *Profile* sheet to give a visual presentation of how the setting is doing for each health issue.

Completing the CFA: Qualitative Analysis

On the right side of each page, space is provided for recording specific information gathered from your walk-through of the health settings, as well as from informants' interviews (practitioners, administrative staff, patients). The principal aim of this component (Step 3 in Figure 1) is to identify specific issues that can be used as input for setting improvement priorities. To facilitate a 'balanced' analysis of organizational strengths and limitations, begin by asking about 'Points of Pride'. This signals the intention of fostering a nonblaming and constructive commitment to continuous improvement.

It is important to ask open-ended questions, that is, ones which cannot be answered 'yes' or 'no'. Encourage participants to describe their own perspectives and experiences. Listed below are some open-ended questions that you can use as guides.

Points of Pride:
1. What aspects about this _____ (critical function) are being done well?
2. Describe aspects that you think are particularly unique, novel, or innovative?
3. What stands out? What do you think your organization does best with this function?

Areas Needing Improvement:
1. Which aspects, in your view, require improvement with this function?
2. What areas do you feel are being ignored and/or declining in quality?
3. Describe one area that would benefit most from attention.

Suggestions for Improvement:
1. What are your suggestions for improvement with this function?
2. What is the most important aspect to focus on first?
3. What barriers will have to be addressed?

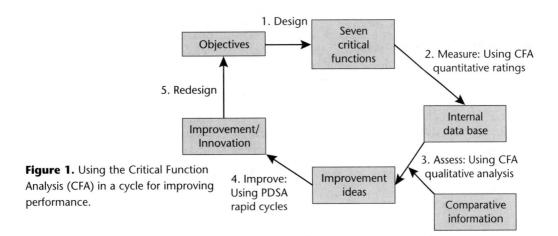

Figure 1. Using the Critical Function Analysis (CFA) in a cycle for improving performance.

1. Professional Development in Behavior Change

Status: **0** = Absent/Minimal **1** = Fair **2** = Good **3** = Excellent

Individual Level	Issue 1	Issue 2
1. Training/continuing education on behavior change and motivation enhancement provided for:		
a) Practitioners	0 1 2 3	0 1 2 3
b) Staff	0 1 2 3	0 1 2 3
c) Administrators	0 1 2 3	0 1 2 3
2. Resources available for self-directed learning (e.g., books, audio/video tapes, workshops, distance learning)	0 1 2 3	0 1 2 3
3. Regular meetings to discuss motivation and resistance issues (patient, practitioner and staff perspectives)	0 1 2 3	0 1 2 3
4. Access to expert advice regarding patient motivation, resistance and behavior change strategies	0 1 2 3	0 1 2 3
5. Reinforcers in place to encourage and recognize practitioners and staff in using motivational approaches	0 1 2 3	0 1 2 3
Organizational Level		
6. Training/continuing education on organizational change, teamwork and continuous improvement provided for:		
a) Practitioners	0 1 2 3	0 1 2 3
b) Staff	0 1 2 3	0 1 2 3
c) Administrators	0 1 2 3	0 1 2 3
7. Learning resources on organizational change (e.g., books, audio/video tapes, workshops, distance learning courses)	0 1 2 3	0 1 2 3
8. Regular small group meetings to address teamwork and continuous improvement issues	0 1 2 3	0 1 2 3
9. Access to advice regarding organizational change and continuous improvement	0 1 2 3	0 1 2 3
10. Reinforcers in place to encourage and recognize practitioners and staff in using continuous improvement protocols	0 1 2 3	0 1 2 3
11. Access to learning resources and advice on the use of information technology	0 1 2 3	0 1 2 3
TOTAL		

1. Professional Development in Behavior Change

Points of Pride:

Areas Needing Improvement:

Suggestions for Improvement:

2. Priming and Prompting

Status: **0** = Absent/Minimal   **1** = Fair   **2** = Good   **3** = Excellent

Materials-Related, Location-Related	Issue 1	Issue 2
1. Posters, promotional materials and mission statement visible and accessible to patients/clients:		
a) In reception/waiting areas	0 1 2 3	0 1 2 3
b) In clinical areas (e.g, examining rooms)	0 1 2 3	0 1 2 3
2. Pamphlets and self-directed learning material made available to patients/clients:		
a) In waiting areas	0 1 2 3	0 1 2 3
b) In clinical areas (e.g, examining rooms)	0 1 2 3	0 1 2 3
3. Patient/client prompting/reminder system (telephone, mail)	0 1 2 3	0 1 2 3
4. Specific priming/prompting materials (e.g. seasonal newsletter)	0 1 2 3	0 1 2 3
5. Computer/Information Technology systems for priming/prompting		
a) Currently in place	0 1 2 3	0 1 2 3
b) Planning for future	0 1 2 3	0 1 2 3
Practitioner and Staff-Related		
6. System for practitioner prompts (e.g., flagging records, practice tools)	0 1 2 3	0 1 2 3
7. Pamphlets, learning material provided by practitioners to patients during clinical encounters	0 1 2 3	0 1 2 3
8. Responsibility assigned for		
a) Ordering/stocking material	0 1 2 3	0 1 2 3
b) Updating and seeking new material	0 1 2 3	0 1 2 3
9. Evidence of role modelling of healthy behavior by practitioners, staff and administrators	0 1 2 3	0 1 2 3
TOTAL		

2. Priming and Prompting

Points of Pride:

Areas Needing Improvement:

Suggestions for Improvement:

3. Identification of Risk Behaviors

Status: **0** = Absent/Minimal **1** = Fair **2** = Good **3** = Excellent

Clinical Encounter-Based	Issue 1	Issue 2
1. Risk factor assessment (form) integrated into intake process	0 1 2 3	0 1 2 3
2. Risk factor assessments (form) repeated over time	0 1 2 3	0 1 2 3
3. Case-finding during patient contacts	0 1 2 3	0 1 2 3
4. Use of validated screening methods (e.g., CAGE or AUDIT for alcohol problems)	0 1 2 3	0 1 2 3
5. Standardization of assessment (e.g., use of specific questionnaires, structured interviews, computerized assessments)	0 1 2 3	0 1 2 3
6. Performance of diagnostic tests to assess severity of a risk behavior or related complications	0 1 2 3	0 1 2 3
7. Reinforcers in place to encourage/assist practitioners to perform risk factor assessments	0 1 2 3	0 1 2 3
8. Follow-up mechanism for contacting nonresponders and no-shows	0 1 2 3	0 1 2 3
Community/Population-Based		
9. Register maintained (age/sex) of chronic diseases and risk behaviors (e.g., diabetes and weight control) of the patient population	0 1 2 3	0 1 2 3
10. Outreach initiatives for special populations at risk	0 1 2 3	0 1 2 3
11. Health and risk factor assessments conducted on population-basis (e.g., mail-out questionnaire)	0 1 2 3	0 1 2 3
12. Reinforcers in place to encourage/assist practitioners and staff in population-based risk identification	0 1 2 3	0 1 2 3
13. Follow-up mechanism for contacting nonresponders (e.g., post cards, repeat surveys)	0 1 2 3	0 1 2 3
TOTAL		

3. Identification of Risk Behaviors

Points of Pride:

Areas Needing Improvement:

Suggestions for Improvement:

4. Continuing Care

Status: **0** = Absent/Minimal   **1** = Fair   **2** = Good   **3** = Excellent

	Issue 1	Issue 2
1. Standards of practice used for this behavior/issue (e.g., clinical guidelines, recommended protocols)	0 1 2 3	0 1 2 3
2. Ongoing records kept in the patients' charts regarding risk behaviors	0 1 2 3	0 1 2 3
3. Motivational approaches used during:		
a) Successive clinical encounters and follow-up	0 1 2 3	0 1 2 3
b) Staff interactions with patients over time	0 1 2 3	0 1 2 3
4. Motivational approaches used during:		
a) shifts in patients' readiness for change	0 1 2 3	0 1 2 3
b) Progress toward goals	0 1 2 3	0 1 2 3
c) Patients' health status	0 1 2 3	0 1 2 3
d) No-shows of appointments	0 1 2 3	0 1 2 3
5. Follow-up organized for the specific behaviors in Step 4:		
a) Individual or groups	0 1 2 3	0 1 2 3
b) By telephone contacts	0 1 2 3	0 1 2 3
6. System for providing additional information/care:		
a) Individual or groups	0 1 2 3	0 1 2 3
b) Via telephone	0 1 2 3	0 1 2 3
c) Via mail	0 1 2 3	0 1 2 3
7. Use of information technology for follow-up assessment and counseling (e.g., e-mail, telephone messaging, fax, Internet)	0 1 2 3	0 1 2 3
8. Tracking patient involvement with places and persons to which they are referred	0 1 2 3	0 1 2 3
TOTAL		

4. Continuing Care

Points of Pride:

Areas Needing Improvement:

Suggestions for Improvement:

5. Linkages and Networks

Status: **0** = Absent/Minimal   **1** = Fair   **2** = Good   **3** = Excellent

		Issue 1	Issue 2
1.	List of services and resource options compiled and available for practitioners	0 1 2 3	0 1 2 3
2.	Informing practitioners and staff of services and resource options:		
	a) Within the health setting	0 1 2 3	0 1 2 3
	b) Outside the setting	0 1 2 3	0 1 2 3
3.	Referral criteria specified and updated for services and resources:		
	a) Within the health setting	0 1 2 3	0 1 2 3
	b) Outside the setting	0 1 2 3	0 1 2 3
4.	Specific advice available for patients regarding services and resources:		
	a) Within the health setting	0 1 2 3	0 1 2 3
	b) Outside the setting	0 1 2 3	0 1 2 3
5.	Linkages developed and maintained with:		
	a) Community health organizations (e.g., home care)	0 1 2 3	0 1 2 3
	b) Public health departments	0 1 2 3	0 1 2 3
	c) Community groups (e.g., women's groups)	0 1 2 3	0 1 2 3
	d) Social Services	0 1 2 3	0 1 2 3
6.	New services and resource options identified on a regular basis	0 1 2 3	0 1 2 3
7.	Technology used to support linkages (e.g., Internet, e-mail, public broadcast)	0 1 2 3	0 1 2 3
	TOTAL		

5. Linkages and Networks

Points of Pride:

Areas Needing Improvement:

Suggestions for Improvement:

6. Options for Help

Status: **0** = Absent/Minimal   **1** = Fair   **2** = Good   **3** = Excellent

		Issue 1	Issue 2
1.	Accommodation to patient's needs and preferences (choice) for assistance	0 1 2 3	0 1 2 3
2.	Family members or friends involved (when appropriate)	0 1 2 3	0 1 2 3
3.	Able to schedule additional time with individual patients if needed	0 1 2 3	0 1 2 3
4.	Additional professional assistance identified and available (e.g., health educator, nutritionist):		
	a) Internal to health setting	0 1 2 3	0 1 2 3
	b) External to health setting	0 1 2 3	0 1 2 3
5.	Range of referral options used:		
	a) Support groups (professionally lead)		
	I) in the health setting	0 1 2 3	0 1 2 3
	II) outside the health setting	0 1 2 3	0 1 2 3
	b) Self help groups/peer education groups	0 1 2 3	0 1 2 3
	c) Community Health Organizations (e.g., home care)	0 1 2 3	0 1 2 3
	d) Community Resources (e.g., diabetic association)	0 1 2 3	0 1 2 3
	e) Public Health	0 1 2 3	0 1 2 3
	f) Social Services	0 1 2 3	0 1 2 3
6.	Access to a broad range of approaches/philosophies (e.g., women-focused, culturally sensitive, harm reduction)	0 1 2 3	0 1 2 3
	TOTAL		

6. Options for Help

Points of Pride:

Areas Needing Improvement:

Suggestions for Improvement:

7. Information Management

Status: **0** = Absent/Minimal   **1** = Fair   **2** = Good   **3** = Excellent

Access	Issue 1	Issue 2
1. Ready access for practitioners to patients' risk factor profiles and health status	0 1 2 3	0 1 2 3
2. Patient access to lifestyle and risk factor assessment results (timely, individualized)	0 1 2 3	0 1 2 3
3. Updating patients' risk factor profiles and health status	0 1 2 3	0 1 2 3
Feedback		
4. Feedback given to practitioners on adherence to practice standards (e.g., clinical guidelines)	0 1 2 3	0 1 2 3
5. Results given to practitioners and staff regarding their aggregate (group) performance in:		
a) Prompting and response to prompting	0 1 2 3	0 1 2 3
b) Identification of risk behavior and complications	0 1 2 3	0 1 2 3
c) Using interventions on patient outcomes	0 1 2 3	0 1 2 3
d) Using options and making referrals	0 1 2 3	0 1 2 3
6. Individualized feedback provided to practitioners and staff on elements described in 5a–d:	0 1 2 3	0 1 2 3
7. Patients' evaluations of care collected and feedback given to practitioners and staff	0 1 2 3	0 1 2 3
System Design and Maintenance		
8. Needs analyses conducted regarding systems and supports for behavior change	0 1 2 3	0 1 2 3
9. Designated personnel and access to expertise for system design, development and implementation	0 1 2 3	0 1 2 3
10. Access to appropriate technology		
a) Hardware (e.g., computers, video players)	0 1 2 3	0 1 2 3
b) Software (e.g., automated prompts and records, voice mail)	0 1 2 3	0 1 2 3
TOTAL		

7. Information Management

Points of Pride:

Areas Needing Improvement:

Suggestions for Improvement:

CFA Scoring Template

1. Professional development   _____   /45* x 100 =   _____

2. Priming/Prompting   _____   /39* x 100 =   _____

3. Identification   _____   /39* x 100 =   _____

4. Continuing care   _____   /45* x 100 =   _____

5. Linkages and networks   _____   /39* x 100 =   _____

6. Options for help   _____   /39* x 100 =   _____

7. Information management   _____   /42* x 100 =   _____

* Maximum Score: pro-rate for any N/A (not applicable) items
(i.e. for each not applicable item subtract 3 from the total possible score).

CFA Profile Template

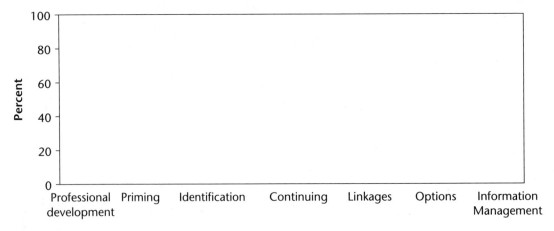

Tips for Administering and Scoring the CFA

Completion of the Critical Functions Analysis normally involves a careful 'walk-through' of the health care setting, as well as selected interviews with key personnel (practitioners, administrators, staff) and patients. The CFA booklet provides a convenient means for recording results from both the quantitative and qualitative components.

Begin by selecting a particular health issue, or set of issues, to analyze. Results can be recorded for up to two health issues in a single CFA booklet. If more than two issues are being addressed, then use additional booklets. Ensure that the assessment date, setting, and health issues are clearly noted on the back side of the front page of the CFA booklet. Also, indicate who is conducting the analysis.

1. Quantitative Ratings

Open the booklet to the first critical function: professional development. On the left side of the page you will see 11 activities and processes to be assessed, with several activities having subcomponents. Make notes (on the booklet or separate sheets) regarding the status of each particular activity/process during a walk-through of the setting, and use these as prompts for questions while interviewing key informants (e.g., practitioners, staff, patients). Once you have completed your data gathering, indicate your numerical evaluation of the status (0, 1, 2, or 3) for each activity/process.

Status: For each item, circle the number which best reflects the current status of the activity or process in the health setting:

0 = **Absent** (or **Minimal**): major improvement needed in all areas

1 = **Fair:** some processes in place but improvement clearly needed in a number of areas

2 = **Good:** organization does very well in all areas, or is extremely strong in some but not as strong in others

3 = **Excellent:** in all aspects

N/A = not applicable to this setting (write this in the next to the numerical ratings).

Observations: Make simple notes regarding the rationale for your assessment of each item. Describe any notable features, missing elements, strengths, and weaknesses in such a way that they can be embellished upon in the qualitative **Points of Pride, Areas Needing Improvement** and **Suggestions for Improvement** sections. When an item deals with two or more activities or processes, specify to what your rating is referring. For example, under the second critical function of Priming and Prompting, item 1 states "Posters, promotional materials, and mission statement visible and accessible to patients/clients". You might note:

a) Are posters, promotional materials and mission statement all present or just some of these? Specify which are present.

b) Are they visible as well as accessible, or just one of the two? Are they both visible and accessible but to differing degrees?

Scoring: Use the *Scoring Template* to compute the score for each function, and then plot these scores on the *Profile Template* to facilitate interpretation and communication.

I) Determine: the number of items that are applicable to (valid for) this health issue

II) Compute: $\underline{\text{Total Score Received}}$ X 100 = % Score

   Total Score Possible
   (number of valid items x 3)

III) Plot the % scores for the seven critical functions on the profile sheet to give a visual presentation of how the setting is doing with this health issue. An example of a profile plot for the Lakeside case study is given in Figure 12.3.

IV) Compute an Overall Score based on the numeric average of the seven critical function % score. Then, plot this Overall Score on the Profile Sheet.

Scoring Example: Assume that a particular health issue was rated as follows for the critical function, Priming and Prompting:

1a)	3	Excellent	5a)	2	Good
1b)	2	Good	5b)	1	Fair
2a)	3	Excellent	6)	0	Absent
2b)	0	Absent	7)	2	Good
3)	3	Excellent	8a)	1	Good
4)	2	Good	8b)	0	Absent
			9)	1	Fair

All 13 processes applied to (were valid for) this health issue and setting. Score is 20/39 X 100 = 51%.

2. Qualitative Analysis

For each critical function, space is provided for recording information gathered from your walk-through, as well as from informants' interviews (practitioners, administrators, staff, patients). The aim is to identify specific areas for improvement that can be used as input for setting priorities (discussed in Chapter 13). To facilitate a 'balanced' analysis of organizational strengths and limitations, begin by asking about 'Points of Pride'. This helps foster a nonblaming and constructive approach to quality improvement. Ask open-ended questions, such as those suggested in the CFA booklet. Ask interviewees to describe their own perspectives and experiences. Encourage them to be specific.

References

Abrams, D.B., Orleans, C.T., Niaura, R.S., Goldstein, M.G., Prochaska, J.O., & Velicer, W. (1996). Integrating individual and public health perspectives for treatment of tobacco dependents under managed care: A combined stepped-care and matching model. *Annals of Behavioral Medicine*, 18, 290–304.

Adams, D. (1998). *The long dark tea-time of the soul*. Toronto, Canada: Stoddart Publishing. (Published in Great Britain by William Heinemann).

Aday, L.A., Begley, C.E., Lairson, D.R., & Slater, C.H. (1998). *Evaluating the health care system: effectiveness, efficiency and equity* (2nd ed.). Chicago, Illinois: Health Administration Press.

Adlaf, E., Frank, J., & Smart, R. (1997). The Ontario Student Drug Use Survey: 1997-1997. Toronto: Addiction Research Foundation.

Adlaf, E., Ivis F., & Paglia, A (1999). *Drug Use Among Ontario Students 1977-1999: Finding from the OSDUS [Ontario Student Drug Use Survey]*. Toronto, Canada: Addiction Research Foundation.

Agency for Healthcare Research and Quality. (2001). *Quality research for quality Health Care*. Agency for Healthcare Research and Quality. U.S. Agency for Healthcare Research and Quality. (www.ahcpr.gov)

Agency for Healthcare Policy and Research. (1996). *Smoking Cessation*. Clinical practice guideline, No. 18. *Agency for Healthcare Policy and Research, No. 96 – 0692*. [Online]. Available: http://www.surgeongeneral.gov/tobacco/default.htm

Ajzen, I. (1991). The theory of planned behavior. *Organizational Behavior and Human Decision Processes*, 50, 179–211.

Ajzen, I., & Fishbein, M. (1980). *Understanding Attitudes and Predicting Social Behavior*. Inglewood Cliffs, NJ: Prentice–Hall.

Albert, T. (2000). More doctors following trend to unionise. American Medical News Nov. 27, 2000. American Medical Association.

Alemi, F., Mosavel, M., Stephens, R.C., Ghadiri, A., Krishnaswamy, J., & Thakkar, H. (1996). "Electronic self-help and support groups." *Medical Care, 34* (Suppl.), 10, OS32-OS44.

Allen, J., Lowman, C., & Miller, W. R. (1996). Perspectives on precipitants of relapse. *Addiction, 91*, S3-S4.

Allsop, S., Saunders, B., Phillips, M., & Carr, A. (1997). A trial of relapse prevention with severely dependent male problem drinkers. *Addiction, 92*, 61–74.

Alter, D.A., Naylor, C.D., Austin, P., & Tu, J.V. (1999). Effects of socio-economic status on access to invasive cardiac procedures and on mortality after acute myocardial infarction. *The New England Journal of Medicine*, 341, 1359–1367.

American Board of Internal Medicine. (1998). *Project Professionalism*. Philadelphia: American Board of Internal Medicine.

American Medical Association. (2001a). Expanding health insurance: The AMA proposal for reform. Chicago: Author.

American Medical Association. (2001b). House of Delegates Policy: Managed Competition. H-165.944. Chicago, IL: AMA.

Anderson, G.F., & Poullier, J-P. (1999). Health care spending, access and outcomes: trends in industrialized countries. *Health Affairs, 18*, 178–192.

Anderson, L.A., Jaines, G.R., & Jenkins, C. (1998). Implementing preventive services: To what extent can we change provider performance in ambulatory care? A review of the screening, immunization and counselling literature. *Annals of Behavioral Medicine, 20*, 161–167.

Anderson, R., Franckowiak, S., Snyder, J., Bartlett, S., & Fontaine, K. (1998). Can inexpensive signs encourage the use of stairs? Results from a community intervention. *Annals of Internal Medicine, 129*, 363–369.

Annis, H. (1990). Relapse to substance abuse: Empirical findings within a cognitive-social learning approach. *Journal of Psychoactive Drugs, 22*, 117–123.

Annis, H.M., & Davis, C.S. (1991). Relapse prevention. *Alcohol Health and Research World, 15*, 204–212.

Annis, H., Schober, R., & Kelly, E. (1996). Matching addiction outpatient counseling to client readiness for change: The role of structured relapse prevention counseling. *Experimental and Clinical Psychopharmacology, 4,* 1–9.

Anonymous. (1999). Special Issue on Managed Care. *Journal of Health Politics, Policy and Law,* 24 (5),

Argyris, C., Putnam, R., & Smith, D. (1985). *Action Science.* San Francisco: Jossey-Bass.

Ashenden, R., Silacy, C., & Weller, D. (1997). A systematic review of the effectiveness of promoting lifestyle change in general practice. *Family Practice, 14,* 160–176.

Ayanian, J.Z., Weissman, J.S., Schneider, E.C., Ginsberg, J.A., & Zaslavsky, A.N. (2000). Unmet health needs of uninsured adults in the United States. *Journal of American Medical Association, 284,* 2061–2069.

Babor, T.F. (1994). Avoiding the horrid and beastly sin of drunkenness: Does dissuasion make a difference? *Journal of Consulting and Clinical Psychology, 62,* (6), 1127–1140.

Bailar, J., & Smith, E. (1986). Progress against cancer. *The New England Journal of Medicine, 314,* 1226–1232.

Balas, A., Jaffrey, F., Kuperman, G., Boren, S., Brown, G., Pinciroli, F., & Mitchell, J. (1997). Electronic communication with patients. Evaluation of distance medicine technology. *Journal of American Medical Association, 278,* 152–159.

Bandura, A. (1977). Self-efficacy: Toward a unifying theory of behavioral change. *Psychological Review, 84,* 191–215.

Bandura, A. (1986). *Social foundations of thought and action: A social cognitive theory.* Englewood Cliffs, N.J.: Prentice-Hall.

Bandura, A. (1991). Self-efficacy mechanism in physiological activation and health-promoting behavior. In J. Madden IV (Ed.), *Neurobiology of learning, emotion and affect* (pp. 229–270). New York: Raven.

Bandura, A. (1997). *Self-efficacy. The exercise of control.* New York: W.H. Freeman & Company.

Baranowski, T. (1990). Reciprocal determinism at the stages of behavior change: An integration of community, personal and behavioral perspectives. *International Quarterly of Community Health Education, 10,* 297–327.

Baranowski, T., Perry, C.L., & Parcel, G.S. (1997). How individuals, environments, and health behavior interact: social cognitive theory. In K. Glanz, F.M. Lewis, & B.K. Rimer (Eds.) *Health behavior and health education: Theory, research and practice.* San Francisco: Jossey-Bass.

Barefoot, J.C., & Schroll, M. (1996). Symptoms of depression, acute myocardial infarction, and total mortality in a community sample. *Circulation, 93,* 1976–1980.

Barinaga, M. (1997). How Much Pain for Cardiac Gain? *Science, 276,* 1324–1327.

Bartlett, E.E. (1995). Cost-benefit analysis of patient education. *Patient Education and Counselling, 26,* 87–91.

Batalden, P., Nelson, L., & Roberts, J. (1994). Linking outcomes measurment to continual improvement: The serial 'V' way of thinking about improving clinical care. *Joint Comission Journal on Quality Improvement, 20,* 167.

Batalden, P., & Nolan, T. (1993). Knowledge for the leadership of continual improvement in healthcare. *AUPHA manual of health services management.* Rockville, MD: Aspen Publishers.

Batalden, P., & Stoltz, P. (1993). A framework for the continual improvement of health care: Building and applying professional and improvement knowledge to test changes in daily work. *Journal of Quality Improvement, 19,* 424–447.

Becker, M. (1992). A medical sociologist looks at health promotion. *Journal of Health and Social Behaviour, 34,* 1–6.

Becker, M., & Janz, N. (1990). Practicing health promotion: The doctor's dilemma. *Annals of Internal Medicine, 113,* 419–422.

Beer, M., Eisenstat, R., & Spector, B. (1990, November/December). Why change programs don't produce change. *Harvard Business Review,* 128–166.

Bemowski, K., & Stratton, B. (1998). *101 Good ideas: How to improve just about any process.* Milwaukee, WI: American Society for Quality, Press.

Bental, D., Cawsey, A., & Jones, R. (1999). Patient information systems that tailor to the individual. *Patient Education and Counselling, 36,* 171–180.

Berkman, L., & Breslow, L. (1983). *Health and ways of living*. New York: Oxford University Press.

Berlow, D. (1960). *The process of communication: An introduction to theory and practice*. New York: Holt, Rinehart & Winston.

Berwick, D. (1989). Sound board. Continuous improvement as an ideal in health care. *The New England Journal of Medicine, 320*, 53–56.

Berwick, D. (1996). A primer on leading the improvement of systems. *British Medical Journal, 312*, 619–22.

Berwick, D. (1998). Developing and testing changes in delivery of care. *Annals of Internal Medicine, 128*, 651–656.

Berwick, D., Godfrey, A., & Roessner, J. (1990). *Curing health care*. San Francisco: Jossey-Bass.

Berwick, D., & Nolan, T. (1998). Physicians as leaders in improving health care: A new series in annals of internal medicine. *Annals of Internal Medicine, 128*, 289–292.

Bien, T., Miller, W., & Boroughs, J. (1993). Motivational interviewing with alcohol outpatients. *Behavioral and Cognitive Psychotherapy, 21*, 347–356.

Bien, T.H., Miller, W.R., & Tonigan, J.S. (1993). Brief interventions for alcohol problems: a review. *Addiction, 88*, 315–336.

Biermann, J.S., Golladay, G.J., Greenfield, M.L. V.H., & Baker, L. H. (1999). Evaluation of cancer information on the Internet. *Cancer, 86*, 381–390.

Blane, D., Brunner, E.J., & Wilkinson, R.D. (1996). *Social organization and health*. London, Routledge.

Blendon, R., Leitman, R., & Morrison, I. (1990). Satisfaction with health systems in ten nations. *Health Affairs, 9*, 185–192.

Block, B. (1996, October). Using an automated tracking system to improve patient care. *Family Practice Management*, 47–54.

Blum, R., Beuhring, T., Wunderlich, M., & Resnick, M. (1996). Don't ask, they won't tell: the quality of adolescent health screening in five practice settings. *American Journal of Public Health, 86*, 1767–1772.

Bobadilla, J.L., Cowley, P., Musgrave, P., & Saxenian, H. (1994). Design, content and financing of an essential national package of health services. *Bulletin of the World Health Organization, 72* (4): 653 – 662.

Bodenheimer, T. (2000). California's beleaguered physician groups: Will they survive? *The New England Journal of Medicine, 342*, 1064–1068.

Boon, H., & Verhoef, M.J. (2001). Complementary and alternative medicine: A Canadian perspective. In Edzard (Ed.). *Desk top reference on complementary / alternative medicine for physicians*. London: Churchill-Livingstone, pp. 362–73.

Boore, J.P.R. (1978). *Prescription for recovery: The effect of pre-operative preparation of surgical patients on post-operative stress, recovery and infection*. London: Royal College of Nurses.

Borkman, T.J. (1999). *Understanding self-help/mutual aid*. New Brunswick, NJ: Rutgers University Press.

Botelho, R.J. (2001). *Becoming a motivational practitioner*. (www.MotivateHealthyHabits.com).

Botelho, R.J., Skinner, H.A., Williams, G.C., & Wilson, D. (1999). Patients with alcohol problems in primary care: Understanding their resistance and motivating change. *Primary Care, 26*, 279–298.

Botvin, G., & Botvin, E. (1997). School-based programs. In J. Lowinson, P. Ruiz, R. Millman, & J. Langrod (Ed.), *Substance abuse: A comprehensive textbook*, Baltimore: Williams & Wilkins.

Boult, C., Altmann, M., Gilbertson, D., Yu, C., & Kane, R. (1996). Decreasing disability in the 21st century: The future effects of controlling six fatal and nonfatal conditions. *American Journal of Public Health, 86*, 1388–1393.

Brassard, M., & Joiner, B. (1995). *The team memory jogger*. Metheun, MA: GOAL/QPC.

Brassard, M., & Ritter, D. (1994). *The memory jogger II. A pocket guide of tools for continuous improvement and effective planning*. Metheun, MA: GOAL/QPC.

Brehm, S.S., & Brehm, J.W. (1981). *Psychological reactance: A theory of freedom and control*. New York: Academic Press.

Brennan, T.A., & Berwick, D.M. (1996). *New rules: Regulation, markets, and the quality of American health care*. San Francisco: Jossey-Bass.

Brennan, T.A., Leape, L.L.,& Laird, N.M. (1991). Incidence of adverse events and negligence in hospitalized patients: results of the Harvard Medical Practice Study I. *New England Journal of Medicine, 324,* 370–376.

Breslow L, Breslow N. (1993). Health practices and disability: Some evidence from Alameda County. *Preventive Medicine, 22*(1), 86–95.

Bridges-Webb, C. (1987). General practitioner services. *Australian Family Physician,* 16, 898.

British Columbia Medical Association. (1995). *CAPITATION: A wolf in sheep's clothing?* Vancouver, Canada. Author.

British Medical Journal (1999a). American Medical Association launches new internet "supersite". *British Medical Journal, 319,* 1217.

British Medical Journal (1999b). DrKoop.com criticised for mixing information with advertising. *British Medical Journal, 319,* 727.

Brown, A., & Armstrong, D. (1995). Telephone consultations in general practice: an additional or alternative service? *British Journal of General Practice, 45,* 673–675.

Brown, J., & Miller, W. (1993). Impact of motivational interviewing on participation and outcome in residential alcoholism treatment. *Psychology of Addictive Behaviors, 7,* 211–218.

Brown, D'Emidio-Caston, & Pollard. (1997). Students and substances. Social power in drug education. *Educational Evaluation and Policy Analysis, 19,* 65–82.

Brownell, K.D., Marlatt, G.A., Lichtenstein, E.R., & Wilson, G.T. (1986). Understanding and preventing relapse. *American Psychologist, 41,* 765–782.

Brundtland, G.H. (2000). *Overcoming antimicrobial resistance. World Health Report on Infectious Diseases 2000.* Geneva, Switzerland: World Health Organization.

Brunner, E., White, I., Thorogood, M., Bristow, A., & Curle, D. (1996). Can dietary interventions change diet and cardiovascular risk factors? A meta-analysis of randomized controlled trials. *American Journal of Public Health, 87,* 1415–1422.

Bryson, J. (1995). *Strategic planning for public and non-profit.* San Francisco: Jossey-Bass.

Bryson J.M., & Alston, F.K. (1996). *Creating and implementing your strategic plan.* San Francisco: Jossey-Bass.

Bull, F., Kreuter, M., & Scharff, D. (1999). Effects of tailored, personalized and general health messages on physical activity. *Patient Education and Counselling, 36,* 181–192.

Bunker, J.P., Frazier, H.S., & Mosteller, F. (1994). Improving health: measuring effects of medical care. *Milbank Quarterly; 72,* 225–258.

Burns D, Pierce JP. (1992). *Tobacco use in California 1990-1991.* Sacramento: California Department of Health Services.

Calfas, K., Long, B., Sallis, J., Wooten, W., Pratt, M., & Patrick, K. (1996). A controlled trial of physician councelling to promote the adoption of physical activity. *Preventive Medicine, 25,* 225–233.

Campbell, M., DeVellis, B., Strecher, V., Ammerman, A., DeVellis, R., & Sandler, R. (1994). *American Journal of Public Health, 84,* 783–787.

Canadian Federal, Provincial and Territorial Advisory Committee on Population Health. (1994). Strategies for Population Health, Investing in the Health of Canadians. Prepared for the meeting of the provincial ministers of health, September 1994.

Canadian Medical Association (2000c). My office has become my prison. *Canadian Medical Association Journal, 163.*

Canadian Medical Association. (2000a). CMA survey shows fee-for-service not dead yet. *Canadian Medical Association Journal, 163*(5), 607. Toronto: Canadian Medical Association.

Canadian Medical Association. (2000b). *Looking at the future of health, health care and medicine: The CMA Futures Project.* Toronto: Canada. Author.

Canadian Medical Association Journal (2000). Nearly a quarter of Canadians health online for health info. *Canadian Medical Association Journal, 163,* 1328.

Canadian Medical Association. (2001). *1999 Pre-budget consultations.* Canadian Medical Association.

2000 CMA physician resource questionnaire results. (2000). *Canadian Medical Association Journal.* [Online]. Available: http://www.cma.ca/cmaj/index.htm

Canadian Task Force on the Periodic Health Examination. (1994). *The Canadian guide to clinical preventive health care.* Ottawa, Canada: Canada Communication Group-Publishing.

Cancer Care Ontario. (2000). *An ounce of prevention: Ontario's cancer prevention blueprint*. Toronto, Canada: Cancer Care Ontario. (www.cancercancer.on.ca)

Campbell, M.K., DeVellis, B.M., Strecher, V.J., Ammerman, A.S., DeVellis, R.F., & Sandler, R.S. (1994). Improving dietary behavior: The effectiveness of tailored messages in primary care settings. *American Journal of Public Health, 84*(5), 783–787.

Carey, R.G., & Lloyd, R.C. (2001). *Measuring quality improvement in health care: A guide to statistical process control applications*. Milwaukee, WI: American Society for Quality Press.

Carrol, J., Broadhead, R. (1999). *Canadian Internet handbook, 2000: lightbulbs to yottabits*. Toronto, Canada: Stoddart.

Carroll, K.M. (1996). Relapse prevention as a psychosocial treatment: A review of controlled clinical trials. *Experimental and Clinical Psychopharmacology, 4*, 46–54.

Cartwright, A., & Anderson, R. (1977). *Patients and their doctors*. London: Royal College of General Practitioners.

Charlton, J., & Velez, R. (1986). Some international comparisons of mortality amenable to medical intervention. *British Medical Journal, 292*, 295–301.

Chassin, M.R., Galvin, R.W., & The National Roundtable on Health Care Quality, (1998). The urgent need to improve healthcare quality. *Journal of American Medical Association, 280*, 1000–1005.

Chassin, M.R., Kosecoff, J., Park, R.E. (1987). Does inappropriate use explain geographic variations in the use of health services? A study of three procedures. *Journal of the American Medical Association, 253*, 2533–2537.

Cheung, P., Hungin, A., Verrill, J., Russell, A., & Smith, H. (1997). Are the Health of the Nation's targets attainable? Postal survey of general practitioners' views. *British Medical Journal, 314*, 1250–1251.

Chirrey, S., & McGowan, P. (1999). Self-Help in Canada: Resource mapping report to the canadian health network. Report by the Self-Help Resource Centre of Greater Toronto and University of BC to Canadian Health Network, Health Canada, [Online]. Avalaible: *http://www.selfhelp.on.ca/backgrounder.html*

Clark, M., Ghandour, G., Miller, N.H., Taylor, C.B., Bandura, A., & DeBusk, R.F. (1995). *Development and testing of a computer-based system for dietary management of hyperlipidemia*. Manuscript unpublished.

Clemmer, J. (1992). *Firing on all cylinders: The service/quality system for high-powered corporate performance*. Toronto, Canada: Macmillan Canada.

Clemmer, T., Spuhler, V., Berwick, D., & Nolan, T. (1998). Cooperation: the foundation of improvement. *Annals of Internal Medicine, 128*, 1004–1009.

Coburn, D., Rappolt, S., & Bourgeault, I. (1997). Decline vs retention of medical power through restratification: An examination of the Ontario case. *Sociology of Health & Illness, 19*, 1–22.

Cohen, S. (1983). Potential barriers to diabetes care. *Diabetes Care, 5*, 499–500.

Coiera, E. (1998). Information epidemics, economics, and immunity on the internet. *British Medical Journal, 317*, 1469–1470.

Colby, S., Monti, P., Barnett, N., & Rohsenow, D. (1998). Brief motivational interviewing in a hospital setting for adolescent smoking: A preliminary study. *Journal of Consulting and Clinical Psychology, 66*, 574–578.

College of Family Physicians of Canada. (2000). *The postgraduate family medicine curriculum: An integrated approach*. Ottawa, Canada: College of Family Physicians of Canada.

Collins, K., Shoen, C., & Sandman, D. (2001). The commonwealth fund survey of physician experiences with managed care. *Health Care Quality*, 1997.

Collins, R.L., Morsheimer, E.T., Shiffman, S., Paty, T.A., Gnys, M., & Papandonatos, G.D. (1998). Ecological momentary assessment in behavioral drinking moderation trading program. *Experimental and Clinical Psychopharmacology, 6*(3), 306–315.

Conner, D.R. (1995). *Managing at the speed of change*. New York: Villard Books.

Connors, G., Maisto, S., & Donovan, D. (1996). Conceptualizations of relapse: A summary of psychological and psychobiological models. *Addiction, 91*, S5-S13.

Cook, D., & et al. (1996). Residents' experiences of abuse, discrimination and sexual harassment during residency training. *Canadian Medical Association Journal, 154*, 1657–1665.

Cottrell, R.R., Girvan, J.T., & McKenzie, J.F. (1999). *Principles and Foundations of Health Promotion and Education*. Boston: Allyn & Bacon.

Crabtree, B.F., Miller, W.L., Aita, V.A., Floke, S.A., & Stange, K.C. (1998). Primary care organization and preventive services delivery: A qualitative analysis. *Journal of Family Practice, 46,* 403–409.

Crow, J.F. (2000). Two centuries of genetics: A view from half-time. *Annu.Rev.Genomics Hum. Genet., 01,* 21–40.

Crump, W., & Pfeil, T. (1995). A telemedicine primer. *Archive Family Medicine, 4,* 796–803.

Cullinane, P.M, Hypolite, K., Zastawney, A.L., & Friedman, R.H. (1994). Telephone linked communication-activity counseling and tracking for older patients. *Journal of General Internal Medicine, 9,* 86.

Curry, S.J., Wagner, E.H., & Grotaus, L.C. (1991). Evaluation of intrinsic and extrinsic motivation interventions with a self-help smoking cessation program. *Journal of Consulting and Clinical Psychology, 59,* 318–324.

Cyber Dialogue (2000a). Major cyber trends for 2000: Taking the "E" out of e-commerce. [Online]. Available online: www.cyberdialogue.com.

Cyber Dialogue (2000b). *Ethics Survey of Consumers Attitudes about Health Web Sites,* 2nd Ed. (September, 2000). Produced in cooperation with California Health Care Foundation and Internet Healthcare Coalition. [Online]. Available: www.cyberdialogue.com

Daugherty, S.R. (1998). Learning, satisfaction, and mistreatment during medical internship: a national survey of working conditions. *Journal of the American Medical Association, 279,* 1194–1199.

Davis, D., O'Brien, M.A.T., Freemantle, N., Wolf, F.M., Mazmanian, P., & Taylor-Vaisegy, A. (1999). Impact of formal continuing medical education. *Journal of American Medical Association, 282,* 867–874.

Davis, D., Thompson, M., Oxman, A., & Haynes, R. (1992). Evidence for the effectiveness of CME: a review of 50 randomized controlled trials. *Journal of the American Medical Association, 268,* 1111–1117.

DeBusk, R.F., Miller, N.H., Superko, H.R., Dennis, C.A., Thomas, R.J., Lew, H.T. et al. (1994). A case-management system for coronary risk factor modification after acute myocardial infarction. *Annals of Internal Medicine, 120*(9), 721–729.

DeCastro, A.M. (2000). Literature and medicine on-line medical students essays. [Online]. Available: *http://www.endeavor.med.nyu.edu/lit-med/syllabi.for.web/decastro.umkc.essay.html*

Deci, E.L., & Ryan, R. M. (1985a). *Intrinsic motivation and self-determination in human behavior.* New York: Plenum.

Deci, E., & Ryan, R. (1985b). The general causality orientations scale: Self-determination in personality. *Journal of Research in Personality, 19,* 109–134.

Deci, E.L., & Ryan, R.M. (1990). A motivation approach to self: Integration in personality. In R. Dienstbier (Ed.), *Nebraska symposium on motivation, Vol. 38. Perspectives on motivation* (pp. 237–288). Lincoln, NE: University of Nebraska Press.

Decter, M.B. (2000). *Four strong winds: Understanding the growing challenges to health care.* New York: Stoddart Publishing.

DeFriese, G., & Fielding, J. (1990). Health risk assessment and the clinical practice. In R. Goldbloom & R. Lawrence (Eds.), *Preventing disease: Beyond the rhetoric* (pp. 460–466). New York: Springer-Verlag.

Delamothe, T. (2000). Quality of websites: kitemarking the west wind. *British Medical Journal, 321,* 843–844.

Deming, E.E. (1986). *Out of the Crisis.* Cambridge: Center for Advanced Engineering Study, MA: Institute of Technology.

Dever, G.E.A. (1997). *Improving outcomes in public health practice: Strategy and methods.* Aspen Publishers.

Dickery, L.L., & Kamerow, D.B. (1994). The put prevention into practice campaign: Office tools and beyond. *Journal of Family Practice, 89* (4), 321 – 323.

Diestbier (Ed.). *Nebraska symposium on motivation: Perspectives on motivation.* (pp. 237–288). Lincoln: University of Nebraska Press.

Dietrich, A., Woodruff, C., & Carney, P. (1994). Changing office routines to enhance preventive care. The preventive GAPS approach. *Archives of Family Medicine, 3,* 176–183.

Dijkstra, A., & De Vries, H. (1999). The development of computer-generated tailored interventions. *Patient Education and Counselling, 36,* 193–203.

Dimeff, L.A.,& Marlatt, G.A. (1998). Preventing relapse and maintaining change in addictive behaviors. *Clinical Psychology: Science & Practice, 5*(4), 513 – 525.

Donaldson, M., Yordy, K., & Vanselow, N. (1994). Defining primary care: An interim report. Washington, DC: *National Academy Press.*

Dooley K., & Johnson, T.L. (1995). TQM, chaos and complexity. *Human Systems Management, 14,* 287–302.

Duffin, J. (2001). What goes around, comes around: A history of medical tuition. *Canadian Medical Association Journal, 164,* 50–56.

Dusenbury, L., & Falco, M. (1997). School-based drug abuse prevention strategies: from research to policy and practice. In *Enhancing Children's Wellness,* pp. 47–75. R. Weissberg, T. Gullotta, R. Hampton, B. Ryan, & Adams (Eds.) Thousand Oaks, CA: Sage Publications.

Ebrahim, S., & Smith, D. (1997). Systematic review of randomized controlled trials of multiple risk factor interventions for preventing coronary heart disease. *British Medical Journal, 314,* 1666–1674.

Eisenberg, D.M., Davis, R.B., Ettner, S.L., Appel, S., Wilkey, S., Van Rompay, M., & Kessler, R.C. (1998). Trends in alternative medicine use in the United States, 1990–1998. *Journal of American Medical Association, 280,* 1569–1575.

Eisenberg, J.M., & Power, E.J. (2000). Transforming insurance coverage into quality health care: Voltage drops from potential to delivered quality. *Journal of American Medical Association, 284,* 2100–2107.

Ellickson, P. Schools. (1995) In R. Coombs & D. Ziedonis (Eds.). *Handbook on drug abuse prevention* pp. 93–120. Coombs, R., & Ziedonis, D. (Eds.) Toronto: Allyn & Bacon, p. 93–120.

Emanuel, E.J, & Emanuel, L.L. (1996). What is accountability in health care? *Annals of Internal Medicine, 124,* 229–239.

Entwistle, V.A., Sheldon, T.A., Sowden, A.J., & Watt, I.S. (1996). Supporting consumer involvement in decision making: What constitutes quality in consumer health information? *International Journal for Quality in Health Care, 8* (5), 425–437.

Epps, R.P., & Manley, M.W. (1991). Clinical interventions to prevent tobacco use by children and adolescents. In U.S. Department of Health and Human Services, Public Health Service, National Institutes of Health (Eds.). *How to help your patients stop smoking: A National Cancer Institute manual for physicians.* Bethesda, MD:

Erickson, P.G, Riley, D.M, Cheung, Y.W., & O'Hare, P.A. (Eds.). (1997). *Harm reduction: A new direction for drug policies and programs.* Toronto, Canada: University of Toronto Press.

Ernst, & Young, and the American Quality Foundation. (1992). *International quality study: Health industry report.* Cleveland, OH: Ernst and Young and the American Quality Foundation.

Eskinazi, D.P. (1998). Factors that shape alternative medicine. *Journal of American Medical Association, 280,* 1621–1623.

Essex, B., & Bate, J. (1991). Audit in general practice by a receptionist: A feasibility study. *British Medical Journal, 302,* 573–576.

Evans, G., & Stoddart (1990). Producing health, consuming healthy care. *Social Science and Medicine, 31,* 1347–1363.

Evans, R., Barer, M., & Marmor, T. (1994). *Why are some people health and others not? The determinants of health of populations.* New York: Aldine De Gruyter.

Eysenbach, G., Diepgen, T. L., Muir Gray, J. A., Bonati, M., Impiccatore, P., Pandolfini, C., & Arunachalam, S. (1998). Towards quality management of medical information on the Internet: Evaluation, labelling, and filtering of information. *British Medical Journal, 317,* 1496–1502.

Eysenbach, G., Sa, E.R., & Diepgen, T.L. (1999). Shopping around the internet today and tomorrow: Towards the millennium of cybermedicine. *British Medical Journal, 319,* 1294–1299.

Eysenbach, G., & Diepgen, T.L. (1999). Patients looking for information on the Internet and seeking teleadvice. *Archives of Dermatology, 135,* 151–156.

Eysenbach G., Sa E.R., Diepgen T.L. (1999). Shopping around the internet today and tomorrow: Towards the millennium of cybermedicine. *British Medical Journal, 319,* 1294.

Farkas, A., Pierce, J., Zhu, S., Rosbrook, B., Gilpin, E., Berry, C., & Kaplin, R. (1996). Addiction versus stages of change models in predicting smoking cessation. *Addiction, 91,* 1271–1280.

Feinleib, M. (1996). Editorial: New directions for community intervention studies. *American Journal of Public Health, 86,* 1696–1698.

Ferguson, T. (1991). The health-activated, health-responsible consumer. Rees In A.M. (Ed.), *Managing consumer health information services* (pp. 15–22) Phoenix, AZ: Oryx Press.

Fiore, M., Epps, R., & Manley, M. (1994). A missed opportunity. Teaching medical students to help their patients successfully quit smoking. *Journal of American Medical Association, 271,* 624–626.

Fishbein, M., (1967). *Readings in attitudes, theory and measurement.* New York: Wiley.

Fishbein, M., & Ajzen, I. (1975). *Belief, attitude, intention and behavior: An introduction to theory and research.* Reading, MA: Addison-Wesley.

Flexner, A. (1910). Medical education in the United States and Canada. (Bulletin No. 4). New York: Carnegie Foundation for the Advancement of Teaching.

Frame, P. (1992). *Health maintenance in clinical practice: Strategies and barriers. American Family Physician, 45,* 1192–1200.

Frame, P. (1995). Computerized health maintenance tracking systems: A clinician's guide to necessary and optional features. *Journal of the American Board of Family Practice, 8,* 221–229.

Frame, P., Zimmer, J., Werth, P., Hall, W., & Martens W. (1991). Description of a computerized health maintenance tracking system for primary care practice. *American Journal of Preventive Medicine, 7,* 311–318.

Frame, P., Zimmer, J., Werth, P., Hall, W., & Eberly, S. (1994). Computer-based vs manual health maintenance tracking: a controlled trial. *Archives of Family Medicine, 3,* 581–588.

Frank, J. (1995). The determinants of health: A new synthesis. *Current Issues in Public Health, 1,* 233–240.

Friedman, R., Stollerman, J., Mahoney, D., & Rozenblyum, L. (1997). The virtual visit: Using telecommunications technology to take care of patients. *Journal of the American Medical Informatics Association, 4,* 413–425.

Friedman, R., Kazis, L., Jette, A., Smith, M., Stollerman, J., Torgerson, J., & Carey, K. (1996). A telecommunications system for monitoring and counseling patients with hypertension. Impact on medication adherence and blood pressure control. *American Journal of Hypertension, Ltd., 9,* 285–292.

Freidson, E. (1970). *Profession of medicine: A study of the sociology of applied knowledge.* New York: Dodd and Mead.

Freidson, E. (1994). *Professionalism reborn theory, prophecy and policy.* Cambridge: Polity Press.

Friedly, J. (2000). Speaking of tradition. *Oregon Health Sciences University Medical Student Journal, 1,* 5–15.

Fries, J., Botch, D., Harrington, H., Richardson, N., & Beck, R. (1993). Two-year results of a randomized controlled trial of a health promotion program in a retiree population. *American Journal of Medicine, 94,* 455–462.

Fries, J., Koop, C., Beadle, C., Cooper, P., England, M., Greaves, R., Sokolov, J., Wright, I., & Health Project Consortium. (1993). Reducing health care costs by reducing the need and demand for medical services. *The New England Journal of Medicine, 329,* 321–325.

Gaucher, E., & Coffey, R. (1993). *Total quality in healthcare: From Theory to Practice.* San Francisco: Jossey-Bass Publishers.

Gilbert, J.R., Dudley, T.E., Falvo, Dr, Podell, R.N., & Renner, J. (1997). When your patient is a 'medical news junkie.' *Patient Care Canada, 8* (5), 60–73.

Ginzberg, E., & Ostow, M. (1997). Managed care — a look back and a look ahead. *The New England Journal of Medicine, 336,* 1018–1020.

Glanz, K., Lewis, F.M., Rimer, B.K. (Eds.). (1997). *Health behavior and health education: Theory, research and practice,* 2nd Ed. San Francisco: Jossey-Bass.

Glazier, R.H., Badley, E.M., Gilbert, J.E., & Rothman, L. (2000). The nature of increased hospital use in poor neighbourhoods: Findings from a Canadian inner city. *Canadian Journal of Public Health, 91,* 268–273.

Glynn, T., Manley, M. M., & Bethesda. (1989). How to help your patients stop smoking. *National Institutes of Health US DDHS publication. NIH 89-3064, A National Cancer Institute Manual for Physicians.*

Goedert, J. (1997). HMOs test the Internet. *Health Data Manager, 5*(3), 81–82.

Goldberger, A.L. (1996). Non-linear dynamics for clinicians: Chaos theory, fractals, and complexity at the bedside. *Lancet, 347,* 1312–1314.

Gonzales, R., Steiner, J.F., & Sande, M.A. (1997). Antibiotic prescribing for adults with colds, upper respiratory tract infections, and bronchitis by ambulatory care physicians. *Journal of the American Medical Association, 278,* 901–904.

Graham, K., Annis, H., Brett, P., & Venesoen, P. (1996). A controlled field of group versus individual cognitive-behavioural training for relapse prevention. *Addiction, 91,* 8, 1127–1139.

Graham, W. (1996). Primary care reform: A strategy for stability. *Ontario Medical Review*, 21–27.

Graham, W. (1999). Primary care reform progress report. *Ontario Medical Review*, 21–23.

Greco, P., & Eisenberg, J. (1993). Changing physicians' practices. *The New England Journal of Medicine, 329*, 1271–1274.

Green, L., & Kreuter, M. (1991). *Application of Precede-Proceed in community settings. Health Promotion Planning: An educational and environmental approach.* Mountainview, California: Mayfield.

Greenberg, H. (1998). American medicine is on the right track. *Journal of the American Medical Association, 279*(6), 426–428.

Greenfield, S., Kaplan, S.H., Ware, J.E. Jr., Yano, E.M., & Frank, H.J. (1988). Patients participation in medical care: Effects on blood sugar control and quality of life in diabetes. *Journal of General Internal Medicine,* (3), 448–457.

Gregory, J. (1772). Observations on the duties and offices of a physician. London: Printed for W. Strahan and T. Cadell.

Grigsby, J., & Sanders, J. (1998). Telemedicine: Where it is and where it's going. *Annals of Internal Medicine, 129*, 123–127.

Grumbach, K., Osmond, D., Vranizan, K., Jaffe, D., & Bindman, A.B. (1998). Primary care physicians' experience of financial incentives in managed-care systems. *The New England Journal of Medicine, 339*, 1516–1521.

Grumbach, K. (2000). Insuring the uninsured: time to end the aura of invincibility. *Journal of American Medical Association, 284*, 2114–2116.

Gustafson, D.H., Robinson, T.N., Ansley, D., & Brennan, P.F. (1999). Consumers and evaluation of interactive health communication applications. *American Journal of Preventive Medicine, 16* (1), 23–29.

Hackman, J.R., & Wageman, R. (1995). Total quality management empirical, conceptual, and practical issues. *Administrative Science Quarterly, 40*, 309–342.

Haddix, A.C., Teutsch, S.M., Shaffer, P.A., & Dunet, D.O. (1996). *Prevention effectiveness.* Oxford University Press.

Haddock, T. (2001). Avoiding blindness: Lessons from jungian and buddhist philosophies. Chrysalis: A journal of becoming a physician 2. *Johns Hopkins University School of Medicine Medical Student Journal, 2* [Online] Available: *http://omie.med.jhmi.edu/chrysalis/webengine/webpage.cfm?webpageID=140*

Hahn, D., & Berger, M. (1990). Implementation of a systematic health maintenance protocol in a private practice. *The Journal of Family Practice, 31*, 492–504.

Hamill, P. (1994). *A drinking life: A memoir.* Boston: Little, Brown & Company.

Hammer,M. (1993). *Reengineering the corporation: A manifesto for business revolution.* New York: HarperBusiness

Hancock, T. (1993). The evolution, impact and significance of the healthy cities/healthy communities movement. *Journal of Public Health Policy, 14* (1), 5–18.

Harackiewicz, J.M., Samsone, C., Blair, L.W., Epstein, J.A., & Manderlink, G. (1987). Attributional processes in behavior change and maintenance: Smoking cessation and continued abstinence. *Journal of Consulting and Clinical Psychology, 55*, 372–378.

Harman, P., & King, D. (1985). *Expert systems: Artificial intelligence in business.* New York: John Wiley & Sons.

Harvard Center for Cancer Prevention, Harvard School of Public Health. (1996). Harvard report on cancer prevention. *Cancer Causes and Control*, 7 (Suppl.), s3 – s59.

Health Canada. (1998). *Supporting self-care: Perspectives of nurse and physician educators.* [Online] Available: *http://www.hcsc.gc.ca/hppb/healthcare/supporting.htm.*

Health Canada, Health Promotion and Programs Branch. (1997). *Supporting self-care: The Contribution of Nurses and Physicians.* [Online]. Available: http://www.hwc.ca

Healthy People: The Surgeon General's Report on Health Promotion and Disease Prevention. (1979). Washington, DC: U.S. Public Health Services, U.S. Department of Health, Education, and Welfare publication PHS 79-55071.

Heather, N. (1995). Interpreting the evidence on brief interventions for excessive drinkers: The need for caution. *Alcohol and Alcoholism, 30*, 227–296.

Hester, R. K., & Delaney, D. (1997) Behavioral self-control program for Windows: Results of a controlled clinical trial. *Journal of Consulting and Clinical Psychology, 65,* 686–693.

Hoffman-Goetz, L., & Clarke, J.N. (2000). Quality of breast cancer sites on the World Wide Web. *Canadian Journal of Public Health, 91*(4), 281–284.

House, J., Landis, K., & Umberson, D. (1988). Social relationships and health. *Science, 241,* 540–545.

House of Delegates Policy: Managed Competition. (2001). American Medical Association policy. AMA, Chicago H-165.944.

Hunink, M., Goldman, L., Tosteson, A., Mittleman, M., Goldman, P., Williams, L., Tsevat, J., & Weinstein, M. (1997). The recent decline in mortality from coronary heart disease, 1980–1990. The effect of secular trends in risk factors and treatment. *Journal of the American Medical Association, 277,* 535–541.

Hunt, W.A., Barnett, L.W., & Branch, L.G. (1971). Relapse rates in addiction programs. *Journal of Clinical Psychology, 27,* 455–6.

IDC. (2000). *Email deluge continues with no end in sight.* [Online] Available: (*http://www.idc.com/software/press/PR/SW101000pr.stm*).

IDC Research (2000). Email Usage Forecast and Analysis, 2000-2005 (press report). *http://www.idc.com/software/press/PR/SW101000pr.stm* (accessed February 9, 2001).

Impiccatore, P., Pandolfini, C., Casella, N., & Bonati, M. (1997). Reliability of health information for the public on the world wide web: Systematic survey of advice on challenges for the Internet. *British Medical Journal, 319,* 761–764.

Inlander, C.B. (1991). Trends in medical consumerism. In A.M. Rees, (Ed.), *Managing consumer health information services.* Phoenix, AZ: Oryx Press. pp. 3–14.

Institute for the Future. (2000). *Health and Health Care 2010. The forecast, the challenge.* San Francisco: Jossey-Bass.

Institute for Healthcare Improvement. (1996). *Reducing delays and waiting times throughout the heathcare system.* Boston: Institute for Healthcare Improvement.

Institute of Medicine. (2001). *Crossing the quality chasm: A new health system for the 21st century.* Washington, DC: National Academy Press.

International Union for Health Promotion and Education. (2000). *The evidence of health promotion effectiveness: shaping public health in a new era.* A report for the European Commission. Brussels, Luxemburg. Available from IUHPE, 2 rue Auguste Comet, 92170 Banbes, France, or online at: *www.iuhpe.org*

Jadad, A. R., & Gagliardi, A. (1998). Rating health information on the internet: navigating to knowledge or to Babel? *Journal of American Medical Association, 279,* 611–699.

Jadad, A.R. (1999). Promoting partnerships: challenges for the Internet age. *British Medical Journal, 319,* 761–764

Jadad, A. R., Haynes, R. B., Hunt, D., & Brownman, G. P. (2000). The Internet and evidence-based decision-making: A needed synergy for efficient knowledge management in health care. *Canadian Medical Association Journal, 162.*

Jadad, A.R., & Enkin, M.W. (2000). The new alchemy: Transmuting information into knowledge in an electronic age. *Canadian Medical Association Journal, 162,* 1826–1841.

Jadad, A.R. (2001, January). *Towards e-Health: The promise, perils and paradoxes of telecommunications in the health system.* Nortel Institute for Telecommunications of the University of Toronto and Edward S. Rogers Sr. Department of Electrical and Computer Engineering Distinguished Lecture, presented at Toronto, Canada.

Jaen, R., Stange, K., & Nutting, P. (1994). Competing demands of primary care: A model for the delivery of clinical preventive services. *Journal of Family Practice, 38,* 166–171.

Jenkins, K. (1997). Primary Care Reform: OMA membership survey results. *Ontario Medical Review,* 20–21, 59.

Jimison, H. (1997). Patient-specific interfaces to health and decision-making information. In R. Street, W. Gold & T. Manning (Eds.), *Health promotion and interactive technology,* (pp. 141–156). Nahway, NJ: Lawrence Erlbaum.

Joiner, B. (1994). *Fourth generation management.* New York: McGraw Hill. Oakbrook Terrace, Illinois: Joint commission on accreditation of healthcare organizations.

Joint Commission on Accreditation of Healthcare Organizations. (1994). *Framework for improving performance: From principles to practice*. Oakbrook Terrace, IL. Joint commission on accreditation of healthcare organizations.

Jonas, W.B. (1998). Alternative medicine-learning from the past, examining the present, advancing to the future. *Journal of American Medical Association, 280*, 1616–1618.

Johnston, L., Bachman, J., & O'Malley, P. (2000). *Monitoring the future: National results on adolescent drug use overview of key findings 1999*. Washington. D.C.: NIDA.

Johnston, L.D., O'Malley, P.M., & Bachman, J.G. (2000, December). *Cigarette use and smokeless tobacco use decline substantially among teens*. University of Michigan News and Information Services: Ann Arbor, MI. [Online]. Available: *www.monitoringthefuture.org*

Joseph, J., Breslin, C., & Skinner, H.A. (1999). Critical perspectives on the transtheoretical model and stages of change. In J. Tucker, D. (p. 160–190) Donovan & A. Marlatt (Eds.), *Changing addictive behavior: Moving beyond therapy assisted change*. New York: Guilford.

Juran Institute (1989). *Quality improvement tools*. Wilton, CN: Juran Institute.

Juran, J.M. (1996). *A history of managing for quality: The evolution, trends, and future directions of managing for quality*. Milwaukee, WI: ASQC Quality Press.

Kahan, M., Wilson, L., & Becker, L. (1995). Effectiveness of physician-based interventions with problem drinkers: A review. *Canadian Medical Association Journal, 152*, 851–859.

Kane, B., & Sands, D. (1998). Guidelines for the clinical use of electronic mail with patients. *Journal of American Medical Association, 5*, 104–111.

Kane, B., & Sands, D.Z. for the AMIA Internet Working Group, Task Force on Guidelines for the use of clinic-patient electronic mail. (1998). Guidelines for the clinical use of electronic mail with patients. *Journal of American Medical Association, 5*(1), 104–111.

Kaplan, R.M., Pierce, J.P., Gilpin, E.A., Johnson, M., Bal, D.G. (1993). Stages of smoking cessation: The 1990 California tobacco survey. *Tobacco Control, 2*, 139–144.

Kasebaum, D., & Cutler, E. (1998). On the culture of student abuse in medical school. *Academic Medicine, 73* (11), 1149–1158.

Kassirer, J. (1998). Doctor discontent. *The New England Journal of Medicine*, 339, 1543–1545.

Keegan, D. (2000). Here in Placentia. *Canadian Medical Association Journal, 163*, 1582–1583.

Keeler, E., Manning, W., Newhouse, J., Sloss, E., & Wasserman, J. (1989). The external costs of a sedentary lifestyle. *American Journal of Public Health, 79*, 975–981.

Keller, E.F. (2000). *The century of the gene*. Cambridge, MA: Harvard University Press.

Kelner, M., Wellman, B., Pescosolido, B., & Saks, M. (Eds.). (2000). *Complementary alternative medicine: Challenge and change*. Reading, U.K.: Harwood Academic Press.

Kemper, D., Lorig, K., & Mettler, M. (1993). The effectiveness of medical self-care interventions: A focus on self-initiated responses to symptoms. *Patient Education and Counseling, 21*, 29–39.

Kim, P., Eng, T.R., Deering, M.J., & Maxfield, A. (1999). Published criteria for evaluating health related web sites: Review. *British Medical Journal, 318*, 647–649.

Kobak, K., Taylor, L., Dottl, S., Greist, J., Jefferson, J., Burroughs, D., Mantle, J., Kalzelnick, D., Norton, R., Henk, H., & Serlin, R. (1997). A computer-administered telephone interview to identify mental disorders. *Journal of American Medical Association, 278*, 905–910.

Kohn, L.T., Corrigan, J.M., & Donaldson, M.S. (Eds.). (1999). *To err is human: Building a safer health system*. Institute of Medicine. Washington, DC: National Academy Press.

Kongstvedt, P. (1995). *Essentials of managed care*. Gaithersberg, MD: Aspen.

Koop, C. Everitt. (1995). A personal role in health care reform. *American Journal of Public Health*, 85,759-760.

Kop, W.J. (1997). Acute and chronic psychological risk factors for coronary syndromes: Moderating effects of coronary artery disease severity. *Journal of Psychosomatic Research, 43*,167–181.

Korcok, M. (2001). Number of medical school applicants drops on both sides of border. *Canadian Medical Association Journal, 164*, p.79.

Kotter, J. (1996). *Leading change*. Boston: Harvard Business School Press.

Kottke, T., Gatewood, L., Wu, S., & Park, H. (1988). Preventing heart disease: Is treating the high risk sufficient? *Journal of Clinical Epidemiology, 41*, 1083–1093.

Kottke, T., Brekke, M., & Solberg, L. (1993). Making "time" for preventive services. *Mayo Clin Proceedings, 68*, 785–791.

Kretzmann, J.P., & McKnight, J.L. (1993). *Building communities from the inside out: A path toward finding and mobilizing a communities' assets.* Chicago, IL: ACTA Publications.

Krishna, S., Balas, A., Spencer, D., Griffin, J., & Austin Boren, S. (1997). Clinical trials of interactive computerized patient education: Implications for family practice. *Journal of Family Practice, 45,* 25–33.

Kyrouz, E.M., & Humphreys, K. (2000). *A review of research on the effectiveness of self help mutual aid groups.* [Online] Available: *www.mentalhelp.net/articles/selfres.htm*

Lalonde, M. (1974). *A new perspective on the health of Canadians.* Ottawa, Canada: Health and Welfare Canada.

Langer, E.J.and Rodin, J. (1976). The effects of choice and personal responsibility for the aged: A field experiment in an institutional setting. *Journal of Personality and Social Psychology, 34,* 191–198.

Langley, G., Nolan, K., Nolan, T., Norman, G., & Provest, L. (1996). *The improvement guide: A practical approach to enhance organizational performance.* San Francisco: Jossey-Bass.

Langley, G., Nolan, K., & Nolan, T. (1994). The foundation of improvement. *Quality Progress, 27,* 81–86.

Law, M., & Tang, J. (1995). An analysis of the effectiveness of interventions intended to help people stop smoking. *Archives of Internal Medicine, 155,* 1933–1941.

Lawrence, S., & Giles, C. L. (1999). Accessibility of information on the web. *Nature, 400,* 107–109.

Lazarsfeld, P., & Merton, R. (1971). Mass communication, taste and organized social action. In W. Schramm, & D.F. Roberts (Ed.). *Process and effects of mass communications,* (pp. 554–578). Urbana, IL: University of Illinois Press.

Lazarus, W., & Lipper, L. (2000). *Creating a children's policy agenda in the digital world: Strategies.* Santa Monica, CA: The Children's Partnership.

Leatt, P., Pink, G., & Naylor, D. (1996). Integrated delivery systems: Has their time come in Canada? *Canadian Medical Association Journal, 154,* 803–809.

Leebov, W., & Ersoz, C. (1998). *The health care manager's guide to continuous quality improvement.* Chicago, IL: American Hospital Publishing, Inc.

Lehoux, P., Battista, R.N., Lance, J.M., (2000). Telehealth: Passing fad or lasting benefits? *Canadian Journal of Public Health, 91*(4), 277–281.

Levin, L. (1987, Summer). Every silver lining has a cloud: The limits of health promotion. *Social Policy,* 57–60.

Lewin, K. (1951). The nature of field theory. In M.H. Marx (Ed.), *Psychological Theory.* New York: MacMillan.

Lewis, S. (1999, October). Toward a general theory of indifference to research evidence. presented at the closing the loop conference, Toronto, Canada.

Lewis, C., Clancy, C., Leake, B., & Schwartz, S. (1991). The counseling practices of internists. *Annals of Internal Medicine, 144,* 54–58.

Lichtenstein, E., & Glasgow, R.E. (1992). Smoking cessation: what have we learned over the past decade? *Journal of Consulting and Clinical Psychology, 60,* 518–527.

Logan, R.K. (1995). *The fifth language.* Toronto, Canada: Stoddart.

Long, B., Calfas, K., Wooten, W., Sallis, J., Patrick, K., Goldstein, M., Marcus, B., Schwenk, T., Chenoweth, J., Carter, R., Torres, T., Palinkas, L., & Health G. (1996). A multisite field test of the acceptability of physical activity counseling in primary care: Project PACE. *American Journal of Preventive Medicine,* 0749–3797/96.

Lurie, N. (2000). Strengthening the U.S. health care safety net. *Journal of American Medical Association, 284,* 2112–2114.

Lynagh, M., Schofield, M., and Sanson-Fisher, R. (1997). School health promotion programs over the past decade: A review of the smoking, alcohol and solar protection literature. *Health Promotion International, 12*(1), 43–59.

Madara, E. (1995, April 20–21). *"More than warm fuzzies for frugal times: Low cost, high impact self-help support groups." Through the patient's eyes: Incorporating the patient's perspective.* Conference proceedings, the Picker Institute, Cambridge, MA.

Madara, E. (1997). The mutual-aid self-help online revolution. *Social Policy, 27* (3), 20–26.

Madara, E., Kalafat, J., & Miller, B.N. (1988). The computerized self-help clearinghouse: Using 'high tech' to promote 'high touch' support networks. *Computers in Human Services, 3,* 39–54.

Madara, E., & White, B.J. (1997). On-line mutual support: The experience of a self-help clearing-house. *Information and Referral: The Journal of the Alliance of Information and Referral Systems, 19,* 91–108.

Managed Care On-Line. Online: *http://www.mcareol.com/factshts/mcolfact.htm*

Manning, W., Keeler, E., Newhouse, J., Sloss, E., & Wasserman, J. (1991). *The costs of poor health habits: A rand study.* Cambridge, MA: Harvard University Press.

Marcus, S.H., & Tuchfeld, B.S. (1993). Sharing information, sharing responsibility: Helping health care consumer make informed decisions. *Conference Proceedings from 17th Annual Symposium on Computer Applications in Medical Care, 17,* 3–7.

Marlatt, G.A., Baer, J.S., & Quigley, L.A. (1995). Self–efficacy and addictive behavior. In A. Bandura (Ed.) *Self–Efficacy In Changing Societies.* Cambridge, UK: Cambridge University Press.

Marlatt, G.A., & Gordon, J.R., (1985). *Relapse prevention: Maintenance strategies in the treatment of addictive behaviors.* New York: Guilford.

Marlatt, G.A., Larimer, M.E., Baer, J. S., & Quigley, L.A. (1993). Harm reduction for alcohol problems: Moving beyond the controlled drinking controversy. *Behavior Therapy, 24,* 461–504.

Marlatt, G.A., & Tapert, S.F. (1993). Harm reduction: Reducing the risks of addictive behaviors. In J. S. Baer, G. A. Marlatt, & R. McMahon (Eds.), *Addictive behaviors across the lifespan* (pp.243–273). Newbury Park, CA: Sage.

Marlatt, G.A. (1998). *Harm reduction: Pragmatic strategies for managing high-risk behaviors.* New York: Guilford Press.

Marshall, K.G. (1996a). Prevention. How much harm? How much benefit? The ethics of informed consent for preventive screening programs. *Canadian Medical Association Journal.* 155 (4),377–83.

Marshall, KG. (1996b). Prevention. How much harm? How much benefit? Influence of reporting methods on perception of benefits. *Canadian Medical Association Journal,* 54 (10), 1493 – 1499.

Marshall KG. (1996c). Prevention. How much harm? How much benefit? Physical, psychological and social harm. *Canadian Medical Association Journal,155* (2),169 – 176.

Marshall, K.G. (1996d). Prevention. How much harm? How much benefit? Ten potential pitfalls in determining the clinical significance of benefits. *Canadian Medical Association Journal.* 154(12),1837–1843.

McAfee, T., Wilson, J., Dacey, S., Sofian, N., Curry, S., & Wagener, B. (1995). Awakening the sleeping giant: Mainstreaming efforts to decrease tobacco use in an HMO. *HMO Practice, 9,* 138–143.

McBeth, A.J., & Schweer, K.D. (2000). *Building healthy communities: The challenge of health care in the 21st century.* Boston: Allyn & Bacon.

McGinnis, J.M. (1994). The role of behavioral research in national health policy. In S. Bloomenthal, K. Mathews, & S. Weiss (Eds.), *New Research Frontiers in Behavioral Medicine: Proceedings of the National Conference.* Bethesda, MD: National Institutes of Health, Health and Behavior Coordinating Committee.

McGinnis, M., & Foege, W. (1993). Actual causes of death in the United States. *Journal of the American Medical Association, 270,* 2207–2212.

McGinnis, M., & Lee, P. (1995). Healthy people 2000 at mid decade. *Journal of the American Medical Association, 273;* 1123–1141.

McIlvain, H., Crabtree, B., Gilbert, C., Havranek, R., & Backer, E. (1997). Current trends in tobacco prevention and cessation in Nebraska physicians' offices. *Journal of Family Practice, 44,* 193–202.

McPhee, S., Bird, J., Fordham, K., Rodnick, J., & Osborn, E. (1991). Promoting cancer prevention by primary care physicians: Results of a randomized, controlled trial. *Journal of the American Medical Association, 266,* 538–544.

McVea, K., Crabtree, B., Medder, J., Susman, J., Lukas, L., McIlvain, H., Davis, C., Gilbert, C., & Hawver, M. (1996). An Ounce of Prevention? Evaluation of the 'Put Prevention into Practice' Program. *The Journal of Family Practice, 43,* 361–369.

Mechanic, D. (2000). Managed care and the imperative for a new professional ethic. *Health Affairs, 19* (5), 100–111.

Medder, J., Susman, J., Gilbert, C., Crabtee, B., McIlvain, H., Davis, C., & Hawver, M. (1997). Dissemination and implementation of put prevention into family practice. *American Journal Of Preventive Medicine,* 13, 345–351.

Medical Post. (2000). *The Medical Post 2000 National Survey of Doctors.* Toronto, Canada: Author.

Michaud, C.M., Murray, C.J.L., & Bloom, B.R. (2001) Burden of disease—Implications for future research. *Journal of American Medical Association, 285,* 535–539.

Mischel, W. (1973). Toward a cognitive social learning reconceptualization of personality. *Psychological Review, 80,* 252–283.

Mischel, W., & Shoda, Y. (1995). A cognitive-affective system theory of personality: Reconceptualizing situations, dispositions, dynamics, and invariance in personality structures. *Psychological Review, 102,* 246–268.

Migneault, J.P., Pallonen, U.E., Velicer, W.F. (1997). Decisional balance and stage of change for adolescent drinking. *Addictive Behaviors, 21,* 1–13.

Milio, N. (1996). *Engines of empowerment: Using information technology to create healthy communities and challenge public policy.* Chicago, IL: Health Administration Press.

Miller, J.G. (1978). *Living systems.* New York: McGraw-Hill.

Miller, S.M., Shoda, Y., & Hurley, K. (1996). Applying cognitive-social theory to health-protective behavior: Breast self-examination in cancer screening. *Psychological Bulletin, 119,* 70–94.

Miller, T., & Galbraith, M. (1995). Injury prevention counseling by pediatricians: A benefit-cost comparison. *Pediatrics, 98,* 1–4.

Miller, W.R. (1985). Motivation for treatment: A review with special emphasis on alcoholism. *Psychological Bulletin, 98,* 84–107.

Miller, W.R. (1996). What is a relapse? Fifty ways to leave the wagon. *Addiction, 91,* S15–S27.

Miller, W.R., Benefield, R.G., & Tonigan, J.S. (1993). Enhancing motivation for change in problem drinking: a controlled comparison of two therapist styles. *Journal of Consulting and Clinical Psychology, 61,* 455–461.

Miller, W., Crabtree, B., McDaniel, R., & Stange, K. (1998). Understanding change in primary care practice using complexity theory. *Journal of Practice, 46,* 369–376.

Miller, W.R., & Rollnick, S. (1991). *Motivational interviewing: Preparing people to change addictive behavior.* New York: Gilford Press.

Minkler, M. (1997). *Community organizing and community building for health.* New Brunswick, NJ: Rutgers University Press.

Minkler, M., & Wallerstein, N. (1996). Improving health through community organization and community building. In *Health behavior and health education: Theory, research and practice* (p.). K. Glanz, F. Lewis, & B. Rimer (Eds.), San Francisco: Jossey–Bass.

Mitretek Systems IQ Tools. (2001). Online: *http://hitiweb.mitretek.org/iq.htm*

Mittman. R, & Cain. M. (1999) *The Future of the Internet in Health Care.* 1–41.

Montaña, D.E., Kasprzyk, D., & Taplin, S.H. (1997). The theory of reasoned action and the theory of planned behavior. *Health behavior and health education: Theory, research, and practice,* 2nd ed. (chapter 5, pp. 85–110). San Francisco, L.A.: Jossey-Bass.

Monti, P.M., Colby, S.M., Barnett, N.P., Spirito, A., Rohsenow, D.J., Myers, M., Wollard, R., & Lewander, W. (1999). Brief intervention for harm reduction with alcohol-positive older adolescents in a hospital emergency department. *Journal of Consulting and Clinical Psychology, 67,* 989–994.

Morrissey, J. (1997). HMOs enter Internet age. Plans begin electronic interaction with enrollees. *Modern Healthcare, 27* (14), 140, 142–144.

Moser, A.E., & Annis, H.M. (1996). The role of coping in relapse crisis outcome: A prospective study of treated alcoholics. *Addiction, 91*(8), 1101–1113.

Murphy, H.B.M. (1980). Hidden barriers to the diagnosis and treatment of alcoholism and other alcohol misuses. *Journal of Studies in Alcohol, 41,* 417–428.

National Cancer Institute. (1989). *How to help your patients stop smoking: A National Cancer Institute manual for physicians* (NIH Publication No. 89-3064). Bethesda, MD: National Institutes of Health.

National Research Council, Committee on Enhancing the Internet for Health Applications. (2000). *Networking health: Prescription for the Internet.* Washington, DC: National Academy Press.

National Telecommunications and Information Administration (1999). Falling through the Net: Defining the digital divide. Washington, DC: U.S. Department of Commerce.

Negotia, U.N. (1985). *Expert systems and fuzzy systems.* Menlo Park, CA: Benjamin.

Nelson, E., & Mohr, J. (1996). Improving health care, Part 1: The clinical value compass. *Joint Commission Journal on Quality Improvement, 22,* 243–258.

Nelson, E., Splaine, M., Batalden, P., & Plume, S. (1998). Building measurement and data collection into medical practice. *Annals of Internal Medicine, 128,* 460–466.

Nelson, L., & Burns, F. (1984). High performance programming: A framework for transforming organizations. In J. Adams (Ed.), *Transforming work. A collection of organizational transformational readings* (pp. 226–242). VA: Miles River Press.

Newhouse, J. (1993). *Free for all: Lessons from the Rand health insurance experiment.* Cambridge, MA: Harvard University Press.

Nilasena, D.S., Lincoln, M.J., Turner, C.W., Warner, H.R., Foerster, V.A., Williamson, J.W., & Stults, B.M. (1994). Development and implementation of a computer-generated reminder system for diabetes preventive care. *American Medical Informatics Association, 18,* 831–835.

Noble, H.B. (1999, September 5). Hailed as a Surgeon General, Koop is faulted on web ethic. *New York Times,* E-Medicine Supplement, p. .

Noonan, W.C., & Moyer, T.B. (1997). Motivational interviewing: a review. *Journal of Substance Misuse, 2,* 8–16.

Norman, C.D., & Skinner, H.A. (2000). Where is the consumer in the evaluation of online consumer health information? *Canadian Psychology, 41*(2a), 34.

NUA. (2000). How many people are on line? [Online]. Available: *http://www.nua.ie/surveys/how_many_online/index.htm*

Nyquist, A-C., Gonzales, R., Steiner, J.F., Sande, M.E. (1998). Antibiotic prescribing for children with colds, upper respiratory tract infections, and bronchitis. *Journal of the American Medical Association, 279,* 875 – 877.

O'Brien, J.L., Shortell, S.M., Foster, R.W., Carman, J.M., Hugues, E.F., Boerstler, H., & O'Connor, E.J. (1994). A framework for advancing continuous quality improvement: some results and lesson from ten comparative case studies. Working paper, Center for Health Services and Policy Research and the J.L. Kellogg Graduate School of Management, Northwest University, Evanston, IL.

Ockene, J.K., Kristeller, J., Goldberg, R. et al. (1991). Increasing the efficacy of physician delivered smoking interventions: A randomized clinical trial. *Journal of General Internal Medicine, 6,* 1–8.

Oka, T. & Borkman, T. (2000). The history, concepts and theories of self-help groups: From an international perspective. *Japanese Journal of Occupational Therapy, 34* (7), 718–722. (*http://www.shgj.net/2000/jjot*).

O'Loughlin, J.L., Paradis, G., Gray-Donald, K., & Renauld, L. (1999). The impact of a community-based heart disease prevention program in a low-income, inner-city neighborhood. *American Journal of Public Health, 89,* 1819–1826.

Olson, J.M. (1992). Psychological barriers to behavior change. *Canadian Family Physician, 38,* 309–319.

Ontario College of Family Physicians. (2000, July 19). Implementation strategies: Too many hours, too much stress, too little respect. Toronto, Canada: Author.

O'Reilly, M. (1998). Ontario's attempt at primary care reform hits another snag. *Canadian Medical Association Journal, 159,* 1398–1400.

Orford, D.R., Kraemer, H.C., Kazdin, A.E., Jensen, P.S., & Herrington, R. (1998). Lowering the burden of suffering from child psychiatric disorder: Trade offs among clinical, targeted, and universal interventions. *J.AM. Acad. Child Adolesc. Psychiatry, 37,* 686–694.

Orleans, C. (1988). Effectiveness of self–help quit smoking strategies. In T. Glynn (chair), *Four national cancer institute-funded self-help smoking cessation trials: interim results and emerging patterns.* Symposium conducted at the annual meeting of the Association for the Advancement Of Behavior Therapy, New York.

Orleans, C., Schoenback, V., & Wagner, E. (1991). Self-help quit smoking interventions: Effects of self-help materials, social support instructions, and telephone counseling. *Journal of Consulting and Clinical Psychology, 59,* 439–448.

Ornstein, S., Garr, D., Jenkins, R., Rust, P., & Arnon, A. (1991). Computer-generated physician and patient reminders. Tools to improve population adherence to selected preventive services. *Journal of Family Practice, 6,* 55–60.

Ornstein, S., Garr, D., & Jenkins, R. (1993). A comprehensive microcomputer-based medical records system with sophisticated preventive services features for the family physician. *Journal of American Board of Family Practice, 6,* 55–60.

Osler, W. (1930). *Aequanimitas, with Other Addresses to Medical Students, Nurses and Practitioners of Medicine,* with three additional addresses, (2nd ed.). London: H.K. Lewis.

Pallonen, U.E., Prochaska, J.O., Velicer, W.F., Prokhorov, A.V., & Smith, N.F. (1998). Stages of acquisition and cessation for adolescent smoking: An empirical integration. *Addict Behavior, 23,* 303–324.

Palmer, P.J. (1998). *The courage to teach.* San Francisco: Jossey-Bass.

Paperny, D. (1997). Computerized health assessment and education for adolescent HIV and STD prevention in health care settings and schools· *Health Education & Behavior, 24,* 54–70.

Patrick, K., & Koss, S. (1995). *Consumer health information (White Paper).* Washington, DC:

Patrick, K., Sallis, J., Long, B., Calfas, K., Wooten, W., Health, G., & Pratt, M. (1994). A new tool for encouraging activity. *The Physician and Sports Medicine, 22.* 11.

Patterson, G.A., & Forgatch, M.S. (1985). Therapist behavior as a determinant for client noncompliance: a paradox for the behavior modifier. *Journal of Consulting and Clinical Psychology, 53,* 846–851.

Pelletier, K.R. (1993). A review and analysis of the health and cost-effective outcome studies of comprehensive health promotion and disease prevention programs at the worksite: 1991–1993 update. *American Journal of Health Promotion; 8,* 50–62.

Pelletier, K.R. (1996). A review and analysis of the health and cost-effective outcome studies of comprehensive health promotion and disease prevention programs at the worksite: 1993–1995 update. *American Journal of Health Promotion, 10,* 380–388.

Perz, C., DiClemente, C., & Carbonari, J. (1996). Doing the right thing at the right time? The interaction of stages and processes of change in successful smoking cessation. *Health Psychology, 15,* 462–468.

Pifalo, V., Hollander, S., Henderson, C.L., DeSalvo, P., & Gill, GP. (1997). The impact of consumer health information provided by libraries: The Delaware experience. *Bulletin of the Medical Libraries Association, 85* (1), 16–22.

Pincus, C. (1995). Have doctors lost their work ethic? *Medical Economics, 72,* 24.

Plsek, P. (1994). Tutorial: planning for data collection. Part II: designing the study. *Quality Management in Health Care, 2,* 73–81.

Plsek, P.E. (1997). *Creativity, innovation, and quality.* Milwaukee, WI: ASQ Quality Press (American Society for Quality).

PriceWaterhouseCoopers. (1999a) *Health Cast 2010: Small world, bigger expectations.* USA: PriceWaterhouseCoopers. (www.pweglobal.com/healthcare)

PriceWaterhouseCoopers. (1999b). *Health insider.* Toronto, Canada: PriceWaterhouseCoopers' Canadian Healthcare Practice.

Prigogine, I., & Stengers, I. (1984). *Order out of chaos.* New York: Bantam Books.

Prilleltensky, I. (1994). Empowerment in mainstream psychology: Legitimacy, obstacles and possibilities. *Canadian Psychology, 35*(4), 358–375.

Prochaska, J., DiClemente, C., & Norcross, J. (1992). In search of how people change. Applications to addictive behaviors. *American Psychologist, 47,* 1102–1114.

Prochaska, J.O., DiClemente, C.C. (1983). Stages and processes of self-change of smoking: Toward an integrative model of change. *Journal of Consulting and Clinical Psychology, 51*(3), 390–395.

Prochaska, J.O., DiClemente, C.C., Velicer, W.F., & Rossi, J.S. (1993). Standardized, individualized, interactive and personalized self-help programs for smoking cessation. *Health Psychology; 12*(4), 399–405.

Prochaska, J.O., Redding, C.A., & Evers, K.E. (1997). The transtheoretical model and stages of change. In K. Glanz, F.M. Lewis, and B.K. Rimer, (Eds) *Health behavior and health education: Theory, research and practice.* San Francisco: Jossey-Bass.

Prochaska, J.O., Velicer, W., DiClemente, C.C., & Fava, J. (1988). Measuring processes of change: Applications to the cessation of smoking. *Journal of Consulting & Clinical Psychology, 56*(4), 520–528.

Prochaska, J.O., Velicer, W.F., Rossi, J.S., Goldstein, M.G., Marcus, B.H., & Rakowski, W. et al. (1994). Stages of change and decisional balance for 12 problem behaviors. *Health Psychology, 13*(1), 39–46.

Promoting Health / Preventing Disease: Objectives for the Nation. (1980). Washington, DC: U.S. Public Health Service.

Rachlis, M.R., & Kushner, C. (1994). *Strong medicine*. Toronto, Canada: Harper Collins Publishers.

Raeburn, J., & Rootman, I. (1998). *People-centred health promotion*. Toronto, Canada: Wiley.

Rakowaski, W., Ehrich, B., M.G., Reimer, B.K., Pearlman, D.N., Clark, M.A., Velicer, W.F., & Woolverton, H. (1998). Increasing mammography among women aged 40–64 by use of a stage-matched, tailored intervention. *Preventive Medicine, 27*, 748–756

Ramelson, H., Freidman, R., & Ockene, J. (1999). An automated telephone-based smoking cessation education and counseling system. *Patient Education and Counseling, 36*, 131–144.

Raphael, D. (2000). Health inequalities in Canada: Current discourses and implications for public health action. *Critical Public Health, 10*, 193–216.

Ravaja, N., Kauppinen, T., & Keltikangas–Jarvinen, L. (2000). Relationships between hostilityand physiological coronary heart disease risk factors in young adults: The moderating influence of depressive tendencies. *Psychological Medicine*, 30, 381–393.

Reeder, L.G. (1972). The patient-client as a consumer: Some observations on the changing professional-client relationship. *Journal of Health and Social Behaviour, 13*, 406–412.

Reid, J. (1996). *A telemedicine primer: understanding the issues*. Billings, MT:Innovative Medical Communication.

Reilly, P.R. (2000). Public concern about genetics. *Annual Review of Genomics and Human Genetics, 1*, 485–506.

Richard Ivey School of Business. (1997, September). Leading the management of change: A study of 12 Ontario hospitals. London: Canada.

Richmond, R., & Heather, N. (1990). General practitioner interventions for smoking cessation: Past results and future prospects. *Behaviour Change, 7*(3), 110–119.

Richmond, R., Heather, N., Wodak, A., Kehoe, L., & Webster, I. (1995). Controlled evaluation of a general practice-based brief intervention for excessive drinking. *Addiction, 90*, 119–132.

Ridley, M. (1999). *Genome*. New York: Perennial.

Ritvo, P.G., Irvine, J., Lindsay, E., Kraetschmer, N., Blair, N., & Shnek, Z. (1997). A critical review of research related to family physician-assisted smoking cessation interventions. *Cancer Prevention & Control, 1*(4), 289–304.

Rivara, F.P., Rogers, L. W., Thompson, D.C. et al. (1994). The Seattle children's bicycle helmet campaign: Changes in helmet use and head injury admissions. *Pediatrics, 1993*, 567–569.

Robbins, A., & Freeman, P. (1999). How organized medical care can advance public health. *Public Health Reports, 114*, 120–129.

Robert Wood Johnson Foundation. (1994). Annual report. Princeton. NJ: The Robert Wood Foundation.

Robinson, B., Gjerdingen, D., & Houge, D. (1995). Obesity: A move from traditional to more patient-orientated management. *Journal of the American Board of Family Practice, 8*, 99–108.

Robinson, T.N., Patrick, K., Eng, T.R., & Gustafson, D. for the Science Panel on Interactive Communication and Health (1998). An evidence-based approach to interactive health communication: A challenge to medicine in the information age. *Journal of American Medical Association, 280*, 1264–1269.

Roemer, M.I. (1984). The value of medical care for health promotion. *American Journal of Public Health, 74*, 243–248.

Rollnick, S., Mason, P., & Butler, C. (1999). *Health behavior change: A guide for practitioners*. Edinburgh, Scotland: Churchill Livingstone.

Rosen, C.S. (2000). Is the sequencing of change processes by stage consistent across health problems? A meta-analysis. *Health Psychology, 19*, 593–604.

Rosenstock, I.M. (1974). Historical origins of the health belief model. *Health Education Monographs, 2*, 328–335.

Rosenstock, I.M., Strecher, V.J., & Becker M.H. (1988) Social learning theory and the health belief model. *Health Education Quarterly, 15*, 175–183.

Rosser, W. (1996). Approach to diagnosis by primary care clinicians and specialists: Is there a difference? *Journal of Family Practice, 42*, 139–144.

Rosser, W., McDowell, I., & Newell, C. (1991). Use of reminders for preventive procedures in family medicine. *Canadian Medical Association Journal, 145*(7), 805–812.

Royal College of Physicians and Surgeons of Canada. (2000). *Skills for the new millennium: Report of the societal needs working group*. Ottawa, Canada: Author.

Russell, L. (1993). The role of prevention in health reform. *The New England Journal of Medicine*, 352–354.

Russell, M.A.H., Wilson, C., Taylor, C. et al. (1979). The effect of general practitioners' advice against smoking. *British Medical Journal, 2*, 231–234.

Ryan, R., & Deci, E. (2000). Self-determination theory and the facilitation of intrinsic motivation, social development, and well-being. *American Psychologist, 55*(1), 68–78.

Ryan, R.M., & Frederick, C.M. (1997). On energy, personality, and health: subjective vitality as a dynamic reflection of well–being. *Journal of Personality, 65*, 529–565.

Ryan, R., Plant, R., & O'Malley, S. (1995). Initial motivations for alcohol treatment: Relations with patient characteristics, treatment involvement and dropout. *Addictive Behaviors, 20*, 279–297.

Sandvik, H. (1999). Health information and interaction on the internet: A survey of female urinary incontinence. *British Medical Journal, 319*, 29–32.

Sanson-Fisher, R.W., Webb, G.R., & Reid, A.L. (1986). The role of the medical practitioner as an agent for disease prevention. *Better Health Commission: Looking Forward to Better Health, 3*, 201–212.

Saunders, B., Wilkinson, C., & Philips, M. (1995). The impact of a brief motivational intervention with opiate users attending a methadone programme. *Addiction*, 90, 415–424.

Scheffler, R. (1999). Physician collective bargaining: A turning point in U.S. medicine. *Journal of Health Politics, Policy and Law, 24*, 1071–1076.

Schmid, T.L., Jeffrey, R.W., & Hellerstedt, W.L. (1989). Direct mail recruitment to house-based smoking and weight control programs: A comparison of strengths. *Preventive Medicine, 18*, 503–517.

Scholtes, P. (1988). *The Team Handbook*. Madison, WI: Joiner Associates.

Scott, C., Neighbor, W., & Brock, D. (1992). Physicians' attitudes toward preventive care services: A seven-year prospective cohort study. *American Journal of Preventive Medicine, 8*, 241–248.

Seely-Brown, J., & Duguid, P. (2000). *The social life of information*. Cambridge, MA: Harvard Business School Press.

Senge P.M. (1990). *The fifth discipline: The art and practice of learning organization*. New York: Doubleday.

Senge, P., Kleiner, R., Roberts, C., Ross, R.B., Roth, G., & Smith, B. (1999). *The dance of change: The challenges to sustaining momentum in learning organizations*. New York: Doubleday.

Senge, P.M., Kleiner, A., Roberts, C., Ross, R.B., & Smith, B.G. (1994). *The fifth discipline field book: Strategies and tools for building a learning organization*. New York: Doubleday.

Shea, S., DuMoughel, W., & Bahamonde, L. (1996). A meta-analysis of 16 random controlled trials to evaluate computer-based clinical reminder systems for preventive care in the ambulatory setting. *Journal of the American Medical Informatics Association, 3*, 399–409.

Shedroff, N. (1999). Information interaction design: A unified field theory of design. In R. Jacobson (Ed.), *Information design* (pp. 267–292). Cambridge, MA: MIT Press.

Sheehy, D. (2000). Reflections from the edge. *Canadian Medical Association Journal, 163*, 1612.

Shenk, D. (1997). *Data smog*. San Francisco, CA: HarperEdge.

Shepard, R. (1994). Exercise and reduced health-care costs: A substantial dividend of primary preventive programs? *Journal of Cardiopulmonary Rehabilitation, 14*, 161–165.

Sheppard, S., Charnock, D., & Gann, B. (1999). Helping patients access high quality health information. *British Medical Journal, 319*, 764–766.

Shiffman, R.N., Liaw, Y., Brandt, C.A., & Corb, G.J. (1999). Computer–based guideline implementation Systems: a systematic review of functionality and effectiveness. *JAMIA, 6*, 104–114.

Shiffman, S., Fisher, L., Paty, J., Gnys, M., Hickcox, M., & Kassel, J. (1994). Drinking and smoking: a field study of their association. *Annals of Behavioral Medicine*, 16(3), 203–209.

Shiffman, S., Paty, J., Gnys, M., Kassel, J., & Elash, C. (1995). Nicotine withdrawal in chippers and regular smokers: Subjective and cognitive effects. Health Psychology, 14, 301–309.

Shiffman, S., Paty, J., Gyns, M., Kassel, J., & Hickcox, M. (1996). First lapses to smoking: Within-subjects analysis of real-time reports. *Journal of Consulting and Clinical Psychology, 64*, 366–379.

Shortell, S., Gillies, R., & Devers, K. (1995). Reinventing the American hospital. *Milbank Quarterly, 73*, 131–160.

Shortell, S., Levin, D., O'Brien, J., & Hughes, E. (1995). Assessing the evidence on CQI: Is the glass half empty or half full? *Hospital & Health Services Administration, 40,* 226–246.

Shortliffe, E. (1998). Health care and the next generation Internet. *Annals of Internal Medicine, 129,* 138–140.

Shortt, S.E.D. (1999). *The doctor dilemma.* Montreal & Kingston, Canada: McGill-Queen's University Press.

Silversin, J., & Kornacki, N.J. (2000). *Leading physicians through change.* Tampa, FL: American College of Physician Executives.

Simon, S.R., Pan, Richard, J.D., Sullivan, A.M., Clark-Chiarelli, N., Connelly, M.T., Peters, A.S.; Singer, J.D., Inui, T.S., & Block, S.D. (1999). Views of managed care: A survey of students, residents, faculty, and deans at medical schools in the United States. *The New England Journal of Medicine, 340,* 928–936.

Single, E., Robson, L., Xie, X., & Rehm, J. (1996). *The costs of substance abuse in Canada. Highlights of a major study of the health, social and economic costs associated with the use of alcohol, tobacco and illicit drugs.* Toronto, Canada: Canadian Centre on Substance Abuse.

Skinner C.S., Strecher V.J., Hospers H. (1994). .Physicians' recommendations for mammography: Do tailored messages make a difference? *American Journal of Public Health; 84,* 43–49.

Skinner, H.A., McIntosh, M., & Palmer, W. (1985a). Lifestyle assessment: Applying microcomputers in family practice. *British Medical Journal, 290,* 212–214.

Skinner, H.A., McIntosh, M., & Palmer, W. (1985b). Lifestyle assessment: Just asking makes a difference. *British Medical Journal, 290,* 214–216.

Skinner, H.A. (1994). *Computerized lifestyle assessment.* Toronto, Canada: Multi-Health Systems.

Skinner, H.A. (1993). Early identification of addictive behaviors using a computerized lifestyle assessment. In J.S. Baer, G.A. Marlatt, & R.J. McMahon (Eds.). *Addictive behaviors across a lifespan: Prevention, treatment and policy issues* (p.). Newbury Park, CA: Sage.

Skinner, H.A., & Bercovitz, K.L. (1997). *Person-centred health promotion* (Report series). Toronto, Canada: Centre for Health Promotion, University of Toronto and participACTION.

Skinner, H.A., Maley, O., Smith, L., Chirrey, S., & Morrison, M. (2001, on press). New Frontiers: Using the Internet to engage teens in substance abuse prevention and treatment. In P. Monte & S. Colby (Eds.), *Adolescence, alcohol, and substance abuse: Reaching teens through brief interventions.* New York: Gilford Press.

Skinner, H.A., Morrison M., Bercovitz, K., Haans, D., Jennings, M.J., Magdenko, L., Polzer, J., Smith, L., & Weir, N. (1997). Using the Internet to engage youth in health promotion. *International Journal of Health Promotion & Education, 4,* 23–25.

Smith, D.E., Kratt, P.P., Heckemeyer, C.M., & Mason, D.A. (1997). Motivational interviewing to improve adherence to a behavioral weight–control program for elder obese women with NIDDM. *Diabete Care,* vol. 20, 1, 52–54.

Sobel, D. (1995). Rethinking medicine: Improving health outcomes with cost-effective psychosocial interventions. *Psychosomatic Medicine, 27,* 234–244.

Soet, J., & Bausch, C. (1997). The telephone as a communication medium for health education. Health Education & Behavior, 24, 759–772.

Soet, J.E., & Basch, C.E. (1997). The telephone as a communication medium for health education. *Health Education & Behavior,* 24, 759–772.

Sokolov, J.J. (1992a). National health care reform: a corporate perspective. *Compensation Benefits and Management,* Spring, 1–6.

Sokolov, J.J. (1992b). Building a prototype for the nineties. *Heathcare Forum J,* Spring, 36–42.

Solberg, L.I., Kottke, T.E., Conn, S.A., Brekker, M.L., Calomeni, C.A., & Conboy, K.S. (1997). Delivering clinical preventive services is a systems problem. *Annals of Behavioral Medicine, 19,* 271–278.

Solomon, J. (1992). National health care reform: a corporate perspective. *Compels Benefits Manage, spring,* 1–6.

Somerville, M. (2000). *The ethical canary: Science, society and the human spirit.* Toronto, Canada: Penguin Books.

Sox H.C. (1994). Preventive health services in adults. The *New England Journal of Medicine, 330* (22), 1589–95.

Stacey, R.D. (1996). *Complexity and creativity in organizations.* San Francisco: Berrette-Koehler.

Stange, K. (1996). One size doesn't fit all. Multimethod research yields new insights into interventions to increase prevention in family practice. *The Journal of Family Practice, 43,* 358–360.

Starfield, B. (1992). *Primary care. Concept, evaluation, and policy.* New York: Oxford University Press.

Starfield, B. (1994). Primary care: Is it essential? *Lancet, 344,* 1129–1133.

Starfield, B. (1996). Public health and primary care: A framework for proposed linkages. *American Journal of Public Health, 86,* 1365–1369.

Starr, P. (1982). *The social transformation of american medicine.* New York: Basic Books.

Stewart, M., Brown, J., Weston, W., McWhinney, I., McWilliam, C., & Freeman, T. (1995). *Patient-centered medicine-transforming the clinical method.* Thousand Oaks, CA: Sage.

Stokols, D. (1992). Establishing and maintaining health environments: Toward a social ecology of health promotion. *American Psychologist, 47,* 6–22.

Stone, A., & Shiffman, S. (1994). Ecological momentary assessment (EMA) in behavioral medicine. Annals of Behavioral Medicine, 16, 199–202.

Strecher, V., Kreuter, M., Den Boer, D., Kobrin, S., Hospers, H., & Skinner, C. (1994). The effects of computer-tailored smoking cessation messages in family practice settings. *Journal of Family Practice, 39,* 262–270.

Strecher, V.J., & Rosenstock, I.M. (1997). The health belief model. In K. Glanz, F.M. Lewis, & B.K., Rimer (Eds.), *Health behavior and health education: Theory, research, and practice.* (2nd ed.). San Francisco: Jossey-Bass.

Strecher, V. (1999). Computer-tailored smoking cessation materials: A review and discussion. *Patient Education and Counseling, 36,* 107–117.

Street, R., & Rimal, R. (1997). Health promotion and interactive technology: A conceptual framework. In R. Street, W. Gold, & T. Manning (Eds.), Health Promotion and Interactive technology (pp. 1–18). Mahawah NJ: Lawrence Erlbaum.

Szilagyi, P.G., Boardley, C., Vann, J.C., Chelmineski, A., Kraus, R.M., Margolis, P.A., & Rodewald, L.E. (2000). Effect of patient reminder-recall interventions on immunization rates: A review. *Journal of American Medical Association, 284,* 1820–1827.

Tague, N.R. (1995). *The Quality Toolbox.* Milwaukee, WI: American Society for Quality, ASQ Quality Press.

Taylor, C.D., Polich, S.M., Peterson, C.E., Sloss, E.M. (1987). *User's guide to HIE data* (HIE Reference Series, vol.3). Santa Monica, CA: RAND Corporation.

Tengs, T., Adams, M., Pliskin, J., Gelb Safran, D., Siegal, J., Weinstein, C., & Graham, J. (1995). Five hundred life-saving interventions and their cost-effectiveness. *Risk Analysis, 15,* 369–390.

Thayer, L. (1988). How does information inform? In B.D. Ruben (Ed.) *Information and Behavior* (vol.2). New Brunswick, NJ: Transaction Press.

The Institute for the Future. (2000). Health and Health Care 2010. The forecast, the challenge. San Francisco: Jossey-Bass Publishers.

Thompson, R.S. (1996). What have HMOs learned about clinical prevention services? An examination of the experience at group health cooperative of Puget Sound. *The Millbank Quarterly, 74,* 469–509.

Thomas, R., Cahill, J., & Santilli, L. (1997). Using an interactive computer game to increase skill and self-efficacy regarding safer sex negotiation. Field test results. *Health Education and Behavior, 24,* 71–86.

Thompson, R., McAfee, T., Stuart, M., Smith, A., Wilson. J., & Handley, M. (1995a). A review of clinical prevention services at group health cooperative of Puget Sound. *American Journal of Preventive Medicine, 11,* 409–416.

Thompson, R., Taplin, S., McAfee, T., Mandelson, M., & Smith, A. (1995b). Primary and secondary prevention services in clinical practice. *Journal of the American Medical Association, 273,* 1130–1135.

Tobler, N., & Stratton, H. (1997). Effectiveness of school-based drug prevention programs: A meta-analysis of the research. *Journal of Primary Prevention, 8*(1): 71–128.

Todd, J., Seekins, S., Krichbaum J., & Harvey, L. (1991). Health access America: Strengthening the U.S. health care system. *Journal of the American Medical Association, 265,* 2503–2506.

Turner, A., Singleton, N., & Easterbrook, S. (1997). Developing sexual health software incorporating user feedback: A British experience. *Health Education & Behavior, 24,* 102–120.

U.S. Centers for Disease Control and Prevention. (1999). *Morbidity and Mortality Weekly Report* (MMWR), 48

a. Changes in the public health system. p. 1141–1147.

b. Control of Infectious Diseases. p.621–629.

c. Decline and deaths from heart disease and stroke. p. 649–656.

d. Family planning. p. 1073–1080.

e. Fluoridation of drinking water to prevent dental caries. p. 933–940.

f. Healthier mothers and babies. p.849–857.

g. Impact of vaccines universally recommended for children. p.243–248.

h. Improvements in workplace safety. p.461–469.

i. Motor-vehicle safety. p. 369–374.

j. Safer and healthier foods. p. 905–913.

k. Ten great public health achievements United States, 1900-1999. p. 241–243.

l. Tobacco use. p. 986–993.

U.S. Centers for Disease Control and Prevention and National Center for Health Statistics. (1994). Current estimates from the National Health Survey, 1992. DHHS Publication Series 10, No. 189). Washington, D.C.:

U.S. Centers for Disease Control and Prevention (1999m). An ounce of prevention: What are the returns? *American Journal of Preventive Medicine.*

U.S. Department of Health, Education and Welfare. Healthy People: The surgeon generals report on health promotion and disease prevention. PHS publication no. 79-55071. Bethesda, Md: U.S. Department of Health, Education, and Welfare, Public Health Service, 1979.

U.S. Department of Health and Human Services. Promoting health and preventing disease: Health objectives for the nation. Washington. D.C.: U.S. Government printing office, 1980.

U.S. Department of Health and Human Services. *Healthy people 2000: National health promotion and disease prevention objectives.* (DHHS Publication No. PHS 91-50213). Washington, DC: U.S. Government printing office, 1991.

U.S. Department of Health and Human Services. (2000). Healthy people 2010: understanding and improving health. Washington, D.C.: U.S. department of health and human services, government printing office. Also available at: www.health.gov/healthypeople.

Velicer, W.F., DiClemente, C.C. (1993). Understanding and intervening with the total population of smokers. *Tobacco Control, 2,* 95–96.

Velicer, W.F., DiClemente, C.C., Prochaska, J.O., Brandenburg, N. (1985). Decisional balance measure for assessing and predicting smoking status. *Journal of Personality & Social Psychology, 48,* 1279–1289.

Velicer, W.F., DiClemente, C.C., Rossi, J.S., Prochaska, J.O. (1990). Relapse situations and self-efficacy: An integrative model. *Addictive Behaviors, 15,* 271–283.

Velicer W.F., Fava, J.L., Prochaska, J.O., Abrams, D.B., Emmons, K.M., Pierce, J.P. (1995). Distribution of smokers by stage in three representative samples. *Preventive Medicine, 24,* 401–411.

Velicer, W.F., Prochaska, J.O., Fava., J.L., LaForge., R.G., & Rossi, J.S. (1999). Interactive versus non-interactive interventions and dose-response relationships for stage-matched smoking cessation programs in a managed care setting. *Health Psychology, 18,* 21–28.

Velicer, W.F., Prochaska, J.O., Rossi, J.S., & Snow, M.G. (1992). Assessing outcome in smoking cessation studies. *Psychological Bulletin, 111,* 23–41.

Velicer, W.F., Prochaska, J.O., Rossi, J.S, DiClemente, C.C. (1996). A criterion measurement model for addictive behaviors. *Addictive Behaviors, 21,* 555–584.

Vicente, K. (2001, February). *Designing technology that works for people.* Presentation at the University of Toronto's Knowledge Media Design Institute's Humanizing Technology Spring Lecture Series, Toronto, Canada.

Vickery, D., Dalmer, H., Lowry, D., Constantine, M., Wright, I., & Loren, W. (1983). Effect of a self-care education program on medical visits. *Journal of American Medical Association, 250,* 2952–2956.

Vickery, D., & Fries, J. (1993). *Take care of yourself (5th ed.),* Reading, MA: Addison-Wesley.

Waitzkin, H. (1984). Doctor-patient communication. *Journal of American Medical Association, 252,* 2441.

Waitzkin, H. (1991). *The politics of medical encounters.* New Haven, CT: Yale University Press.

Waldrop M.M. (1992). *Complexity: The emerging science at the edge of order and chaos.* New York: Simon and Schuster.

Wallace, P.G., Brennan, P.J., & Haines, A.P. (1987). Are general practitioners doing enough to promote healthy lifestyle? Findings of the medical research council's general practice research framework study on lifestyle and health. *British Medical Journal: 294*, 940–942.

Wallace P., Cutler, S., & Haines, A. (1988). Randomized controlled trial of general practitioner intervention in patients with excessive alcohol consumption. *British Medical Journal, 297*, 663–668.

Wallace, PG, & Haines, AP. (1984). General practitioners and health promotion: What patients think. *British Medical Journal: 289*, 534–536.

Wallerstein, N. (1992). Powerlessness, empowerment and health: Implications for health promotion programs. *American Journal of Public Health, 6*, 197–205.

Walsh, J., & McPhee, S. (1992). A systems model of clinical preventive care: An analysis of factors influencing patient and physician. *Health Education Quarterly, 19*, 157–175.

Ward, K., & Hawthorne, K. (1994). Do patients read health promotion posters in the waiting room? A study in one general practice. *British Journal of General Practice, 44*, 583–585.

Wasson, J., Gaudette, C., Whaley, F., Sauvigne, A., Baribeau, P., & Welch, G. (1992). Telephone care as substitute for routine clinic follow-up. *Journal of the American Medical Association, 267*, 1788–1793.

Waterman DA. (1986). A Guide to Expert Systems. Redding, MA: Addison-Wesley.

Waterman, D.H. (1987). *The Renewal Factor*. New York: Bantam.

Watzlawick, P., Weakland, J., & Fisch, R. (1974). *Change*. New York: Norton.

Wechsler, H., Levine, S., Idelson, R.K., Rohman, M., & Taylor, J.O. (1983). The physician's role in health promotion: A survey of primary-care practitioners. *The New England Journal of Medicine, 308*, 97–100.

Weinberg, A., & Andrus, P.L. (1982). Continuing medical education: Does it address prevention? *Journal of Community Health, 7*, 211–214.

Weinstein, N.D. (1993). Testing for competing theories of health-protective behavior. Health Psychology, 12, 324–333.

Weiss, S. (1984). Health hazard/health risk appraisals. In J. Matarazzo, S. Weiss, J. Herd, & N. Miller (Eds.), *Behavioral health: A handbook of health enhancement and disease prevention* (pp. 275–294). New York: John Wiley & Sons.

Wells, K.B., Hays, R.D., Burnam, M.A., Rogers, W., Greenfield, S., & Ware, J.E. (1989). Detection of depressive disorder for patients receiving prepaid or fee-for-service care: results from the medical outcomes study. *Journal of the American Medical Association, 262*, 3298–3302.

Westberg, E., & Miller, R. (1999). The basis for using the Internet to support the information needs of primary care. *JAMIA, 6*, 6–25.

Wheeler, D. (1993). *Understanding variation: The key to managing chaos*. Knoxville, TN: SPC Press.

White, D.G., (1991). Wearing a wife-assault-prevention button: Impact on a family practice. *Canadian Medical Association Journal, 145*(8), 1005–1012.

White, K. (1991). *Healing the schism: Epidemiology, medicine, and the public's health*. New York: Springer-Verlag.

Whitelaw, S., Baldwin, S., Bunton, R., & Flynn, D. (2000). The status of evidence and outcomes in stages of change research. *Health education research: Theory and practice, 15*, 707–718.

Wigle, D., Mao, Y., Semenciw, M., McCann, C., & Davies, J. (1990). Premature deaths in Canada: Impact, trends and opportunities for prevention. *Canadian Journal of Public Health, 81*, 376–381.

Wilkinson, R., & Marmot, M. (1998). *The solid facts: Social determinants of health*. Geneva: World health organization.

Wilkinson, R.G. (1996). *Unhealthy societies: From inequality to well-being*. New York: Routledge.

Williams, G.C., & Deci, E.L.(1996). Internalization of biopsychosocial values by medical students: A test of self-determination theory. *Journal of Personality and Social Psychology, 70*, 767–679.

Williams, G.C., Deci, E.L., & Ryan, R.M. (1998). Building healthcare partnerships by supporting autonomy: promoting maintained behavior change and positive health outcomes. In A. Suchman et al. (Eds), *Partnerships in healthcare*. (pp.60–87). Rochester, NY: University of Rochester Press.

Williams, G.C., Freedman, Z.R., & Deci, E.L. (1998). Supporting autonomy to motivate glucose control in patients with diabetes. *Diabetes Care, 27*, 1644–1651.

Williams, G.C., Grow, V.M., Freedman, Z., Ryan, R.M., & Deci, E.L. (1996). Motivational predictors of weight loss and weight-loss maintenance. *Journal and Personality and Social Psychology, 70*, 115–126.

Williams, G.C., Rodin, G.C., Ryan, R.M., Grolnick, W.S., & Deci, E.L. (1998). Autonomous regulation and long-term medication adherence in adult outpatients. *Health Psychology, 17*, 269–276.

Willms, D., Best, A., Wilson, D., Gilbert, R., Taylor, W., Lindsay, E., Singer, J., & Arbuthnot Johnson, N. (1991). Patients' perspectives of a physician-delivered smoking cessation intervention. *American Journal of Preventive Medicine, 7*, 95–100.

Wilson, A., McDonald, P., Hayes, L., & Cooney, J. (1992). Health promotion makes a difference in the general practice consultation: A minute makes a difference. *British Medical Journal, 304*, 227–230.

Winett, R.A., Moore, J.F., Wagner, J.L., Hite, L.A., Leahy, M., & Neubauer, T.E. (1991). Altering shoppers' supermarket purchases to fit nutritional guidelines: An interactive information system. *Journal of Applied Behavior Analysis, 24*(1), 95–105.

Winkler, M.A., Flanagin, A., Chi-Lum, B., White, J., Andrews, K., Kennett, R.L., DeAngelis, C.D., & Musacchio, R.A. (2000). Guidelines for medical and health information sites on the Internet. *Journal of American Medical Association, 283*,(12), 1600–1606.

World Health Organization. (1978). Alma Ata 1978: Primary Health Care (Rep. No.1). Geneva: World health organization.

World Health Organization (1986). *Ottawa charter for health promotion*. Ottawa, Canada: Canadian Public Health Association.

World Health Organization (1992). *Reflections on progress: a framework for the healthy cities project review*. Copenhagen: WHO Europe.

World Health Organization. (2000). The World Health Report 2000. Health systems: improving performance. Geneva, Switzerland: World Health Organization.

Worrall, G., Chaulk, P., & Freake, D. (1997). The effects of clinical practice guidelines on patient outcomes in primary care: A systematic review. *Canadian Medical Association Journal, 156*, 1705–1712.

Wurman, R. S. (2001). *Information anxiety 2*. Indianapolis, In QUE.

Zimmerman, B., Lindberg, C., & Plsek, P. (1998). *Edgewear: Insights from complexity science for health care leaders*. Irving, TX: VHA Inc.

Zweben, A., & Fleming, M.F. (1999). Brief interventions for alcohol and drug problems in J.A. Tucker, D.M. Donovan, & G.A. Marlatt (Eds), *Changing addictive behavior: Bridging clinical and public health strategies* (pp. 251–282). New York: Guilford Press.

Index

Page numbers followed by *f* indicate a figure; followed by *t* indicate a table.

ABIM (American Board of Internal Medicine), 106
Abrams, D. B., 36, 37
action phase, 135
ACTSS: Success Factors for Organizational Improvement, 154, 174, 175, 176*f*-180
Aday, L. A., 61
addictive behavior, 129*t*
affective dimension
    described, 177
    Westbourne case study on, 180-181
Agency for Health Care Policy and Research website, 54-55
AHCPR panel, 68
AHCPR Tobacco Cessation Guideline website, 68
Alameda County Project (1983), 44
Alcoholics Anonymous, 324
Alemi, F., 324
Alston, F. K., 185
Alter, D. A., 24
AMA (American Medical Association), 96, 102, 103-104
American Academy of Family Physicians smoking cessation kit, 73
American Association of Medical Colleges, 7
American College of Surgeons, 77
American Medical Informatics Association AMIA, 269-270, 329-330
Anderson, L. A., 71
Annis, H., 145
antibiotics overuse, 20-21
Aristotle, 83
Ashenden, R., 54, 55
Ask-Advise-Assist approach, 137, 286
assessment
    capacity for organization improvement, 179-180
    Computerized Lifestyle Assessment tool for, 265
    EMA (Ecological Momentary Assessment) tool for, 273
    GHC process of outcomes, 91
    of PTC system outcomes, 283-284
autonomous behavior, 58-59, 130*f*, 132*f*-133
avoid argumentation, 58

Babor, T. F., 54
Baer, J. S., 129
Baker, R., 81
Balas, A., 269
Bandura, A., 126, 130
Bartlett, E. E., 31
Batalden, P., 175, 222
Bausch, C., 275
Becker, M., 5
Beer, M., 70
Begley, C. E., 61

behavioral intention, 125-126
behavior change. *See* health behavior change; organizational behavior change
Bercovitz,, 47, 120, 297
Berger, M., 70
Berkman, L., 44
Berwick, D., 80, 81, 160, 178
bicycle safety campaign, 85*f*, 86
Bien, T., 54
biotechnological advances, 19
Bisognano, Maureen, 81
Block, B., 208
Borkman, T. J., 28, 210
Botelho, R. J., 56, 159, 174, 199, 278
Boult, C., 25
breast cancer
    applying Social Cognitive Theory to, 127*t*
    screening for, 84, 85*f*
Breslin, C., 140, 337, 339
Breslow, L., 44
Brewster, J., 337, 339
Brock, D., 51
Bryson, J. M., 184, 185, 186, 188
Building Motivation guide worksheet, 111
buttons (health promoting), 205-206

Cain, M., 258
Califano, J., 45
CAM (complementary and alternative medicine), 29-30
Canada
    adoption of population health framework by, 48
    causes of premature deaths in, 43*f*
    pilot projects for health care reform in, 100
    reform proposals for health care of, 104-105
Canadian Medical Association Journal, 98
Canadian Medical Association's Futures Project, 106
Cancer Care Ontario (Canada), 39-40
Cancer Prevention in Community Practice Project, 71
Cancer Prevention Research Center website, 284
Carbonari, J., 139
Carroll, K. M., 145
CDC (U.S. Center for Disease Control and Prevention), 31, 92
CFA (Critical Functions Analysis)
    described, 155, 156, 199
    linking improvement cycles with, 237-239
    smoking cessation case study on, 213-220, 214*f*, 215*t*
    using tools of, 212*f*-213
CFA Scoring Template, 221
CFPC (College of Family Physicians of Canada), 101, 104
change
    how people, 134*f*

Stages of Change concept and, 56, 135, 136*t*, 137-140, 282
study on reducing dietary fat intake, 139*f*
Transtheoretical Model on, 56, 119, 134, 135-140, 282, 297-298
See also health behavior change; organizational behavior change
change motivation
    about choices and, 168-169
    built for improvement, 160-161
    case study on, 167-168
    computer systems used for, 278-292
    Decision Balance worksheet and, 111, 117, 166*f*-167, 173, 282
    dynamics of, 113-114
    as first Five-Step Model step, 151-153
    motivational interviewing (MI), 56, 57-58, 134, 140-143
    prototypes listed for, 159
    strategies for enhancing, 141*t*
    theories on, 123-133
    as trait vs. state, 140
    two essential components of, 118*f*
    understanding, 118-119
    why one acts primer on, 119-123
    See also organizational behavior change
change resistance
    defining the "problem", 117
    dynamics of, 113-114
    mismatches in readiness for change and, 116*f*-117
    poor communication and, 115-116
    understanding, 114-118
Charlton, J., 44
Charter for Action (2000), 46
CHIS (Consumer Health Information Services), 316
Clinical Prevention Guidelines (Agency for Health care Policy and Research website), 54-55
Clinical Value Compass
    data collecting using, 234-236
    described, 224-225
    tips on using, 226*t*
CLIP (Cholesterol Lowering Intervention Program), 285
CMA (Canadian Medical Association), 103, 106
CME (continuing medical education), 68
Cochrane Library website, 55, 262-265
Codman, E., 76, 77
compact, 117
Complexity and Creativity in Organizations (Stacey), 342
Computerized Lifestyle Assessment, 265
Conner, D., 174
consequentialist framework, 320-321
Consumer's Guide to Online Health Information, 323*t*
contemplation stage, 135
continuing care, 208-209, 218, 269

399